Challenging Concepts in Anaesthesia

Titles in the Challenging Concepts in series

Anaesthesia (Edited by Dr Phoebe Syme, Dr Robert Jackson, and Professor Tim Cook)

Cardiovascular Medicine (Edited by Dr Aung Myat, Dr Shouvik Haldar, and Professor Simon Redwood)

Emergency Medicine (Edited by Dr Sam Thenabadu, Dr Fleur Cantle, and Dr Chris Lacy)

Infectious Disease and Clinical Microbiology (Edited by Dr Amber Arnold and Professor George Griffin)

Interventional Radiology (Edited by Dr Irfan Ahmed, Dr Miltiadis Krokidis, and Dr Tarun Sabharwal)

Neurology (Edited by Dr Krishna Chinthapalli, Dr Nadia Magdalinou, and Professor Nicholas Wood)

Neurosurgery (Edited by Mr Robin Bhatia and Mr Ian Sabin)

Obstetrics and Gynaecology (Edited by Dr Natasha Hezelgrave, Dr Danielle Abbott, and Professor Andrew Shennan)

Oncology (Edited by Dr Madhumita Bhattacharyya, Dr Sarah Payne, and Professor Iain McNeish)

Oral and Maxillofacial Surgery (Edited by Mr Matthew Idle and Group Captain Andrew Monaghan)

Respiratory Medicine (Edited by Dr Lucy Schomberg and Dr Elizabeth Sage)

Challenging Concepts in Anaesthesia:
Cases with Expert Commentary

Edited by

Dr Phoebe Syme,
Anaesthetic Registrar, University Hospitals Bristol UK.

Dr Robert Jackson, MB BS, BSc (Hons), MRCP, FRCA, FFICM,
Consultant in Anaesthesia and Intensive Care Medicine, Derriford Hospital, Plymouth UK.

Professor Tim Cook, BA (Cantab. Hons), MBBS (Hons), FRCA, FFICM,
Consultant in Anaesthesia and Intensive Care Medicine, Royal United Hospital, Bath UK.
Macintosh Professor of Anaesthesia, Royal College of Anaesthetists.

Series editors

Dr Aung Myat, BSc (Hons), MBBS, MRCP,
BHF Clinical Research Training Fellow, King's College London British Heart Foundation Centre
of Research Excellence, Cardiovascular Division, St Thomas' Hospital, London UK.

Dr Shouvik Haldar, MBBS, MRCP,
Electrophysiology Research Fellow and Cardiology SpR, Heart Rhythm Centre, NIHR Cardiovascular
Biomedical Research Unit, Royal Brompton & Harefield NHS Foundation Trust, Imperial College London UK.

Professor Simon Redwood, MD, FRCP,
Professor of Interventional Cardiology and Honorary Consultant Cardiologist, King's College London British
Heart Foundation Centre of Research Excellence, Cardiovascular Division, St Thomas' Hospital, London UK.

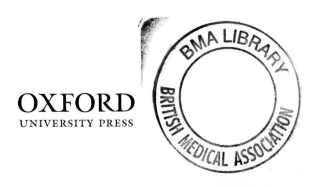

OXFORD
UNIVERSITY PRESS

OXFORD
UNIVERSITY PRESS

Great Clarendon Street, Oxford, OX2 6DP,
United Kingdom

Oxford University Press is a department of the University of Oxford.
It furthers the University's objective of excellence in research, scholarship,
and education by publishing worldwide. Oxford is a registered trade mark of
Oxford University Press in the UK and in certain other countries

Published in the United States of America by Oxford University Press
198 Madison Avenue, New York, NY 10016, United States of America

British Library Cataloguing in Publication Data
Data available

Library of Congress Control Number: 2013944917

ISBN 978-0-19-968627-8

Printed in Great Britain by
Ashford Colour Press Ltd, Gosport, Hampshire

FOREWORD

Tell me and I forget. Teach me and I remember. Involve me and I learn.

(Benjamin Franklin)

People learn in different ways. As a preclinical medical student in the last millennium in an ancient university some 50 miles northwest of London, I experienced two very distinct forms of education: didactic 'talking-head' lectures and small group tutorials. I could not learn anything from lectures, although I found them a very useful form of relaxation, almost always falling asleep within five minutes of the start of the lecture. Tutorials largely comprised my colleagues impressing my tutor with the extent of their knowledge, and me making an even greater impression on him with the seemingly unfathomable depth of my ignorance. My clinical training saw me in a short white coat amidst a row of similarly clad medical students looking for all the world like a flock of sheep that was dumbly following a consultant on a seemingly endless ward round. This was the era of 'teaching by humiliation' and, although some of my peers responded well to the fear of the consultant bearing down on them and shouting at them with gleeful and taunting derision, it didn't work for me. In desperation, I turned to textbooks, but these were mostly frightful things in those days. Chapter upon chapter of closely packed, sterile prose addressing abstract concepts such as the Loop of Henle, the Blood-Brain Barrier and Non-Acute Sclerosing Panencephalitis—things that I found impossible to relate in any real way to my hoped-for future work as a doctor.

You will by now have gathered that I managed to qualify—but only just. My lamentable efforts at acquiring information from the educational techniques then available to me did not see me reach the upper slopes of academia in my year, and it was for this reason that I started my medical career in the most forgettable hospitals in the gloomiest parts of South West London—I will not name names. However, it was in these drear institutions that my world of learning changed almost in an instant. I actually started to learn, and the reason that I started to learn was because the patients in front of me were real people with real names and real problems. When the facts on offer made sense in the context of an individual that I could see or at very least envisage, they came to life, and as they came to life, I found that I could retain the information. I became involved. I learned.

It is for these reasons that I take great pleasure in writing a foreword for *Challenging Concepts in Anaesthesia*. It does what no book did for me while I was learning my trade—it engages the reader with cases that he or she may have encountered or may yet encounter in a way that truly involves. The patients are real, living and breathing—or wheezing and bleeding—people, with an interesting variety of critical conditions with which a career in anaesthesia will inevitably bring you into contact. Each case is succinctly outlined, and the learning made available around the case description is broken up into digestible and interesting chunks: 'Learning Points', 'Clinical Tips', and 'Expert Comments'. What's more, the experts commenting on these cases are real experts—proper clinicians whose experience and expertise is recognized both nationally and internationally, not head-in-the-cloud academics armed with a USB memory

stick full of lectures, a passport, a platinum air miles card and only a vague recollection of what a patient actually looks like. The list of contributors is a veritable Who's
Who of modern clinical anaesthesia. In addition to this, the cases themselves are well
chosen not only to characterize commonly encountered challenging situations, but
also to raise and allow discussion of topics of current clinical interest such as goal-
directed therapy, depth of anaesthesia monitoring, cardiopulmonary exercise testing
and the impact of coronary artery stents on anaesthetic care. *Challenging Concepts in
Anaesthesia* offers a format that brings learning to life.

If only it were possible to hurl this book into some form of time warp such that
it appeared in the tremulous hands of a pimply and disaffected, white-coated youth
in the mid-1980s. Okay, let's be honest—the early 1980s. All right then, the late
1970s—whatever.

Enjoy the book. I certainly did.

Dr William Harrop-Griffiths MA MB BS FRCA
Consultant Anaesthetist, Imperial College Healthcare NHS Trust, London
Honorary Senior Lecturer, Imperial College, London

ACKNOWLEDGEMENTS

I would like to thank my husband and parents for their support and encouragement throughout the preparation of this manuscript.

—Phoebe Syme

To Katie, Henry, and Sam. Thank you for your patience, and encouraging me to finish the book...

—Robert Jackson

Thanks for the constant patience of my family and the enduring support of them and my excellent colleagues in Bath.

—Tim Cook

Chapter 4, Case 4.1

We would like to thank Mr Donald Macarthur, Consultant Neurosurgeon, Neurosurgery Training Programme Director and Honorary Consultant Lecturer at the University of Nottingham, for the pictures.

CONTENTS

CONTRIBUTORS

Dr Vassilis Athanassoglou
Anaesthetic Registrar,
Nuffield Department of Anaesthetics,
Oxford, UK

Professor Mark C. Bellamy
Professor of Critical Care Anaesthesia,
St James' University Hospital,
Leeds, UK

Dr David Bogod
Consultant Anaesthetist,
Nottingham University Hospitals NHS Trust,
Nottingham, UK

Dr David Cain
Anaesthetic Registrar,
University College London,
London, UK

Dr Jeremy Cashman
Consultant in Anaesthesia and Pain Management,
St George's Hospital,
London, UK

Dr Michael DeVile
Consultant in Anaesthesia and Intensive Care Medicine,
Ashford & St Peter's Hospitals NHS Foundation Trust,
Surrey, UK

Dr Erica Dibb-Fuller
Locum Consultant Anaesthetist,
University Hospital Southampton,
Southampton UK

Dr Mark Edwards
Locum Consultant in Anaesthesia,
University Hospital Southampton,
Southampton, UK

Dr Abigail Fell
Specialist Registrar Anaesthesia,
Northampton General Hospital,
Northampton, UK

Professor Pierre Foex
Nuffield Department of Anaesthetics,
John Radcliffe Hospital,
Oxford, UK

Dr Nikki Freeman
Anaesthetic Registrar,
Torbay Hospital South Devon Healthcare NHS
  Foundation Trust,
Torquay, UK

Dr Chris Frerk
Consultant Anaesthetist,
Northampton General Hospital,
Northampton, UK

Dr Mark Hamilton
Consultant and Honorary Senior Lecturer in Anaesthesia
  and Intensive Care Medicine,
St George's Hospital,
London, UK

Dr Rachel Homer
Consultant Paediatric Anaesthetist,
Leeds Children's Hospital,
Leeds, UK

Dr Paul Howell
Consultant Anaesthetist,
St Bartholomew's, Royal London and Homerton
  Hospitals,
London, UK

Dr Dom Hurford
Consultant Anaesthetist,
Royal Glamorgan Hospital,
Llantrisant, Wales

Dr Paul James
Registrar in Anaesthesia and Critical Care Medicine,
North East Midlands School of Anaesthesia,
Nottingham, UK

Dr Robert Jackson
Consultant in Anaesthesia and Intensive
  Care Medicine,
Derriford Hospital,
Plymouth, UK

Dr William Key
Consultant Anaesthetist,
South Devon Healthcare NHS Foundation Trust,
Torquay, UK

Dr Michele Kigozi
Anaesthetic Registrar,
St George's Hospital
London, UK

Dr Simon Law
Consultant in Pain Medicine and Anaesthesia,
Gloucester Hospitals NHS Trust,
Gloucester, UK

Dr Alex Middleditch
Registrar in Anaesthesia and Critical Care,
Bristol School of Anaesthesia,
Bristol, UK

Dr Timothy E. Miller
Assistant Professor of Anesthesiology,
Duke University Medical Center,
Durham, North Carolina, USA

Dr Iain Moppett
Clinical Associate Professor,
School of Medicine, University of Nottingham;
Consultant Anaesthetist,
Queen's Medical Centre,
Nottingham, UK

Professor Paul Myles
Director,
Department of Anaesthesia and Perioperative Medicine,
Alfred Hospital and Monash University Melbourne,
Melbourne, Australia

Dr Mary Newton
Consultant Anaesthetist,
The National Hospital for Neurology and Neurosurgery,
London, UK

Dr Barry Nicholls
Consultant in Anaesthesia and Pain Management,
Musgrove Park Hospital,
Taunton, UK

Dr Jerry Nolan
Consultant in Anaesthesia and Intensive Care Medicine,
Royal United Hospital,
Bath, UK

Dr Paul Older
Senior Lecturer,
University of Melbourne,
Melbourne, Australia;
Honorary Consultant,
Department of Anaesthesia, Western Hospital,
Melbourne, Australia

Associate Professor Michael Parr
Director of Intensive Care,
Liverpool and Macquarie University Hospitals,
Sydney, Australia;
Associate Professor,
University of New South Wales, University of Western Sydney, and Macquarie University,
Sydney, New South Wales, Australia

Dr Anil Patel
Consultant Anaesthetist,
Royal National Throat, Nose and Ear Hospital,
London, UK

Dr Davina Ross-Anderson
Consultant Anaesthetist,
Royal London Hospital,
London, UK

Dr Caroline Sampson
Registrar in Anaesthesia and Intensive Care Medicine,
Queen's Medical Centre,
Nottingham, UK

Dr Louise Savic
Anaesthetic Registrar,
Leeds Teaching Hospitals NHS Trust,
Leeds, UK

Dr Phoebe Syme
Anaesthetic Registrar,
University Hospitals Bristol,
Bristol, UK

Dr Steve Tolchard
Consultant Anaesthetist,
Southmead Hospital,
Bristol, UK

Dr Hugo Wellesley
Consultant Anaesthetist,
Great Ormond Street Hospital,
London, UK

Dr Kathy Wilkinson
Consultant Anaesthetist,
Norfolk and Norwich University Hospital,
Norwich, UK

ABBREVIATIONS

AAA	abdominal aortic aneurysm	ETAC	end-tidal anaesthetic agent concentration
AAGA	accidental awareness during general anaesthesia	EVAR	endovascular aneurysm repair
AAGBI	Association of Anaesthetists of Great Britain and Ireland	EVD	external ventricular drain
		FAST	focused assessment with sonography for trauma
ABC	Airway Breathing Circulation	FBC	full blood count
ACC	American College of Cardiology	FFP	fresh frozen plasma
ACEI	angiotensin-converting enzyme inhibitor	FiO_2	fraction of inspired oxygen
ACT	activated clotting time	fLMA	flexible laryngeal mask airway
AFOI	awake fibreoptic intubation	GA	general anaesthesia
AHA	American Heart Association	GCS	Glasgow Coma Scale
ALP	alkaline phosphatase	HDU	high-dependency unit
ALT	alanine aminotransferase	HES	hydroxyethyl starch
APS	acute pain service	HIV/AIDS	human immunodeficiency virus/acquired immune deficiency syndrome
APTT	activated partial thromboplastin time		
APTTR	activated partial thromboplastin time ratio	HR	heart rate
AT	anaerobic threshold	IABP	intra-aortic balloon pump
BMI	body mass index	IBW	ideal body weight
BMS	bare metal stents	ICP	intracranial pressure
BP	blood pressure	ICS	intraoperative cell salvage
CABG	coronary artery bypass grafting	ICU	intensive care unit
CBF	cerebral blood flow	ID	internal diameter
CICV	'can't intubate–can't ventilate/oxygenate' situation	LAD	left anterior descending artery
		LBM	lean body mass
CIN	contrast-induced nephropathy	LCx	left circumflex artery
$CMRO_2$	cerebral metabolic requirement for oxygen	LMA	laryngeal mask airway
CNB	central neuraxial blockade	LP	lumbar puncture
CNS	central nervous system	LV	left ventricular
CPET	cardiopulmonary exercise test	MAC	minimum alveolar concentration
CPP	cerebral perfusion pressure	MAP	mean arterial pressure
CPR	cardiopulmonary resuscitation	MET	metabolic equivalent of task
CSF	cerebrospinal fluid	MI	myocardial infarction
CT	computed tomography	MILS	manual in-line stabilization
CVP	central venous pressure	MRI	Magnetic Resonance Imaging
DAPT	dual antiplatelet therapy	NEC	necrotizing enterocolitis
DAS	Difficult Airway Society	NMBA	neuromuscular blocking agent
DCI	delayed cerebral ischaemia	NNT	number needed to treat
DES	drug-eluting stents	NPSA	National Patient Safety Agency
ECG	electrocardiogram	NSAID	non-steroidal anti-inflammatory drug
ED_{50}	effective dose for 50% of patients	ODM	oesophageal Doppler monitor
EEG	electroencephalogram	ODP	operating department practitioner
ENT	ear, nose and throat	OOHCA	out-of-hospital cardiac arrest
ERC	European Resuscitation Council	OHS	obesity hypoventilation syndrome

OSA	obstructive sleep apnoea	SDH	subdural haemotoma
PaCO$_2$	partial pressure of arterial carbon dioxide	S$\bar{v}$O$_2$	mixed venous oxygen saturation
PACU	post-anaesthesia care unit	ScvO$_2$	central venous oxygen saturation
PaO$_2$	partial pressure of arterial oxygen	SIADH	syndrome of inappropriate antidiuretic hormone
PCA	patient-controlled analgesia		
PCI	percutaneous coronary intervention	SpO$_2$	blood oxygen saturation as measured by pulse oximetry
PEEP	positive end-expiratory pressure		
PONV	postoperative nausea and vomiting	ST	specialty trainee
PRC	packed red cells	TAP	transversus abdominis plane
PT	prothrombin time	TBI	traumatic brain injury
PTSD	post-traumatic stress disorder	TBW	total body weight
PVB	paravertebral block	TCD	transcranial Doppler
RA	regional anaesthesia	TIMI	thrombolysis in myocardial infarction
RAE	Ring Adair and Elwyn tracheal tube	TIVA	total intravenous anaesthesia
Re	Reynolds number	UKOSS	UK Obstetric Surveillance System
ROSC	return of spontaneous circulation	VF	ventricular fibrillation
RSI	rapid sequence induction	WFNS	World Federation of Neurological Surgeons
SAD	supraglottic airway device		
SAH	subarachnoid haemorrhage	WHO	World Health Organization

Table 0.1 *Challenging Concepts in Anaesthesia* Mapped to Royal College of Anaesthetists CPD Matrix January 2013

1

Scientific Principles	Emergency Management and Resuscitation	Airway Management	Pain Medicine	Patient Safety	Legal Aspects of Practice	IT Skills	Education and Training	Healthcare Management
Physiology and biochemistry (1A01) **2.1* 3.1* 3.2***	Anaphylaxis (1B01)	Airway assessment (1C01) **1.1* 1.2* 3.2***	Assessment of acute pain (1D01) **7.1*, 7.2***	Infection control (1E01)	Consent (1F01)	Use of patient record systems (1G01)	Roles and responsibilities of clinical supervisors (1H01)	Critical incident reporting (1I01)
Pharmacology and therapeutics (1A02) **9.1***	Can't intubate, can't ventilate (1B02) **1.2* 5.2***	Basic airway management (1C02) **1.1* 1.2***	Management of acute pain (1D02) **7.1* 7.2***	Level 2 and Level 3 child protection training (1E02)	Mental capacity and deprivation of liberty safeguards (1F02)	Basic search methodology (1G02)	Personal education and learning (1H02)	Team leadership and resource management (1I02)
Physics and clinical measurement (1A03) **2.2***	Basic life support (all age groups and special situations) (1B03) **9.2***			Protection of vulnerable adults (1E03)	Data protection (1F03)			Human factors in anaesthetic practice (1I03)
	Advanced life support (relevant to practice) (1B04) **9.2***			Blood product checking protocols (1E04)	Equality and diversity (1F04)			Understanding of complaints process (1I04)
				Venous thromboembolism prophylaxis (1E05)	Ethics (1F05)			Quality improvement (1I05)

*indicates case numbers

General	Obstetrics	ICM	Paediatrics	Pain Medicine	Neuro	Regional Anaesthesia	Education and Training
Advanced airway management (2A01) **1.1* 1.2***	Analgesia for labour (2B01)	Assessment of the critically ill patient (2C01) **4.2*, 8.1*, 9.2***	Assessment and initial management of the critically ill child (2D01)	Advanced management of perioperative pain (2E01) **7.1* 7.2***	Initial management of brain injury (traumatic or spontaneous intracranial haemorrhage) (2F01) **4.1* 4.2***	Indications, benefits and risks of RA (2G01) **7.1* 7.2***	Work-place based assessment (2H01)
Principles of assessment and management of major trauma (including burns) (2A02) **4.2* 8.1***	General anaesthesia for elective and emergency LSCS (2B02) **5.1* 5.2***	Initiation and management of ventilatory support (2C02)	Perioperative care of children (2D02) **6.1* 6.2***	Management of acute non-surgical pain (2E02) **7.2***	Initial management of spinal injured patients (2F02)	Principles of performing local, regional and neuraxial techniques (2G02) **7.1* 7.2***	Educational supervisor training (2H02)
Preoperative assessment and preparation for surgery (2A03) **2.2* 2.3* 9.1***	Regional anaesthesia for elective and emergency LSCS (2B03) **5.1***	Diagnosis and management of shock, infection and sepsis (2C03)	Vascular access techniques (2D03)	Basic assessment and management of chronic pain (2E03)	Management of patients with neuro trauma for imaging (2F03) **4.2***	Use of nerve/plexus location techniques (2G03)	
Advanced patient monitoring techniques (2A04) **2.1* 2.2***	Regional anaesthesia complications in the pregnant patient (2B04)	Support of threatened and failing organ systems (2C04) **9.2***	Fluid management for children (2D04)			Recognition and management of side effects and complications of regional anaesthesia (2G04) **7.2***	
Fluid management and blood product usage (2A05) **2.1*, 5.1***	Management of obstetric emergencies (2B05) **5.1* 5.2***	Sedation techniques for ICU patients (2C05)	Analgesia for children (2D05) **6.2*, 7.2***				
Perioperative emergencies (2A06) **1.1*, 1.2*, 5.1*, 6.2*, 9.1***	Assessment of the critically ill parturient (2B06)	End of life issues and organ donation (2C06)	Sedation techniques for children (2D06)				
Perioperative management for surgical specialties not listed elsewhere (2A07) **3.2***	Principles of newborn resuscitation (2B07)	Management of the ICU (2C07)	Team working between DGHs and PIC retrieval teams (2D07)				
Anaesthetic management for non-operative procedures (2A08) **6.1* 9.2***							
Anaesthesia for non-obstetric procedures in the pregnant patient (2A09)							

Sedation techniques for adults (2A10)				
Patient transfer skills (2A11)				
Developments in allied clinical specialties (relevant to practice) (2A12)				

3

	Case Number			
Airway management (3A01)	1.1*	1.2*		
ENT, maxillo-facial and dental surgery (3A02)	6.2*			
General, urological and gynaecological surgery (3A03)	2.1*	2.3*	3.1*	
Hepatobiliary surgery (3A04)				
Vascular surgery (3A05)	2.1*	2.3*		
Day surgery (3A06)	6.2*			
Sedation practice (3A07)				
Orthopaedic surgery (3A08)				
Regional anaesthesia (3A09)	7.1*	7.2*		
Trauma management (including prehospital care) (3A10)	4.2*	8.1*		
Transfer medicine (3A11)				
Ophthalmic (3A12)				
Bariatric (3A13)	3.2*			
Military anaesthesia (3A14)				
Obstetrics (3B00)	5.1*	5.2*		
Adult ICM (3C00)	4.1*	4.2*	8.1*	9.2*
Paediatrics and paediatric ICM (3D00)	6.1*	6.2*		
Pain medicine (3E00)	7.1*	7.2*		
Neuro (including neuro critical care) (3F00)	4.1*	4.2*		
Cardiothoracic (3G00)				
Plastic/burns (3H00)				
Other clinical (3I00)				
Other non-clinical (3J00)				

Reproduced with kind permission from the Royal College of Anaesthestists.

Table 0.2 *Challenging Concepts in Anaesthesia* Mapped to FRCA basic level units of training

Challenging Concepts in Anaesthesia Chapter: / Unit of Training	1.1 Partial airway obstruction: planning for a suspected difficult airway	1.2 Management of unanticipated failed intubation	2.1 Intraoperative fluid balance: what to measure?	2.2 Accidental awareness during general anaesthesia	2.3 Cardiopulmonary exercise testing: utility in major surgery	3.1 Prolonged laparoscopic surgery	3.2 Anaesthesia for bariatric surgery	4.1 Radiological coiling for cerebral aneurysm	4.2 Anaesthesia in the head-injured patient	5.1 Obstetric haemorrhage: planning a safe delivery	5.2 Category 1 caesarean section: treating mother and child	6.1 Magnetic resonance imaging and the neonate	6.2 Paediatric tonsillectomy	7.1 A case for paravertebral blockade?	7.2 Achieving postoperative pain control	8.1 Multiple trauma and the anaesthetist	9.1 Coronary stents and anaesthesia	9.2 Post-arrest percutaneous coronary intervention: the role of the anaesthetist
Preoperative assessment	X	X		X	X	X	X	X	X	X	X	X	X	X			X	
Premedication				X							X		X		X			
Induction of general anaesthesia	X	X	X	X	X	X	X	X	X	X	X	X	X			X	X	X
Intraoperative care including sedation	X	X	X	X	X	X	X	X	X	X	X	X	X	X	X	X	X	X
Postoperative and recovery room care	X	X	X	X		X	X	X	X	X	X	X	X			X	X	X
Introduction to anaesthesia for emergency surgery		X	X				X	X	X	X	X		X			X	X	
Transfer medicine									X									X
Management of respiratory and cardiac arrest																	X	X
Control of infection														X				
Academic and research				X	X													
Airway management	X	X					X	X			X		X				X	
Critical incidents	X	X		X			X		X	X			X			X	X	X
Day surgery						X						X	X					
General, urological and gynaecological surgery			X		X	X	X									X	X	
Head, neck, maxillo-facial and dental surgery	X											X						
Intensive care medicine			X					X	X								X	X
Non-theatre												X					X	X
Obstetrics										X	X							
Orthopaedic surgery															X	X		
Sedation				X														
Paediatrics including child protection												X	X					
Pain medicine				X										X	X			
Regional				X					X	X				X	X		X	
Trauma and stabilization									X						X	X		
Anatomy	X	X					X	X	X					X				
Physiology and biochemistry			X		X	X	X	X	X			X	X				X	X	X
Pharmacology		X							X				X			X	X	
Physics and clinical measurement			X	X	X			X										
Statistical methods																		

Reproduced with kind permission from the Royal College of Anaesthetists.

CHAPTER 1

Airway management

Partial airway obstruction: planning for a suspected difficult airway

Davina Ross-Anderson

Ⓒ Expert Commentary Anil Patel
CPD Matrix Code: *1C01, 1C02, 2A01, 3A01*

Case history

A 74-year-old man presented to the emergency department at midday complaining of a 6 h history of increasingly difficult and noisy breathing. He had recently been seen in the ear, nose and throat (ENT) outpatient department, having been referred by his general practitioner for investigation of a hoarse voice. Five years previously he had undergone a surgical resection of a small squamous cell carcinoma of the floor of the mouth and had received curative radiotherapy to the area. He had continued to smoke, with a history of 45 pack-years, and consumed ~50 units of alcohol per week. He was prescribed digoxin for rate control of atrial fibrillation.

On arrival at the hospital he was alert, but unable to speak in full sentences. He was noted to have marked inspiratory stridor and tracheal tug. He had a respiratory rate of 24 with a prolonged inspiratory phase and oxygen saturations of 88% on room air, rising to 96% breathing oxygen at 15 L/min via a facemask with reservoir bag. On auscultation of the chest a quiet wheeze was heard throughout. Except for rate-controlled atrial fibrillation, confirmed on electrocardiogram (ECG), cardiovascular examination was unremarkable. A chest X-ray showed clear lung fields bilaterally, with moderate hyperexpansion consistent with emphysema. There was no evidence of pulmonary infection. Arterial blood gas analysis was performed (Table 1.1).

After review by the ENT and anaesthesia on-call teams, he was transferred to the high-dependency unit (HDU) for monitoring, repeated nebulized adrenaline, and continued humidified oxygen therapy, while plans were made to investigate and resolve the symptoms. Heliox therapy was considered as a next-line therapy in the case of further airway deterioration.

The medical records from the patient's outpatient visit 10 days previously were obtained. He had undergone a flexible nasendoscopy at the clinic appointment. There was a hand-drawn picture of the view obtained showing a grey ulcerated mass attached to the left vocal cord, reaching the midline and partial vocal cord paralysis on the

Table 1.1 Arterial blood gas on 15 L/min oxygen via facemask with reservoir bag

pH	7.45
pCO_2	4.6 kPa
pO_2	10.8 kPa
HCO_3^-	28.2 mmol/L

> ⊗ **Learning point** Differential diagnosis of upper airway obstruction
>
> The differential diagnosis of upper airway obstruction is broad and may be classified as shown in Table 1.2.
>
> **Table 1.2 Differential diagnosis of upper airway obstruction**
>
> | | |
> |---|---|
> | Tumour | Benign or malignant tumour of any anatomical part of the upper airway and surrounding structures causing compression, luminal obliteration or vocal cord palsy |
> | | Extrinsic compression from mediastinal masses |
> | Infective | Retropharyngeal abscess |
> | | Acute tonsillitis |
> | | Ludwig angina |
> | | Epiglottitis |
> | | Laryngotracheobronchitis (croup) |
> | | Diphtheria |
> | Traumatic | Foreign body |
> | | Haemorrhage (external laryngeal compression or direct contamination) |
> | | Facial trauma |
> | | Laryngeal stenosis |
> | | Burns (chemical or thermal) |
> | | Acute laryngeal injury |
> | Iatrogenic | Laryngotracheal stenosis post intubation/tracheostomy |
> | Angio-oedema | Anaphylaxis |
> | | C1 esterase inhibitor deficiency |
> | Miscellaneous | Vocal cord paralysis |

> ❝ **Expert comment**
> Adrenaline dosing
>
> Different units use different concentrations of nebulized adrenaline ranging from 1 mg to 5 mg in 5 mL. It is important to check your local protocol.

Following the initial management in the emergency department: humidified oxygen (FiO$_2$ 0.6), repeated doses of nebulized adrenaline (1 mL 1:1,000 diluted in 5 mL 0.9% NaCl) and intravenous corticosteroid (dexamethasone 8 mg), the patient reported his breathing to feel easier and accessory muscle use was noticeably reduced, but a quiet inspiratory stridor remained.

> ⊗ **Learning point** Noisy breathing
>
> Obstruction of the airway usually, but not always, causes noisy breathing. If airflow is so restricted as to be almost non-existent, then the noise of breathing may disappear. The timing of airway noise with respiration may help identify the level of the obstruction. Stridor is a harsh, high-pitched sound caused by turbulent airflow past an upper airway obstruction and was originally used only to describe an inspiratory noise. While an expiratory upper airway noise is correctly termed a wheeze, it has become widespread to use the term stridor to describe both inspiratory and expiratory noise arising from a narrow upper airway. It is therefore useful to describe stridor as 'inspiratory stridor' or 'expiratory stridor' to avoid confusion.
>
> An extrathoracic obstruction will generally produce inspiratory stridor due to worsening of the obstruction secondary to the negative intraluminal pressure. An intrathoracic obstruction generally results in expiratory stridor (wheeze) as the increased intrathoracic pressure during active expiration further compresses the obstruction. In severe obstruction a mixed picture can be seen. Other characteristic noises may provide further clues as to the level of obstruction (Table 1.3).
>
> **Table 1.3 Airway noises**
>
> | Level of obstruction | Noise |
> |---|---|
> | Nasopharyngeal | Stertor |
> | Oropharyngeal | Gurgling |
> | Supraglottic | Inspiratory stridor |
> | Glottic | Inspiratory stridor ± expiratory stridor |
> | Subglottic | Inspiratory stridor ± expiratory stridor |
> | Trachea and large bronchi | Expiratory stridor |
> | Small bronchi | Expiratory wheeze |

➕ **Clinical tip** Respiratory muscle conditioning

Patients with chronic obstruction may exhibit no overt signs of airway obstruction despite having airway diameters of a few millimetres which would cause symptoms if occurring acutely. In acute airway obstruction, the requirement of unusually high intrapleural pressure swings to generate adequate minute ventilation causes respiratory muscles to tire. The increased oxygen requirement of the untrained muscles can use up a large proportion of the available oxygen delivery. In chronic obstruction, the increased work of breathing trains the respiratory muscles, so patients are able to produce normal resting minute ventilation through a tiny airway orifice.

⭐ **Learning point** Heliox

'Heliox' is a helium–oxygen mix (supplied in cylinders in a ratio of 79:21 or 70:30 in the UK) used since the 1930s as a temporizing measure in the management of airway obstruction. The physical properties of helium have advantageous effects on gas flow dynamics across a narrowing. There are two effects:

1. Preservation of laminar flow.
2. Reduced resistance during turbulent flow.

Both effects reduce work of breathing and increase alveolar oxygenation.

The important physical characteristic of heliox is reduced density compared to air (or oxygen), while its viscosity is similar.

Obstructing lesions tend to create turbulent flow. Widespread turbulent flow also occurs when gas and flow is such that the Reynolds number (Re) exceeds 2000.

$$Re = \frac{\rho v d}{\eta} = \frac{\text{density of liquid} \times \text{flow velocity} \times \text{orifice diameter}}{\text{viscosity of fluid}}$$

During turbulent flow, density has an important impact on resistance to flow, whereas in laminar flow viscosity is more important. Heliox's lower density improves flow in areas of turbulence such as across an obstruction. Its lower density also leads to a lower Re (for a given flow rate and orifice diameter) so there is a tendency to preserve laminar flow. As flow in the lower airways is laminar, the effect of heliox is minimal there.

Heliox is usually supplied in a 21% oxygen mixture and additional oxygen may need to be supplied from a separate source to prevent hypoxia. However, since helium requires a concentration of >60% to have a significant effect on gas flow, if an FiO_2 of greater than 40% is needed the physical benefits of heliox diminish.

Heliox should only be used to provide the time for other treatments (medical or surgical) to relieve the obstruction [1].

💬 **Expert comment**

Management of potential airway difficulty often needs to carefully balance the urgency of the patient's clinical condition with providing anaesthesia in a planned, well-equipped setting. Airway planning is best achieved with full history and investigation to determine the site and extent of any lesion and the presence of other factors associated with difficult airway management. Useful information can be obtained from old anaesthetic charts, flexible nasendoscopy and imaging (CT or magnetic resonance imaging) but it is important to remember that lesions may have changed considerably between the time of the investigation and a subsequent emergency presentation. In an emergency situation it is often necessary to proceed without the full clinical information.

left side. The records indicated that there had been no obstructive symptoms at that time. The patient had been booked to attend for an elective microlaryngoscopy, biopsy and debulking procedure the following week. The recent computed tomography (CT) showed that the lesion did not extend below the glottis.

Anaesthetic assessment of his airway revealed an upper denture and poor lower dentition; reduced mouth opening to 3 cm, reduced neck extension to 45° due to previous radiotherapy and a Mallampati score of 3 (Figure 1.1). A previous anaesthetic chart for a urological procedure the year before recorded successful insertion of a size 5 laryngeal mask airway (LMA) giving effective positive pressure ventilation. Repeat flexible nasendoscopy in HDU by the ENT team showed a significant size increase in the non-mobile lesion on the left vocal cord, with left-sided supraglottic oedema (Figure 1.2).

An anaesthesia team was assembled, including a consultant and senior trainee experienced in airway management and a senior anaesthetic assistant. The difficult

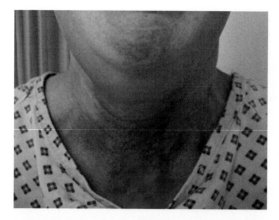

Figure 1.1 Radiotherapy neck with discoloration and 'woody' feel.

⊕ **Clinical tip** Nasal endoscopy

Careful, awake flexible nasendoscopy under topical anaesthesia, by experienced clinicians, provides valuable information regarding the level and site of the airway obstruction. There is a danger, especially in inexperienced hands, of precipitating total airway obstruction. Ideally a senior ENT team member should perform the examination in the presence of the anaesthetist to aid planning of the perioperative management. Flexible nasendoscopy as part of anaesthetic assessment and planning is an under-used technique [2].

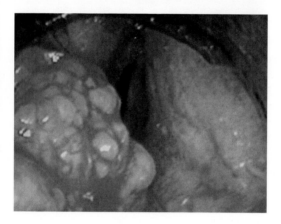

Figure 1.2 View of vocal cords by flexible nasendoscopy.

❝ Expert comment
Defining the difficult airway

It is common to consider the difficult airway as a single entity. In fact, it needs to be viewed as three distinct potential problems:

- difficult facemask ventilation
- difficult direct laryngoscopy
- difficult tracheal tube passage

Ease of supraglottic airway device (SAD) insertion may also be considered as a fourth component, due to its potential importance as a rescue device.

A patient may have any, or all, of these problems which can all result in a failure to oxygenate if not identified and managed promptly and appropriately. It is possible that perfect visualization of the glottis may not be made using direct laryngoscopy, but achieved using either a videolaryngoscope or with flexible fibreoptic intubation.

✪ Learning point The difficult airway trolley

The Difficult Airway Society (DAS) published a list of equipment that should be considered for placement on a difficult airway trolley in 2005 [3]. In addition to the equipment for routine airway management (oropharyngeal and nasopharyngeal airways, laryngeal masks, a range of tracheal tubes, Macintosh laryngoscope blades, gum elastic bougie, stylet and Magill forceps) the list includes the following:

- at least one alternative blade (e.g. straight, McCoy)
- intubating laryngeal mask airway (ILMA™) set (size 3, 4, 5 ILMA with a range of size of ILMA tracheal tubes)
- tracheal tubes: reinforced and microlaryngeal size 5 and 6 mm
- flexible fibreoptic laryngoscope (with portable/battery light source)
- proseal laryngeal mask airway (ProSeal LMA™)
- cricothyroid cannula (e.g. Ravussin) with high pressure jet ventilation system (e.g. Manujet) *or* large bore cricothyroid cannula (e.g. QuickTrach™)
- surgical cricothyroidotomy kit (scalpel with no. 20 blade, tracheal hook, 6/7 mm tracheal and tracheostomy tubes)

In the past few years numerous other airway devices have been produced and their use evaluated. Although any list will be controversial, there are strong arguments for also including the following difficult airway equipment:

- Other SADs for airway rescue or use as an intubation conduit (e.g. i-gel)
- the Aintree intubation catheter to facilitate exchange of SAD for tracheal tube
- a videolaryngoscope with which department members are familiar and trained

airway trolley was available in the operating theatre, with the fibreoptic scope ready for use. The consultant ENT surgeon was on standby to perform a surgical tracheostomy as an emergency. The surgical plan was to perform microlaryngoscopy, biopsy and debulking under suspension laryngoscopy with a microlaryngoscopy tracheal tube to maintain anaesthesia and oxygenation.

It was considered that the patient may be at risk of:

- difficult facemask ventilation due to his dentition and reduced neck extension
- difficult direct laryngoscopy due to his Mallampati score and radiotherapy causing restricted soft tissue movement (Figure 1.2)
- difficult tracheal intubation due to the vocal cord lesion

Using SAD as the primary airway was judged not suitable because of the pathology and the planned surgery.

> ⊕ **Clinical tip** Alternative methods of laryngoscopy
>
> Direct laryngoscopy using a Macintosh, McCoy or Miller blade relies on creating a direct line of sight from the anaesthetist's eye to the patient's glottis. This is often difficult in the case of abnormal airway anatomy and it becomes necessary to look around a corner. Alternative equipment which facilitates this includes videolaryngoscopes (utilizing a channel-on-blade technique or a stylet technique), optical stylets and flexible fibreoptic scopes.

> ❝ **Expert comment**
>
> With end-stage severe airway pathology there may be no method that allows laryngeal visualization. The first laryngoscopy attempt gives the best opportunity for obtaining a view of the larynx. Every subsequent attempt runs the risk of increasing difficulty due to bleeding, oedema and subsequent total airway obstruction. This creates the risk of changing a difficult intubation into a 'can't intubate–can't ventilate/oxygenate' (CICV) situation.

> ✪ **Learning point** The 4th National Audit Project (NAP4) [4, 5]
>
> The report is the result of a year-long prospective study by the Royal College of Anaesthetists and the Difficult Airway Society designed to answer the questions:
>
> - What types of airway device are used during anaesthesia and how often?
> - How often do major complications, leading to serious harm, occur in association with airway management in anaesthesia, in the intensive care units and in the emergency departments of the UK?
> - What is the nature of these events and what can we learn from them, in order to reduce their frequency and consequences?
>
> Among the main findings regarding airway obstruction were:
>
> - poor airway assessment and a failure to alter the airway management technique in response to findings at assessment contributed to poor outcomes.
> - potential difficulties with airway management should be approached using a strategy rather than with a single plan.
> - there was a failure to plan for failure.
> - awake fibreoptic intubation (AFOI) was indicated in many cases, but not used due to deficiencies in skill, confidence, judgement and equipment.
> - repeated attempts at intubation using the same technique led to problems including CICV.

> ❝ **Expert comment** Strategy versus plan
>
> Core training in anaesthesia emphasizes knowledge of the DAS guidelines for unanticipated difficult tracheal intubation, published in 2004 [6]. They have an emphasis on maintaining oxygenation and preventing airway trauma by use of a plan and back-up plans (plan A, B, C, etc). These are essential principles in the management of any airway case, but these guidelines are not intended to be extrapolated to the care of patients with upper airway obstruction (i.e. anticipated difficult intubation). In the case of expected difficulty the main decision-making should involve consideration of the individual clinical circumstances, a team approach with open communication, and the experience and expertise of the anaesthetist and surgeon. In the approach to a difficult airway, anaesthetists should form a co-ordinated logical strategy and communicate this to all who may need to be involved. In this setting a strategy may be defined as a logical sequential series of plans which aim to achieve oxygenation, ventilation, and avoidance of aspiration, and which are appropriate to the patient's specific features and condition. Airway management should not rely on the success of plan A and should be based on a clear strategy that is communicated to all.

⊕ Clinical tip Positive pressure ventilation and the difficult airway

Positive pressure ventilation via tight-fitting facemask or SAD can be an effective method of ventilation in some cases of airway obstruction [7]. During positive pressure ventilation, the walls of the airway are splinted open by the increased intraluminal pressure, in contrast to spontaneous ventilation which creates a sub-atmospheric intraluminal pressure to generate airflow.

However, in some cases facemask ventilation may be impossible (e.g. abnormalities of the facial skeleton) and in others positive pressure ventilation may have an adverse effect of airway obstruction (e.g. a ball-valve obstruction such as a vallecular cyst or pedunculated glottic tumour).

In each case the benefit of applying or avoiding positive pressure ventilation can be better predicted by a full understanding of the anatomy and pathology of the obstruction).

The airway strategy was to conduct awake transtracheal cannulation under local anaesthesia, then perform intravenous induction of anaesthesia with prompt muscle paralysis, perform direct laryngoscopy and intubate the trachea using a microlaryngoscopy tracheal tube. In the event of an inability to intubate after laryngoscopy, the anaesthetist would insert a size 5 classic laryngeal mask and maintain ventilation while preparing for surgical suspension laryngoscopy and transtracheal high frequency jet ventilation. If insertion of the laryngeal mask was unsuccessful the surgeons would perform a surgical tracheostomy (the surgical team would be scrubbed and ready to operate, with all equipment prepared at commencement of induction).

⊕⊕ Expert comment
Choice of technique

There is little consensus among airway anaesthesia experts about the optimum management of the obstructed adult airway, and very little high level evidence to show a preferable technique. Some experts will advocate an approach which is explicitly criticized by other experts in the field. A recent debate about an airway case led to expert choices of inhalational induction, intravenous induction plus neuromuscular blockade and AFOI, when presented with an identical case report [8].

⊕ Clinical tip Awake tracheostomy

Although not chosen here as the primary airway plan, awake tracheostomy performed by an experienced surgeon in some circumstances can be the safest method of airway management in a patient with severe airway obstruction. The ideal position for surgical tracheostomy is supine with the neck extended. In severe compromise this is not possible as the patient may not be able to lie flat due to respiratory compromise, so the surgeon must be confident in performing the surgery with the patient in a semi-recumbent or upright position. Ensure that the patient has been maximally oxygenated prior to starting. The implicit safety of an awake tracheostomy means that the patient must not receive any sedation or anaesthesia while the tracheostomy is performed. This can be difficult for the anaesthetist as awake tracheostomy in a patient who is struggling to breathe is rarely elegant or pleasant for observers. The anaesthetists should be ready to induce anaesthesia immediately once the airway is secured.

✪ Learning point Awake fibreoptic intubation

Awake fibreoptic intubation (AFOI) is an advanced airway management technique which can be useful in the care of some airway problems. Planning for AFOI needs skill, knowledge of site and nature of the obstruction and recognition that it may not be successful. Visualising the route of intubation and using it as a route to pass a tracheal tube while a patient is still fully conscious has many advantages. It is particularly useful in those in whom there may be difficulties with facemask ventilation or with direct laryngoscopy. These patients include those with oral cavity or tongue base lesions, those who have had previous head and neck radiotherapy and those with restricted mouth opening or restricted neck extension. There is debate about the suitability of AFOI in cases of glottic or subglottic narrowing as there is a risk of total airway occlusion. In these situations it may be possible to obtain good visualization of the glottic opening, but not possible to force a tracheal tube through the narrowed lumen. Several of these factors are included in the current case.

The NAP4 report identified 14 failed intubations in 23 fibreoptic intubation attempts in patients with head and neck pathology, of which almost all required a surgical airway. In patients with extensive airway oedema, particularly of an infective origin, the efficacy of topical local anaesthesia will be reduced. In these patients, higher doses of sedation and airway reflex suppression by short-acting opioid such as a remifentanil infusion may be necessary. This needs to be carefully titrated so as not to lose the advantages of a fully awake, spontaneously ventilating, co-operative patient, and carries the risk of oversedation and airway obstruction [9].

⊕ Clinical tip Inhalational induction

The speed of induction of anaesthesia using inhalational agents depends to a certain extent on the minute volume generated by the patient. In cases of airway obstruction, inhalational induction will be extremely slow.

⊗ **Learning point** Inhalational induction

Traditional teaching suggests inhalational induction as a technique for the management of the critically obstructed airway. The theoretical advantage is that a spontaneously breathing patient will be gradually anaesthetized, but that if at any point the airway becomes obstructed and no further gas flow is possible, the inhalational agent present will be redistributed away from the brain, the patient will wake and the airway obstruction will be relieved. Clinical experience, supported by data from NAP4, suggests that this technique is unreliable, and that once airway obstruction has occurred, the patient will desaturate and not waken. In reality, an inhalational induction in a patient with a critically obstructed airway often includes apnoeic periods where hypoxia and hypercapnia ensue. To maintain oxygenation at this point it will be necessary to provide positive pressure ventilation using a bag and mask.

❝ **Expert comment**
Choice of inhalational agent

Traditionally halothane was used for inhalational induction, and the physical properties of sevoflurane are less favourable for this process. The end-tidal concentration of halothane falls more quickly than that of sevoflurane, allowing a faster wake-up.

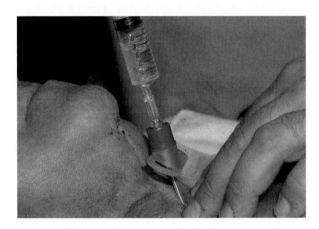

Figure 1.3 Transtracheal cannulation.

On arrival in the anaesthetic room the patient was noted to be unable to lie flat due to shortness of breath and had a quiet inspiratory stridor with a markedly prolonged inspiratory phase and extensive use of accessory muscles. Routine monitoring was started and showed the patient to have SpO_2 of 95% on 15 L/min oxygen by facemask with a respiratory rate of 28 breaths/min, heart rate between 80 and 100 beats/min (atrial fibrillation) and non-invasive blood pressure 145/86.

The patient was asked to extend his neck as far as possible and the skin of the anterior neck was anaesthetized below the level of the second tracheal ring using 2 mL 2% lidocaine. A further 3 mL was injected into the trachea. Transtracheal cannulation was performed by the consultant anaesthetist using a 13G Ravussin cannula designed for this purpose (Figure 1.3). Positioning was confirmed by the aspiration of air into a saline-filled syringe during insertion and by capnography. Equipment for high-frequency jet ventilation was available for use via the transtracheal cannula if necessary.

⊗ **Learning point** Anterior neck access

Anterior neck access to the airway has different requirements and considerations in the elective and the emergency situation.

In an emergency, failure and complication rates of narrow-bore cannulas are high, particularly due to cannula kinking, malposition, barotrauma, and use of unfamiliar or unsuitable equipment. In a head and neck emergency, there is a greater role for formal surgical tracheostomy. NAP4 suggests that anaesthetists should be trained to provide a surgical airway.

(continued)

In the elective situation there is a role for narrow-bore anterior neck access. A Ravussin cannula or similar, designed for tracheal access, can be inserted prophylactically into the cricothyroid membrane or into the upper trachea between the tracheal rings (Figure 1.3). It is then possible to insufflate oxygen at low flow rate or to use high-pressure source ventilation via the cannula. High-pressure source ventilation includes manual low-frequency techniques, such as with a Manujet, and automated techniques, such as high-frequency 'jet' ventilation or oscillation. Having a method of oxygenation available prior to intravenous induction of anaesthesia gives additional time for airway manipulation so that the difficult laryngoscopy is not rushed and is more likely to be successful at first attempt. If high-pressure source ventilation is required via the cannula, the safest technique is likely to be the use of an automated jet ventilator with airway pressure monitoring and pressure-limiting cut-out. However, these are not widely available and manual insufflation with a Sanders or Manujet 'injector' is more common. Whichever technique is used it is vital to ensure that there is a route for exhalation via the upper airway—simple airway manoeuvres or LMA may assist in this. Without a route for expiration there is a very high risk of barotrauma. A narrow-bore cannula can be left in place postoperatively for emergency oxygen therapy if necessary. This technique allows some patients to avoid surgical tracheostomy, with its associated morbidity [10].

✪ Learning point Cormack and Lehane grade

The Cormack and Lehane grade was devised in 1984 to classify difficult intubation, mainly for training purposes (Table 1.4, Figure 1.5) [11]. There have been later modifications proposed to clarify differences in difficulty within a grade (Table 1.5) [12, 13]. The grade refers to the best view obtained with external manipulation of the airway.

Table 1.4 Cormack and Lehane grade at direct laryngoscopy

Grade 1	Most of the glottis is visible
Grade 2	Partial view of the glottis or arytenoids
Grade 3	Only the epiglottis is visible
Grade 4	No laryngeal structures are seen

Reproduced from RS Cormack and J Lehane, 'Difficult tracheal intubation in obstetrics', *Anaesthesia*, 39, 11, pp. 1105–1111, Copyright © 1984, John Wiley and Sons and The Association of Anaesthetists of Great Britain and Ireland, with permission.

Table 1.5 Modifications to Cormack and Lehane grade

Grade 2a	Partial view of the glottis
Grade 2b	Only arytenoids or most posterior part of vocal cords are visible
Grade 3a	Only the epiglottis is visible—and can be lifted
Grade 3b	Only the epiglottis is visible—and cannot be lifted

Grades 2a and 2b Reproduced from Yentis SM, The effects of single-handed or bimanual cricoid pressure on ease of tracheal intubation. *Anaesthesia* 1997; 52: 332–5, with permission from the Association of Anaesthetists of Great Britain & Ireland/Blackwell Publishing Ltd. Grades 3a and 3b Cook TM, Nolan JP, Gabbott DA. Cricoid pressure: are two hands better than one? *Anaesthesia* 1997; 52: 179–80. Cook TM. A new practical classification of laryngoscopy. *Anaesthesia* 2000; 55: 274–9.

After administration of 100% oxygen via a tight-fitting facemask for 3 min, anaesthesia was induced using fentanyl 100 μg, propofol 160 mg, and rocuronium 40 mg. Facemask ventilation with 100% oxygen was possible and anaesthesia was maintained by adding sevoflurane 2–4%. It was still possible to maintain good chest movement after laying the trolley flat. Direct laryngoscopy was attempted using a size 4 Macintosh blade which revealed a Cormack and Lehane grade 3 view of the larynx. This was deemed inadequate for an intubation attempt, so following further facemask ventilation, a second laryngoscopy attempt was made using a straight Miller blade in a paramedian approach, which revealed a grade 2a view of the larynx, and enabled

> ✪ **Learning point** The neuromuscular blockade debate
>
> If the airway management strategy chosen involves an intravenous induction prior to airway manipulation, the decision of whether to then use neuromuscular blockade comes to the fore. Junior anaesthetists are often taught not to administer neuromuscular blockade until they have checked whether bag-mask ventilation is possible; however, many senior anaesthetists do not practise this method of anaesthesia themselves, and there is little evidence to support this view [14]. Intravenous induction and neuromuscular blockade provide the best conditions for a successful first attempt at laryngoscopy and intubation [15]. For routine airway management the administration of neuromuscular blockade almost always makes mask ventilation easier, and can even resolve a 'can't ventilate' situation. Whether the same is true for the obstructed airway has not been demonstrated. Where a technique of induction of anaesthesia with neuromuscular blockade is chosen as the primary plan it is wise to have a clear strategy for managing both difficult or impossible intubation and difficult or failed ventilation.
>
> Sugammadex allows rapid reversal of the neuromuscular blockade of rocuronium and may come to be used by some to create new strategies for difficult airway management; however, sugammadex will only reverse airway obstruction due to pharmacological effects on the airway, not mechanical effects. Use of sugammadex is no substitute for a clear airway strategy including a plan for management of CICV [16].

> ❝ **Expert comment**
> Alternative laryngoscope blade versus videolaryngoscope
>
> Standard laryngoscopy using a Macintosh blade is often the first choice for airway instrumentation, but may not always provide optimum visualization of the glottic inlet. If this occurs, or is expected to occur, then use of an alternative laryngoscope blade or videolaryngoscope can improve the glottic view. Alternative laryngoscope blades, such as McCoy or Miller, cause different forces to be exerted on the airway and therefore different movement of tissue, and can allow a direct, straight line, view of the glottis to be obtained. Videolaryngoscopes allow the anaesthetist to look around the corner, and can bypass the need to increase or change forces applied. It is important in a difficult situation that anaesthetists choose a technique with which they are familiar.

intubation of the trachea using a 5.0 mm inner diameter laser-safe tracheal tube past the vocal cord lesion with no obvious bleeding or trauma.

Surgery proceeded uneventfully to debulk the vocal cord lesion and take biopsies. After the surgery had finished, the position of the transtracheal cannula was checked and confirmed using capnography. Muscle relaxation was reversed using sugammadex and the inhalational anaesthesia discontinued. The patient was positioned in a 45° head-up position and his trachea was extubated once he was fully awake. After extubation, there was very mild stridor, with no use of accessory muscles, and the patient was able to speak in a hoarse voice.

The patient was transferred to the HDU for postoperative care, which involved continuing with intravenous steroid and nebulized saline. The transtracheal cannula was left in position as a precaution but was not needed and was removed 24 h postoperatively.

Discussion

This case of severe airway obstruction is one of many possible difficult airway situations that an anaesthetist can be faced with and highlights the need for a full assessment of the patient, the clinical urgency, the facilities available and the skills of the personnel involved in order to provide safe anaesthesia [18]. A balance must be struck between timely anaesthetic and surgical intervention and proper preparedness. Management of the obstructed airway requires particular skill and co-operation between anaesthetist and surgeon. This is best performed in a fully equipped environment with full surgical, anaesthetic and nursing support. An operating theatre (rather than an anaesthetic room, for instance) is the ideal location. If appropriate facilities and staff are not immediately available then holding measures using nebulized adrenaline, intravenous steroid and heliox can be instituted.

In this case, the airway was likely to be compromised and difficult to manage due to multiple factors, and each had a bearing on the decisions taken. Delineating the anatomical site of obstruction and the nature of the obstruction will help to decide which airway techniques are more likely to be successful, and which should be avoided. Obstruction at the nasopharyngeal or oropharyngeal level is likely to make facemask

> ❝ **Expert comment**
> Emergence
>
> The NAP4 report showed that one-third of adverse perioperative airway events occurred during emergence or recovery. This time needs to be recognized as high risk, and needs equally careful planning as induction. DAS has now developed guidelines for extubation planning [17].

ventilation and direct or videolaryngoscopy difficult or impossible, and these cases are often most suited to an awake fibreoptic technique. If facemask ventilation and laryngoscopy is not anticipated to be difficult, for example in a subglottic lesion, then a direct laryngoscopy view may be enhanced by the use of alternate laryngoscope blades or videolaryngoscopy. Obstructing lesions at the supraglottic and glottic level may be less amenable to a fibreoptic approach due to the risk of complete airway obstruction. It is important to remember that all the other common reasons causing difficult airway management, such as receding or poorly mobile mandible, previous radiotherapy, poor dentition, short thyromental distance, and reduced neck mobility, can also be present in patients with an obstructed airway (indeed several are more likely in this group of patients) and may influence the management strategy. The quality of evidence guiding best management of the obstructed airway is at a low level, and there is often a lack of consensus about an appropriate sequence of interventions.

Inhalational induction of anaesthesia is fraught with difficulty. Most anaesthetists will rarely perform inhalation induction in an adult patient, let alone in adults with obstructed airways, despite being relatively familiar with paediatric inhalational induction. The requirement to gain adequate minute volume for anaesthesia and complete airway relaxation is often difficult in those with severe obstruction due to the flow restriction. The technique may be of help in those with mild airway obstruction.

Fibreoptic intubation is a complex, highly skilled technique and should only be used in a critical airway by those familiar with it, as the risks of total airway obstruction and trauma are higher in inexperienced hands.

Tracheostomy under local anaesthesia may offer a safer alternative to tracheal intubation after induction of anaesthesia, and it should be actively considered in every case of obstructed airway. When surgical airway performed by a surgeon is the back-up plan, preparation should be made so this is instantly available.

Management of all high-risk airways requires an acceptance that the primary chosen technique may fail. Clear back-up planning is mandatory.

A Final Word from the Expert

Every patient with an obstructed airway needs a bespoke airway management strategy. An airway intervention is most likely to be successful when careful planning has been undertaken [19, 20].

Each attempt at laryngoscopy and tracheal intubation reduces the chance of success, both due to the risks of traumatizing the airway structures and due to human factors such as task fixation and (lack of) situation awareness.

An airway anaesthesia expert will have many high-level skills in their repertoire to enable them to deal with the difficult obstructed airway, but all anaesthetists should be able to provide safe airway management for these difficult patients without resorting to techniques with which they are unfamiliar, and recognize that this includes liaison with the surgical team to provide an awake tracheostomy under local anaesthesia.

References

1. McGarvey JM, Pollack CV. Heliox in airway management. *Emerg Med Clin North Am* 2008;26:905–20.

2. Rosenblatt W, Ianus AI, Sukhupragarn W, Fickenscher A, Sasaki C. Preoperative endoscopic airway examination (PEAE) provides superior airway information and may reduce the use of unnecessary awake intubation. *Anesth Analg* 2011;112:602–7.

3. Difficult Airway Society. *Recommended equipment for management of unanticipated difficult intubation;* July 2005. < http://www.das.uk.com/equipmentlistjuly2005.htm >

4. Cook TM, Woodall N, Frerk C. Fourth National Audit Project. Major complications of airway management in the UK: results of the Fourth National Audit Project of the Royal College of Anaesthetists and the Difficult Airway Society. Part 1: Anaesthesia. *Br J Anaesth* 2011;106:617–31.

5. Cook TM, Woodall N, Harper J, Benger J. Fourth National Audit Project. Major complications of airway management in the UK: results of the Fourth National Audit Project of the Royal College of Anaesthetists and the Difficult Airway Society. Part 2: intensive care and emergency departments. *Br J Anaesth* 2011;106:632–42.

6. Henderson JJ, Popat MT, Latto IP, Pearce AC. Difficult Airway Society guidelines for management of the unanticipated difficult intubation. *Anaesthesia* 2004;59:675–94.

7. Nouraei SAR, Giussani DA, Howard DJ, Sandhu GS, Ferguson C, Patel A. Physiological comparison of spontaneous and positive-pressure ventilation in laryngotracheal stenosis. *Br J Anaesth* 2008; 101: 419–-23.

8. Cook TM, Morgan PJ, Hersch PE. Equal and opposite expert opinion. Airway obstruction by a retrosternal thyroid mass: management and prospective international expert opinion. *Anaesthesia* 2011;66:828–36.

9. Mingo OH, Ashpole KJ, Irving CJ, Rucklidge MW. Remifentanil sedation for awake fibreoptic intubation with limited application of local anaesthetic in patients for elective head and neck surgery. *Anaesthesia* 2008;63:1065–9.

10. Ross-Anderson DJ, Ferguson C, Patel A. Transtracheal jet ventilation in 50 patients with severe airway compromise and stridor. *Br J Anaesth* 2011;106:140–4.

11. Cormack RS, Lehane J. Difficult tracheal intubation in obstetrics. *Anaesthesia* 1984;39:1105–11.

12. Yentis SM. The effects of single-handed or bimanual cricoid pressure on ease of tracheal intubation. *Anaesthesia* 1997;52:332–5.

13. Cook TM. A grading system for direct laryngoscopy. *Anaesthesia* 1999;54:496–7.

14. Broomhead RH, Marks RJ, Ayton P. Confirmation of the ability to ventilate by facemask before administration of neuromuscular blocker: a non-instrumental piece of information? *Br J Anaesth* 2010;104:313–17.

15. Calder I, Yentis S, Patel A. Muscle relaxants and airway management. *Anesthesiology* 2009;111:216–17.

16. Curtis R, Lomax S, Patel B. Use of sugammadex in a 'can't intubate, can't ventilate' situation. *Br J Anaesth* 2012;108:612–14.

17. Popat M, Mitchell V, Dravid R, Patel A, Swampillai C, Higgs A. Difficult Airway Society Guidelines for the management of tracheal extubation. *Anaesthesia* 2012;67:318–40.

18. Hung O, Murphy M. Context-sensitive airway management. *Anesth Analg* 2010;110:982–3.

19. Patel A, Pearce A. Progress in the management of the obstructed airway. *Anaesthesia* 2011;66 Suppl 2:93–100.

20. Patel A, Pearce A, Pracy P. Head and neck pathology. In: Cook T, Woodall N, Frerk C editors. *4th National Audit Project of the Royal College of Anaesthetists and the Difficult Airway Society. Major complications of airway management in the United Kingdom.* London: Royal College of Anaesthetists; 2011. p. 143–54.

Management of unanticipated failed intubation

Abigail Fell

⊕ **Expert Commentary** Chris Frerk

CPD Matrix Code: *1C01, 1C02, 1B01, 2A01, 2A06, 3A01*

Case history

A 45-year-old lady was admitted to hospital for elective laparoscopic cholecystectomy.

At the preoperative assessment clinic a past medical history of well-controlled asthma treated with regular salbutamol and becotide inhalers was identified. Her asthma was stable with no history of intensive care admission nor admissions to hospital since she was a teenager. She did not take any other regular medication and had no allergies. She was a non-smoker and denied any history of gastro-oesophageal reflux. Her weight was documented as 84 kg, her body mass index (BMI) was 34 kg/m². She had a normal exercise tolerance and vital signs and routine blood results were unremarkable.

Airway assessment on the day of her admission by the anaesthetic ST5 allocated to the list revealed a Mallampati score of 2 with full range of neck movements (Figure 1.4). She was appropriately fasted.

The anaesthetic plan was discussed with the operating department practitioner (anaesthetic assistant) and included routine intravenous induction of anaesthesia, paralysis with a non-depolarizing muscle relaxant, followed by tracheal intubation with a size 7.0 mm inner diameter (ID) tracheal tube.

On arrival in the anaesthetic room a pre-induction World Health Organization (WHO) check ('sign in') was carried out by the anaesthetic trainee and anaesthetic assistant, in keeping with hospital policy. The patient's identity and proposed operation

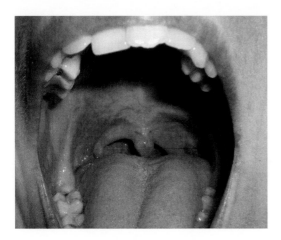

Figure 1.4 Mallampati 2 view (posterior pharyngeal wall visible, including posterior pillars of the fauces but not tip of uvula); the better the view the more likely it is that intubation will be straightforward.

⊗ **Learning point** Prediction of difficult intubation

The Mallampati test [1] is one of several clinical assessment tools developed to attempt prediction of difficulty with tracheal intubation. The orophaynx is inspected while the patient opens the mouth maximally and protrudes the tongue maximally without phonating. It originally consisted of three classes [1]:

Class 1: posterior pharyngeal wall visible, including posterior pillars of the fauces and tip of uvula.
Class 2: posterior pharyngeal wall visible, including posterior pillars of the fauces but not tip of uvula.
Class 3: posterior pharyngeal wall not visible, soft palate visible.

Samsoon and Young modified the classification, adding class 4 when the soft palate is not visible [2].

The implication is that as the Mallampati class increases so does the risk of difficult laryngoscopy (poor laryngeal view). In practice the ability to see the posterior pharyngeal wall identifies an 'easy' or 'difficult' view. Used alone the Mallampati test is an imprecise tool (with a low sensitivity and specificity and a positive predictive value as low as 5%) but combining it with evaluation of other predictors improves the specificity and sensitivity of the preoperative assessment. An assessment that takes account of a variety of anatomical findings is most likely to predict problems accurately [3,4]. The combination of Mallampati class 3 or 4, interincisor distance of ≤4 cm, and a thyromental distance of ≤6.5 cm has been shown to have 85% sensitivity and 95% specificity for difficult tracheal intubation [5].

Preoperative airway assessment will predict many difficult airways; however, despite careful preoperative evaluation, false-negative results will occur and approximately half of difficult intubations are not predicted, so strategies to manage the unanticipated difficult intubation should be pre-formulated and practised [4].

Reproduced from Mallampati SR, Gatt SP, Gugino LD, Desai SP, Waraksa B, Freiberger D, Liu PL. (1985). A clinical sign to predict difficult tracheal intubation: A prospective study. *Canadian Anaesthetists' Society Journal* 32 (4): 429–434, with permission from the Canadian Anaesthesiologists Society.

Expert comment

Airway assessment is an imperfect science but should aim to identify a predetermined cut-off threshold (a 'trigger point') which prompts the anaesthetist to change the primary intubation plan. There is no perfect cut-off point; if the chosen threshold is low the anaesthetist will use an alternate strategy more frequently and (assuming the alternate intubation plan is an effective one, such as AFOI) will encounter fewer unexpected difficult intubations. Conversely if the threshold is high the anaesthetist will use the default strategy more often and will encounter more 'unexpected' difficult intubations.

⊕ **Clinical tip** Size of tracheal tube

Smaller ID tracheal tubes are easier to insert and are associated with less laryngeal and tracheal morbidity. Sizes of 6.0–6.5 mm ID are entirely satisfactory in clinical use [6] and sizes >8.0 (male) and >7.0 (female) should not be used other than in exceptional circumstances (e.g. for the patient who will need prolonged ventilation and weaning on an intensive care unit) [7].

Expert comment

The WHO sign in is a good time to confirm the airway management strategy (including fallback plans in case of unexpected difficulty) with the anaesthetic assistant [8].

⊕ **Clinical tip** Importance of good facemask seal

Maintaining a good facemask seal during preoxygenation provides final confirmation that capnography is connected and functional prior to induction of anaesthesia as well as allowing demonstration of adequate denitrogenation of the lungs.

Expert comment

The dose of atracurium used in this case was <0.5 mg/kg. Inadequate paralysis is associated with suboptimal intubating conditions. Use of a nerve stimulator allows confirmation of full paralysis before laryngoscopy. Regardless of the cause of difficulty in this case it was good practice to avoid persistent intubation attempts in favour of returning to facemask ventilation.

⊗ **Learning point** Incidence of failed intubation

Failure to intubate the trachea occurs in approximately one in 2,000 cases in the non-obstetric population and one in 300 cases in the obstetric population [2]. In the UK a typical hospital can expect between five and 10 failed intubations each year; in the 4th National Audit Project of the Royal College of Anaesthetists and the Difficult Airway Society: major complications of airway management in the UK (NAP4) [8] difficult or delayed intubation, failed intubation and CICV were the primary cause of 39% of serious complications of anaesthetic airway management (leading to death, brain damage, emergency surgical airway or intensive care unit admission) [8].

> **✪ Learning point** Optimizing view at direct laryngoscopy
>
> The best laryngoscopic view is dependent on optimal patient positioning and optimal technique. A frequent problem with laryngoscopy is failure to correctly position the head and neck with the upper cervical spine extended and the lower cervical spine flexed: it is the latter that many forget.
>
> External manipulation of the larynx should be the initial response to a poor view at direct laryngoscopy [4]. Optimal external laryngeal manipulation is described as pressing posteriorly and cephalad over the thyroid, hyoid and cricoid cartilages in an attempt to improve the view, performed initially by the anaesthetist to achieve the best view, and subsequently maintained by the assistant [9]. Alternatively the assistant may apply 'Backwards Upward and to the Right Pressure' (BURP) which opposes the tissue movements caused by laryngoscopy. These manoeuvres are different from cricoid pressure, which, when performed by a blinded assistant, has been shown to impair laryngeal view on ~30% of occasions [10–12].

> **✪ Learning point** McCoy blade
>
> The McCoy is the most widely available alternate blade in the UK. It is known to be useful where the problem with laryngoscopy is caused by limited neck extension (83% of grade 3 views improved compared with the Macintosh) [13]. However, in unselected populations the McCoy only improves the view in 20% of cases [14].

were confirmed against the consent form. Anaesthetic machine and medicines checks were confirmed along with the lack of any history of allergy. The anaesthetist informed the anaesthetic assistant that there was no increased risk of aspiration and confirmed the airway management plan.

The patient was positioned on a tilting trolley with monitoring attached prior to venous cannulation. The patient was then preoxygenated, followed by induction of anaesthesia when the end-tidal oxygen level reached 80%. After administration of fentanyl 100 μg, propofol 200 mg and atracurium 40 mg the patient's lungs were ventilated with isoflurane 1.5% in oxygen without difficulty, using a single-handed facemask technique.

After 3 min of facemask ventilation, direct laryngoscopy was performed using a size 3 Macintosh blade and a grade 3 view was noted (only epiglottis seen), which was not improved by the anaesthetic assistant applying pressure on the front of the neck (Figure 1.5). A single attempt at intubating the trachea was made with the use of a gum elastic bougie. The bougie could not be advanced and the intubation was abandoned in favour of continuing oxygenation of the patient by facemask.

Following repositioning of the head on the pillow a second attempt at intubation was performed, this time using a size 3 McCoy laryngoscope blade in an attempt to improve the view. The view was the same as before but this time the bougie could be advanced easily and the 7.0 mm ID tracheal tube was railroaded.

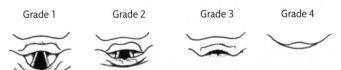

| Grade 1 | Grade 2 | Grade 3 | Grade 4 |

Figure 1.5 Cormack and Lehane classification of laryngeal view. Reproduced from RS Cormack and J Lehane. Difficult tracheal intubation in obstetrics. *Anaesthesia* 39, 11, pp. 1105–1111. Copyright © 1984, John Wiley and Sons and The Association of Anaesthetists of Great Britain and Ireland, with permission.

❝ Expert comment

Lack of a carbon dioxide trace means that the lungs are not being ventilated. Despite this being well known, an overt discussion with the anaesthetic assistant can help correct decision-making in such a situation. Announcing aloud that 'this is a failed intubation' may be helpful to all those present so that the anaesthetic team and surrounding staff have a clear, shared understanding of what they are dealing with.

❝ Expert comment

Using rocuronium rather than atracurium in this case would have given the anaesthetist the additional option of immediate reversal of paralysis with sugammadex and waking the patient up.

❝ Expert comment

When you encounter a difficult airway it is important to remember that you are not alone. In the NAP4 study when airway problems were encountered and senior assistance was requested, help usually arrived in less than 5 min.

❝ Expert comment

Repeating a technique that has failed in the hands of an experienced colleague is not good practice. When intubation fails further attempts have an 80% chance of repeated failure [16]. As well as being unlikely to succeed it 'wastes' one further attempt at laryngoscopy. In this case the consultant sensibly attempted a different intubation technique.

✚ Clinical tip Failed intubation

Placing an SAD following failed intubation is a good plan. As well as 'giving the anaesthetist's hands a rest' it serves as declaration of failure, reducing the temptation to have another look. In this case stopping after two attempts at laryngoscopy left options for the 'help' that had been summoned. When difficulty is encountered during attempts at tracheal intubation, maintenance of oxygenation and avoidance of hypercapnia is paramount. The quality of the airway may deteriorate with multiple intubation attempts, leading to the development of progressive difficulty in ventilating the lungs with a facemask; the final result may be progression to a CICV situation requiring an emergency surgical airway [15]. The DAS guidelines recommend a maximum of four attempts at laryngoscopy in an elective setting and three during rapid sequence induction; some sources suggest that even four attempts are too many.

On connecting the breathing system to the tracheal tube, ventilation was commenced but no carbon dioxide trace was seen on the capnograph. The lack of carbon dioxide was noted by the anaesthetist and the anaesthetic assistant and they agreed that the tube was in the oesophagus. The anaesthetist removed the tube and resumed facemask ventilation. He then discussed with the anaesthetic assistant what they should do next and they agreed that he would place an LMA to 'give his hands a rest' and call for help. A size 5 classic LMA was passed easily and manual ventilation was re-established with a normal capnography trace. The anaesthetic assistant then asked one of the theatre healthcare assistants to contact the consultant anaesthetist on call to come and help urgently with a 'failed intubation'.

Just 2 min later a consultant anaesthetist arrived to help and took over control of the anaesthetic.

After establishing the sequence of events up to that point the consultant asked for the difficult intubation trolley while anaesthesia and oxygenation was maintained via the LMA. Indirect laryngoscopy was then performed using a Pentax video laryngoscope preloaded with a 7.0 mm ID tracheal tube (Figure 1.6).

A full view of the vocal cords was achieved and the trachea was intubated successfully, confirmed under vision with the videolaryngoscope, and subsequently with capnography. The tube was secured in place and the patient was transferred into the operating theatre.

The consultant confirmed that the trainee was happy to manage the anaesthetic from this point but agreed to return for the end of surgery and extubation. Surgery lasted

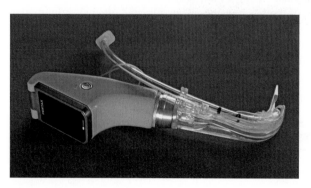

Figure 1.6 The Pentax videolaryngoscope loaded with a 7.0 mm ID tracheal tube. Reproduced with kind permission from Ambu Ltd, copyright Pentax.

> ★ **Learning point** Equipment choices
>
> DAS guidelines advocate alternative intubation devices such as alternate laryngoscopes or the ILMA (Fastrach™, Intavent Direct, UK).
>
> In larger patients the view at laryngoscopy may be improved by using a size 4 Macintosh blade (rather than the more widely used size 3) to ensure that the tip of the blade reaches the base of the vallecula enabling optimal elevation of the epiglottis.
>
> In this case the McCoy blade and a videolaryngoscope were used but other alternatives would have been equally appropriate providing that the anaesthetist had the relevant training and experience in the chosen technique.
>
> The ILMA (Figure 1.7) appears in DAS guidelines for failed intubation and has a high rate of success in expert hands, but the technique is not widely taught. The ILMA has a more rigid, wider tube than the classic LMA [17–20] through which a modified tracheal tube is passed into the trachea; a bar overlying the lower aperture lifts the epiglottis forward, facilitating intubation.
>
> The flexible fibreoptic laryngoscope is the established 'gold standard' for the management of the predicted difficult airway [21] and can also be used in the event of unanticipated difficult intubation. Its effectiveness is compromised in the unconscious or anaesthetized patient [4] and using an SAD as a conduit for fibreoptic intubation in this situation is recognized to make the procedure easier [22].
>
> Intubation through a classic LMA with a small-diameter uncut tracheal tube (6.0 mm for size 4 classic LMA, 7.0 mm for size 5 classic LMA) is possible but when attempted blind has a success rate of <25%. Using an ILMA is reported to give a first-time success rate of tracheal intubation of 75%. To increase the success rate of intubation through an SAD to well above 95% a fibreoptic technique either alone or with an Aintree intubation catheter (Cook Medical, Bloomington, IN, USA) can be used [22–25]. The i-gel (Intersurgical, Wokingham, UK) is as effective as the ILMA as a conduit for fibreoptic intubation [26].
>
>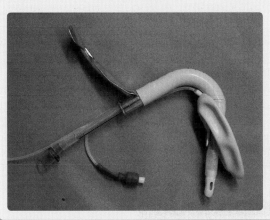
>
> **Figure 1.7** The intubating laryngeal mask airway (ILMA) with purpose-designed tube.
> Reproduced with kind permission from Teleflex.

> ❝ **Expert comment**
>
> There are a number of different videolaryngoscopes on the market which have been reported to rescue failed Macintosh intubations. Unfortunately current evidence does not tell us which videolaryngoscopes perform best and consequently the choice of device remains somewhat controversial.
>
> Success with these devices is (as with all advanced intubation aids) dependent on training and familiarity with their use. Anaesthetists should be experienced in using a videolaryngoscope in elective cases before considering it as a rescue tool in unanticipated failed intubation.

> ❝ **Expert comment**
>
> Failing to intubate is a stressful event and the anaesthetist involved may subsequently underperform for the rest of the anaesthetic. It may have been appropriate for the on-call consultant to remain with the trainee throughout the case.

> ★ **Learning point** Confirmation of tracheal intubation
>
> Waveform capnography is the most reliable method of determining correct tube placement and is defined as the presence of carbon dioxide for a minimum of five successive ventilations. Capnography is now cited by the Association of Anaesthetists of Great Britain and Ireland (AAGBI) as a mandatory tool when conducting general anaesthesia, regardless of location [27].

⭐ **Learning point** Extubation

NAP4 showed that problems at extubation are more likely when difficulty has been encountered at intubation and in these cases a strategy should be in place to ensure oxygenation during and immediately following removal of the tracheal tube. Urgent reintubation is often more difficult than at the start of anaesthesia due to oedema from airway instrumentation, its emergency nature and the rather uncontrolled nature of emergence and extubation which may be associated with hypoxaemia, hypercapnia, haemodynamic instability, patient agitation, and sometimes inadequate preparation or assistance [3]. Planning for problems at extubation necessitates ensuring that all equipment and drugs are available in case they should be needed. NAP4 highlighted several cases of unacceptable delays where this had not occurred. In 2012 DAS produced guidelines for tracheal extubation (Figure 1.8), focusing on where and when it should happen, and how it should be carried out, to ensure avoidance of unnecessary complications [28]. The guidelines emphasize assessment as to whether extubation is likely to be low or high risk. In high-risk situations an awake extubation is strongly recommended with a number of specialized techniques described. All anaesthetists should be familiar with these guidelines [28].

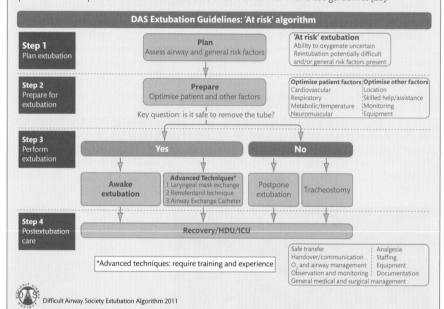

Figure 1.8 Difficult Airway Society extubation guidelines: 'At risk' algorithm. http://www.das.uk.com/guidelines/downloads.html. Reproduced from Popat M, Mitchell V, Dravid R, Patel A, Swampillai C, Higgs A. Difficult Airway Society Guidelines for the management of tracheal extubation. *Anaesthesia* 2012; 67: 318–340, with permission from the Association of Anaesthetists of Great Britain & Ireland/Blackwell Publishing Ltd.

➕ **Clinical tip** Airway problems in recovery

Airway problems are more likely in recovery when problems have occurred intraoperatively. In NAP4 almost one-third of major airway complications associated with anaesthesia occurred either at emergence or in the recovery room. Handover to recovery nurses is especially important and should include signs to look out for, and where help can be obtained. Drugs and equipment that may be required should be readily available in the recovery area.

⭐ **Learning point** Documentation

Following difficulty with intubation, it is important that details of the anaesthetic are documented. This is the responsibility of the anaesthetist involved and should not be delegated to the surgical team [29].

Details of the nature of the problem and how it was dealt with should be recorded on the anaesthetic chart. A letter should also be sent to the patient detailing the problem encountered and how it was resolved [4] with a copy to the general practitioner, in the hospital notes, and stored in the anaesthetic department. The patient should be advised to present this letter at any future hospital admission. The aim is to ensure that any patient with a history of airway difficulty can communicate this (with a detailed history of the event) should any further admission to hospital necessitate general anaesthesia [29]. An example 'Airway Alert' form is available electronically from the DAS website <www.das.uk.com/guidelines/airwayalert.html>, which can be downloaded and modified for local use. A modified example is shown in Figure 1.9. Including the Read code for difficult intubation (SP2y3) in the letter enables the general practitioner to classify the event correctly.

AIRWAY ALERT

XXXX Hospital,
Tel XXXXX
Email XXXXX

Name	....
Date of birth Hospital number	
Home address Telephone	
GP address Tel	

To the patient:

Please keep this letter safe and show it to your doctor if you are admitted to hospital.

Please show this letter to the anaesthetic doctor if you need an operation.

This letter explains the difficulties that were found during your recent anaesthetic and the information may be useful to doctors treating you in the future.

To the GP:

Please copy this letter with any future referral.

READ CODE SP2y3

Summary of Airway Management

Date of operation: ....

Type of operation: ....

		Reasons/comments
Difficult mask ventilation?	**YES/NO**	
Difficult SAD insertion?	**YES/NO**	
Difficult direct laryngoscopy?	**YES/NO**	
Difficult videolaryngoscopy?	**YES/NO**	
Difficult tracheal intubation?	**YES/NO**	
Laryngoscopy grade	1/2a / 2b / 3a / 3b /4	
Extubation		
Further investigation		

Equipment used: ....

Other information: ....

Is awake intubation necessary in the future?

Follow up care (tick when completed)

Copies of letter

YES/NO One copy to patient

YES/NO One copy to GP

YES/NO One copy in case notes

YES/NO One copy in anaesthetic department

YES/NO Spoken to patient

YES/NO Anaesthetic chart complete

YES/NO Information on front of case notes

YES/NO Medic Alert or Difficult Airway

Society referral (Specify)

Name of anaesthetist: ....

Grade: .... Date: ....

If you require further information please contact the Anaesthetic Department.

Figure 1.9 Example template of difficult airway alert letter. Available from The Difficult Airway Society website. http://www.das.uk.com/guidelines/downloads.html. Reproduced with permission from the Difficult Airway Society and David Ball.

45 min and was uneventful, following which the consultant anaesthetist returned as arranged.

Equipment was prepared including the LMA that had been used in the anaesthetic room, the videolaryngoscope and a new 7.0 mm tracheal tube. Suxamethonium 100 mg was drawn into a labelled 2 mL syringe and kept nearby.

Following preoxygenation, neuromuscular blockade was reversed with neostigmine and glycopyrronium, full recovery of motor function was confirmed with train-of-four monitoring, and the patient was extubated awake without complication.

After staying a few minutes in theatre breathing 100% oxygen through a facemask, the patient was transferred to the post-anaesthetic recovery unit and care was handed over to a trained recovery nurse. The intubation difficulties were reported to the nurse and were documented on the anaesthetic chart. Particular instructions were given with regard to observations for stridor or other signs of respiratory distress, and included how to contact the anaesthetist involved and the consultant on call if problems developed, and that the patient should be reviewed by an anaesthetist prior to discharge back to the ward. The laryngeal mask, videolaryngoscope and tracheal tube used for this patient were left with the recovery nurse in case they should be needed.

There were no problems in recovery and following anaesthetic review the patient was discharged to the ward. The anaesthetic registrar visited the patient on the ward the next day and explained what had happened. Before leaving hospital the patient was given a letter explaining the details of the anaesthetic and the airway difficulty. A copy of this letter was placed in an 'airway' folder in the anaesthetic department. Copies were also sent to the patient's general practitioner and filed in the hospital notes (which were tagged with an 'anaesthetic alert sticker') to draw attention to the problem in case the patient required an anaesthetic in the future.

Discussion

The ASA Task Force on difficult airway management defined a difficult airway as 'the clinical situation in which a conventionally trained anesthesiologist experiences difficulty with mask ventilation, difficulty with tracheal intubation, or both' [30]. In modern practice significant difficulty with SAD insertion might also be included.

The Task Force defined difficult laryngoscopy as occurring when 'it is not possible to visualize any portion of the vocal cords with conventional laryngoscopy'. This would equate to a grade 3 or 4 laryngeal view [30].

Difficult intubation was defined by the Task Force as: when an experienced laryngoscopist, using direct laryngoscopy, requires: (1) more than two attempts with the same blade; or (2) a change in the blade or an adjunct to a direct laryngoscope (i.e. bougie); or (3) use of an alternative device or technique following failed intubation with direct laryngoscopy [4].

In the case described it is important to recognize that ventilation was never a problem and that SAD (classic LMA) insertion was straightforward.

All anaesthetists should have: (a) expertise in assessment and recognition of the potentially difficult airway; (b) the ability to formulate a plan (and a clearly structured sequential series of alternatives) for airway management (i.e. a strategy); (c) the skills and experience to use airway adjuncts, particularly those relevant to the unanticipated difficult airway; and (d) familiarity with schemes that outline a sequence of actions designed to maintain oxygenation, ventilation, and patient safety [31–33]. To ensure

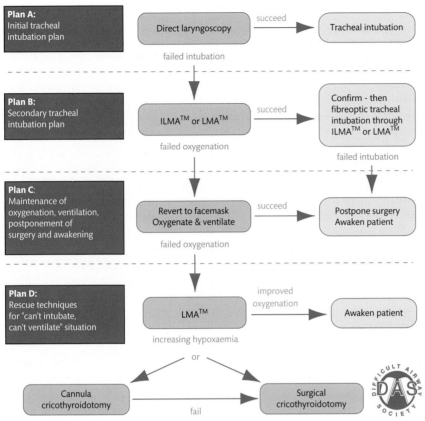

Figure 1.10 Difficult Airway Society guideline for failed intubation 2004. <http://www.das.uk.com/ guidelines/downloads.html>. Reproduced from Henderson JJ, Popat MT, Latto IP, Pearce AC. Difficult Airway Society guidelines for management of the unanticipated difficult intubation. *Anaesthesia* 2004; 59: 675--94, with permission from Blackwell publishing Ltd. Copyright © 2004, John Wiley and Sons.

that all personnel involved perform at their best, it is important to remain calm and follow appropriate algorithms [34]. The DAS guidelines provide one widely used excellent tool (Figure 1.10) [31].

In the unanticipated difficult or failed intubation, the patient is usually anaesthetized and paralysed. Several unsuccessful attempts at intubation may also have been made and it is imperative to call for help as soon as difficulty has been recognized. If the maximum permissible four attempts at intubation have been made the next appropriate step, regardless of the grade of anaesthetist, is to maintain oxygenation and wake the patient up. An awake intubation or tracheostomy can then be planned either after a short period of recovery or on another occasion. However, where muscle relaxation cannot be rapidly reversed, as in the case described, the patient will not be able to be woken quickly: the strategy must therefore include techniques that will ensure oxygenation, ventilation and protection against aspiration.

The case described involved an elective procedure with no increased risk of aspiration. The management of failed intubation during a rapid sequence induction follows a different algorithm where a much higher priority is given to waking the patient up.

A Final Word from the Expert

Difficult laryngoscopy is a relatively frequent occurrence so all anaesthetists should expect to encounter some degree of difficulty with tracheal intubation every now and again throughout their careers. The occasional inability to intubate using a Macintosh laryngoscope should be regarded as a failure of the technique rather than as a personal failure of the anaesthetist, and so it behoves all of us as airway experts to learn and practice alternative intubation techniques that we can use safely when faced with this situation. There are several effective alternatives (fibreoptic intubation, videolaryngoscopy, intubation through an SAD) and to a certain extent it matters less what our alternative technique is, but more that we are skilled in its use and that we recognize when it is appropriate to use it.

All alternative intubation techniques will also fail us occasionally and it is important to remember that failed intubation on its own does not constitute an emergency; it is only when this is associated with inability to oxygenate by facemask and SAD that plan D of the DAS algorithm (emergency surgical airway) becomes necessary. As such, all anaesthetists should be trained and prepared, should it be necessary to secure the airway in this manner without delay.

References

1. Mallampati SR, Gatt SP, Gugino LD, *et al*. A clinical sign to predict difficult tracheal intubation: a prospective study. *Can Anaesth Soc J* 1985;32:429.
2. Samsoon GLT, Young JRB. Difficult tracheal intubation: a retrospective study. *Anaesthesia* 1987;42:487–90.
3. Wilson ME, Spiegelhalter D, Robertson JA, *et al*. Predicting difficult intubation. *Br J Anaesth* 1988;61:211–16.
4. Crosby ET, Cooper RM, Douglas MJ, *et al*. The unanticipated difficult airway with recommendations for management. *Can J Anaesth* 1998;45:757–76.
5. Merah NA, Wong DT, Foulkes-Crabbe DJ, *et al*. Modified Mallampati test, thyromental distance and inter-incisor gap are the best predictors of difficult laryngoscopy in West Africans. *Can J Anaesth* 2005;52:291–6.
6. Koh KF, Hare JD, Calder I. Small tubes revisited. *Anaesthesia* 1998;53:46–50.
7. Farrows S, Farrows C, Soni N. Size matters: choosing the right tracheal tube. *Anaesthesia* 2002;67:815–19.
8. Cook TM, Woodall N, Frerk C. Major complications of airway management in the UK: results of the Fourth National Audit Project of the Royal College of Anaesthetists and the Difficult Airway Society. Part 1: Anaesthesia. *Br J Anaesth* 2011;106:617–31.
9. Adnet F, Racine SX, Borron SW, *et al*. A survey of tracheal intubation difficulty in the operating room: a prospective observational study. *Acta Anaesthesiol Scand* 2001;45:327–32.
10. Levitan RM, Kinkle WC, Levin WJ, *et al*. Laryngeal view during laryngoscopy: a randomized trial comparing cricoid pressure, backward-upward-rightward pressure, and bimanual laryngoscopy. *Ann Emerg Med* 2006;47:548–55.
11. Yentis SM. The effects of single-handed and bimanual cricoid pressure on the view at laryngoscopy. *Anaesthesia* 1997;52:332–5.
12. Snider DD, Clarke D, Finucane BT. The 'BURP' maneuver worsens the glottic view when applied in combination with cricoid pressure. *Can J Anaesth* 2005;52:100–4.
13. Uchida T, Hikawa Y, Saito Y, Yasuda K. The McCoy levering laryngoscope in patients with limited neck extension. *Can J Anaesth* 1997;44:674–6.

14. Frerk C. Laryngoscopy. Is it time to move on from the Macintosh? *Today's Anaesthetist* 2001;**16**:43.

15. Caplan RA, Posner KL, Ward RL, Cheney W. Adverse respiratory events in anesthesia: a closed claims analysis. *Anesthesiology* 1990;72:828–33.

16. Connelly NR, Ghandour K, Robbins L, *et al*. Management of unanticipated difficult airway at a teaching institution over a seven year period. *J Clin Anesth* 2006;18:198–204.

17. Brain AI, Verghese C, Addy EV, *et al*. The intubating laryngeal mask. II: A preliminary clinical report of a new means of intubating the trachea. *Br J Anaesth* 1997;79:699–703.

18. Joo HS, Kapoor S, Rose DK, *et al*. The intubating laryngeal mask airway after induction of general anesthesia versus awake fibreoptic intubation in patients with difficult airways. *Anesth Analg* 2001;92:1342–6.

19. Combes X, Sauvat S, Leroux B, *et al*. Intubating laryngeal mask airway in morbidly obese and lean patients: a comparative study. *Anesthesiology* 2005;102:1106–9.

20. Combes X, Le Roux B, Suen P, *et al*. Unanticipated difficult airway in anesthetized patients: prospective validation of a management algorithm. *Anesthesiology* 2004;100:1146–50.

21. Benumof JL. Management of the difficult adult airway. With special emphasis on awake tracheal intubation. *Anesthesiology* 1991;75:1087–110.

22. Brimacombe J, Berry A. The laryngeal mask airway for obstetric anesthesia and neonatal resuscitation. *Int J Obstet Anesth* 1994;3:211–18.

23. Ansermino JM, Blogg CE. Cricoid pressure may prevent insertion of the laryngeal mask airway. *Br J Anaesth* 1992;69:465–7.

24. Heath ML, Allagain J. Intubation through the laryngeal mask. A technique for unexpected difficult intubation. *Anaesthesia* 1991;46:545–8.

25. Allison A, McCrory J. Tracheal placement of a gum elastic bougie using the laryngeal mask airway [Letter]. *Anaesthesia* 1990;45:419–20.

26. Michalek P, Donaldson W, Graham C, Hinds JD. A comparison of the I-gel supraglottic airway as a conduit for tracheal intubation with the intubating laryngeal mask airway: a manikin study. *Resuscitation* 2009;81:74–77.

27. Anaesthetic Association of Great Britain and Ireland. *Recommendations for standards of monitoring during anaesthesia and recovery*, 4th ed.; 2007. < http://www.aagbi.org/sites/default/files/standardsofmonitoring07.pdf >

28. Popat M, Mitchell V, Dravid R, Patel A, Swampillai C, Higgs A. Difficult Airway Society Guidelines for the management of tracheal extubation. *Anaesthesia* 2012;67:318–40.

29. Barron FA, Ball R, Jefferson P, Norrie J. 'Airway Alerts'. How UK anaesthetists organize, document, and communicate difficult airway management. *Anaesthesia* 2003;58:50–83.

30. Caplan RA, Benumof JL, Berry FA, *et al*. Practice guidelines for management of the difficult airway. A report by the American Society of Anesthesiologists Task Force on Management of the Difficult Airway. *Anesthesiology* 1993;78:597–602.

31. Henderson JJ, Popat MT, Latto IP, *et al*. Difficult Airway Society guidelines for management of the unanticipated difficult intubation. *Anaesthesia* 2004;59:675–94.

32. Benumof JL. Laryngeal mask airway and the ASA difficult airway algorithm. *Anaesthesiology* 1996;84:686–99.

33. Heidgger T, Gerig HJ. Algorithms for management of the difficult airway. *Curr Opin Anaesthesiol* 2004;17:483–4.

34. Lavery GG, McCloskey BV, *et al*. The difficult airway in critical care. *Crit Care* 2008;36:2163–73.

CHAPTER 2

Perioperative care

2.1 Intraoperative fluid balance: what to measure?

David Cain and Mark Edwards

⊕ **Expert Commentary**   Mark Hamilton

CPD Matrix Code: *1A01, 2A04, 2A05, 3A03, 3A05*

Case history

A 65-year-old man was referred to the on-call anaesthetic registrar at 18:00 requiring an urgent laparotomy. He had presented at 17:00 with a 2-day history of vomiting, followed by 4 h of severe abdominal pain. He had a past medical history of hypertension, stable angina, myocardial infarction 5 years previously and type 2 diabetes mellitus. Before this episode he was able to walk up two flights of stairs but became breathless thereafter. His blood pressure had been well controlled 'for years'. A routine echocardiogram previously reported an ejection fraction of 50% and mild diastolic dysfunction. His medications were aspirin 75 mg o.d., bisoprolol 5 mg o.d., ramipril 10 mg nocte, simvastatin 40 mg nocte and metformin 500 mg t.d.s. He was alert but hypotensive and tachycardic (Figure 2.1). He received 2 L of compound sodium lactate (CSL; Hartmann's solution), antibiotics, and his blood pressure improved. CT identified a perforated transverse colon presumed secondary to cancer. There was no evidence of metastatic spread.

He was cool from the elbows and knees down, with capillary refill time of > 4 s and his jugular venous pressure was not visible. An intravenous 16G cannula had already been sited. There was scanty urine in the catheter bag. Observations at his preoperative assessment are detailed in Figure 2.1. Two 250 mL boluses of balanced colloid were prescribed. ECG and chest X-ray were unremarkable. Blood results are shown in Table 2.1. His case was discussed with the ICU team and it was agreed that he would be admitted postoperatively, as a level 2 or 3 patient.

The patient arrived in the anaesthetic room at 19:00. Because of concerns over haemodynamic compromise a decision was made to insert a radial arterial catheter and administer more fluid before induction of anaesthesia. Following administration of 250 mL of colloid the patient's blood pressure improved. An intraoperative lower target for mean arterial pressure (MAP) was set at 65 mmHg. After induction of anaesthesia, tracheal intubation and starting mechanical ventilation, the patient became hypotensive, requiring 300 µg of phenylephrine and a further 250 mL of colloid solution to maintain the target MAP.

A second 16G cannula was sited; intravenous fluid delivered via a fluid warming device was attached. A patient warming blanket was attached, but not turned on because he remained pyrexial. An internal jugular central venous catheter was sited using ultrasound guidance. An oesophageal Doppler monitor (ODM) probe was inserted followed by a nasal temperature probe. A nasogastric tube was sited. Arterial and central venous blood gas samples were taken at 19:45 (Figure 2.1).

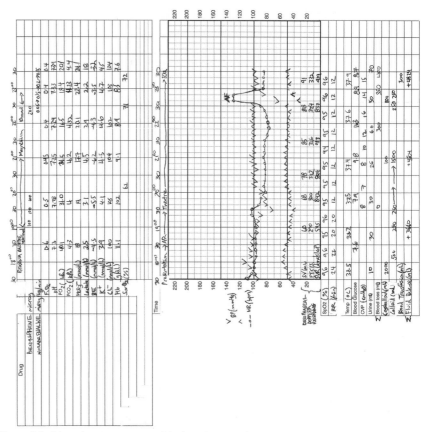

Figure 2.1 Selected perioperative variables from the time of presentation to transfer to the intensive care unit (ICU). CSL, compound sodium lactate/Hartmann's solution; SV, stroke volume; FTc, flow time corrected; SVR, systemic vascular resistance.

> ❝ **Expert comment**
>
> The presenting history is typical of a fluid-depleted patient with multiple comorbidities. Note that the clinical variables show a positive blood pressure and heart rate response to boluses of fluid, but additionally vasopressor is needed as anaesthesia is induced and peripheral dilation occurs.

> ❝ **Expert comment**
>
> The low mean corpuscular volume suggests the possibility of longstanding neoplastic disease, coupled with the high white cell count (WCC) and C-reactive protein indicating an infective process. Severe sepsis can, however, also present with a low WCC. The raised urea and creatinine may reflect acute or chronic kidney disease.

> ✪ **Learning point** Guidelines on intraoperative fluid management
>
> **British Consensus Guidelines on Intravenous Fluid Therapy for Adult Surgical Patients (GIFTASUP) [1]**
>
> The GIFTASUP consensus guidelines statement covers the entirety of the perioperative period. Intraoperative recommendations are:
>
> 1. In patients undergoing some forms of orthopaedic and abdominal surgery, intraoperative treatment with intravenous fluid to achieve an optimal value of SV should be used where possible as this may reduce postoperative complication rates and duration of hospital stay.
> 2. Patients undergoing non-elective major abdominal or orthopaedic surgery should receive intravenous fluid to achieve an optimal value of SV during and for the first 8 h after surgery. This may be supplemented by a low-dose dopexamine infusion.
>
> **NICE [2]**
>
> The ODM should be considered for use in patients undergoing major or high-risk surgery or other surgical patients in whom a clinician would consider using invasive cardiovascular monitoring.

The patient arrived in theatre at 19:55, and surgery commenced at 20:10. The surgical team reported a perforated transverse colon mass with large bowel contents within the peritoneum. They planned resection and Hartmann's procedure. Normokalaemia was maintained using 40 mmol of KCl placed in 100 mL of 0.9% sodium chloride and

Table 2.1 Presenting blood results

Full blood counts			Urea and electrolytes			Liver function tests		
Variable	Mean	Range	Variable	Mean	Range	Variable	Mean	Range
Hb (g/dL)	13.4	(13–18)	Na (mmol/L)	145	(135–145)	Bil (μmol/L)	**18**	(3–17)
MCV (fL)	**75**	(76–96)	K (mmol/L)	4.2	(3.5–5)	ALT (IU/L)	**40**	(3–35)
PLT (×10⁹/L)	320	(150–400)	Urea (mmol/L)	**9.4**	(2.5–6.7)	AST (IU/L)	32	(3–35)
WCC (×10⁹/L)	**19.4**	(4–11)	Cr (μmol/L)	**120**	(60–110)	Alk P (IU/L)	290	(30–300)
Neu %	**82**	(40–75)	Ca (mmol/L)	2.24	(2.12–2.65)			
			Alb (g/L)	40	(35–50)			
			Glucose (mmol/L)	7.5	(3.5–8.5)			
			CRP (mg/L)	**210**	(<10)			

Hb, haemoglobin; Alb, albumin; Bil, bilirubin; MCV, mean corpuscular volume; ALT, alanine transaminase; PLT, platelets; AST, aspartate transaminase; WCC, white blood cell count; Cr, creatine; Alk P, alkaline phosphatase; Neu, neutrophils; CRP, C-reactive protein.

> ✪ **Learning point** Clinical assessment of perioperative fluid balance
>
> Focused clinical examination is the first step in assessing patients' fluid status. Numerous variables—when taken in the context of the clinical scenario—can help confirm a diagnosis of hypoperfusion, although they should be interpreted carefully in isolation (see Table 2.2).
>
> **Table 2.2 Clinical assessment of perioperative fluid balance**
>
> | Clinical measure | Physiological indicator | Notes on interpretation of fluid balance |
> | --- | --- | --- |
> | Heart rate (HR) | Sympathetic/ parasympathetic atrioventricular node balance | • Confounding factors include pain, and drug effects including opioid and beta-blocker administration.
• Cardiac output is the product of HR and SV. HR alone gives limited information concerning cardiac output. |
> | Pulse pressure | Pulse volume and therefore SV | • Pulse pressure is related to pulse volume by arterial compliance.
• Clinical assessment cannot differentiate between changes in compliance and volume. |
> | Blood pressure | Afterload | • Vasoconstriction increases afterload, and therefore blood pressure but reduces SV.
• Blood pressure is typically maintained following ≤30% loss of blood volume.
• A transient rise in diastolic pressure is then followed by a fall in systolic and diastolic pressures with increasing intravascular loss. |
> | Capillary refill | Perfusion of skin | • Assess at a site superior to the heart in order to avoid venous refill. Of limited value in cold patients.
• Warming blankets make skin temperature an unreliable sign. |
> | Conscious state | Perfusion of brain | • Alteration in consciousness is a non-specific and late sign of volume loss.
• Multiple factors influence cognition and alertness. |
> | Urine output | Kidney perfusion | • Typical target 0.5–1 mL/kg/h.
• Hypoperfusion is only one cause of reduced urine output. Other causes include the physiological stress response, blocked catheter, urinary tract obstruction and intrinsic renal disease. |
> | Peripheral oedema | Oncotic pressure, endothelial permeability | • Oedema may be the result of low oncotic pressure or capillary leak in addition to intravascular fluid excess
• Oedema may be an unavoidable consequence of adequate intravascular volume expansion. |

> ⑯ **Expert comment**
>
> It is crucially important that these patients are not only recognized to be at high risk of a poor perioperative outcome but that their postoperative care is equally well planned. The patient is dehydrated, acidaemic with a raised lactate and about to undergo major emergency surgery. In this case an intensive care admission is mandatory. The Physiological and Operative Severity Score for the enUmeration of Mortality and morbidity (POSSUM) is commonly used within the perioperative literature for comparative audit of surgical outcome data [3, 4]. Although not designed for individualized risk prediction, it may be used to provide an estimate of surgical risk. Here the estimated POSSUM mortality is 5–15%, and morbidity >50%.

> ⑯ **Expert comment**
>
> An acute change in intrathoracic pressure caused by mechanical ventilation can reduce venous return and lead to low cardiac output and blood pressure in fluid-depleted patients. Fluid administration and vasopressors may be required to reverse these effects.

infused centrally over 2 h. As there was ongoing suspicion of hypovolaemia, warmed fluid boluses of 250 mL Gelofusine® (B. Braun Medical Ltd, Sheffield, UK) were infused over 15 min intervals, with the aim of increasing ODM stroke volume (SV) by 10%. After 2.5 L, SV failed to increase beyond 90 mL. At this point, central venous pressure (CVP) had reached 16 cmH₂O, and rose by 6 cmH₂O with the final fluid challenge, while the visible variation in arterial line systolic pressure with ventilation (swing) had disappeared. The patient remained oliguric despite apparent euvolaemia and

> **✪ Learning point** Fluid resuscitation protocols
>
> These may be divided into 'recipe' or 'individualized' approaches. Recipe-based models prescribe mL/kg body weight/h, arbitrarily sub-classified into 'wet' or 'dry' protocols by the volume prescribed. There are some suggestions in limited, retrospective trials that dry protocols are associated with improved outcomes after elective oesophagectomy and elective liver resection surgery [5–7]. However, recipe-based approaches fail to account for individual variation between patients and their preoperative state. The majority of clinical trials concerning fluid resuscitation have been performed in elective surgery. This is due to the added difficulties associated with studying non-elective surgery. Nonetheless it is non-elective surgical patients who, because of established physiological upset and disturbances in fluid balance, are at the greatest risk and who are likely to benefit the most from optimization of fluid status. Individualized approaches aim to measure and optimize suitable physiological targets, such as oxygen delivery ($\dot{D}O_2$).
>
> Research in this area historically employed the pulmonary artery catheter (PAC, see Learning point, The evolution of goal-directed therapy). The majority of recent work has used the ODM. Collectively these data suggest that flow-based cardiac output monitors improve postoperative morbidity in high-risk patient groups, if they are used appropriately [8, 9]. The term 'high risk' has been variously defined, but typically applies to patients with a predicted mortality, by POSSUM or similar scoring system, of >5–10%. The high mortality rate and associated resource utilization and costs of care make this group an ideal target for improvements in healthcare provision. Newer devices are available (see Expert Comment, Examining the evidence—do we need monitors to guide intraoperative fluid administration?) which are methodologically appealing but currently lack a robust evidence base.
>
> Repetitive application of fluid challenges to indices of cardiac filling or SV aims to place the patient at the peak of the Frank–Starling curve. The caveat with this approach is that it does not consider whether the increase in cardiac output was necessary; administering a fluid challenge to healthy volunteers will increase their cardiac output without any benefit. The alternative to targeting optimization of $\dot{D}O_2$ is targeting cellular oxygen usage ($\dot{V}O_2$). Although $\dot{V}O_2$ is, in principle, an attractive goal for fluid resuscitation it is difficult to directly manipulate.

> **⑥ Expert comment**
> Examining the evidence—do we need monitors to guide intraoperative fluid administration?
>
> Clinical studies of fluid resuscitation cannot demonstrate that a monitor improves care, but rather that a bundle of care which incorporates a monitor may do so. This bundle also includes a protocol, a fluid, a specified patient population and institutional factors that may not be immediately apparent. All of these must be considered before the results are extrapolated beyond the confines of the original trial.
>
> Some have questioned the necessity of the monitor within these protocols, suggesting that unmonitored prescription of the relevant therapies identified within these trials would generate the same improvements. The principle of a fluid monitor is to guide the prescription of the 'correct amount'. Given the potential for inappropriate therapy to cause harm, removal of the monitor from the protocol would appear counterintuitive. This debate may be partly answered through a recipe-based study with fluid volumes/therapies derived from individualized studies.

> **➕ Clinical tip** The timing of fluid resuscitation
>
> Early fluid resuscitation is physiologically compelling in elective as well as emergency surgery. Although the impact of the timing of fluid resuscitation upon surgical outcome has not been investigated prospectively, subgroup analysis of a study into goal-directed therapy (GDT) for elective colorectal surgery patients has indicated a possible benefit from early resuscitation [10]. Here fluid therapy was administered according to an oesophageal Doppler-guided protocol in the treatment group, and at the discretion of the anaesthetist in the control group. The treatment group had a reduced length of stay, and improvements in a number of other secondary end-points. While there was only a small difference between the overall volumes of fluid the two groups received, the treatment group received the majority of administered fluid within the first quarter of surgery.
>
> (continued)

Initial trials of GDT incorporated preoperative admission to intensive care for optimization before the surgical insult [11]. Despite the possible benefits, this approach has significant resource implications and is rarely practised. In the acute setting preoperative optimization must not be at the expense of delaying surgical control of sepsis; a compromise between adequate pre-anaesthetic resuscitation and surgical timing must be found. Pearse et al. demonstrated that goal-directed care can also achieve benefit when instituted after surgery [12]. Randomized controlled trials examining a combination of intra- and postoperative GDT are underway (POMO, <http://www.controlled-trials.com/ISRCTN76894700>; Optimise, <http://www.controlled-trials.com/ISRCTN04386758>)

⊗ **Learning point** Manipulation of global oxygen delivery

$$\dot{D}O_2 = CO \times CaO_2$$

Global oxygen delivery ($\dot{D}O_2$) is the product of cardiac output (CO) and the oxygen content of arterial blood (CaO_2). Protocols targeting $\dot{D}O_2$ typically include the use of blood transfusion and inotropic medications. A growing body of evidence suggests that the number of units of blood transfused is directly correlated with a range of negative postoperative outcomes [13]. This may be due to sicker patients inherently receiving more blood. Reports also indicate an association between the age of red blood cells and increased morbidity [14]. The majority of resuscitation protocols target haemoglobin levels >8.0 g/dL. This may be raised if there is an increased risk of bleeding.

Inotropic medications may be used when cardiac output is insufficient and unresponsive to fluid resuscitation. In some trials these medications are introduced early to minimize the risk of oedema. Whereas inotropes may improve physiological markers of cardiac output and perfusion, this is at the expense of short- and long-term complications, such as arrhythmias and myocyte death. Adrenergic agents increase myocardial oxygen demand and have myriad systemic effects owing to the wide distribution of adrenoreceptors [15]. Although many goal-directed studies reporting beneficial effects have incorporated inotropic infusions in their protocols, the number of patients who actually receive them is small. These studies can rarely be used as justification for the generalized use of inotropes.

⊕ **Clinical tip** CVP changes and ventilation

During unsupported spontaneous ventilation the CVP falls during inspiration. This relationship is reversed during positive pressure ventilation, and the magnitude of CVP rise is dependent upon lung compliance. Larger rises will be observed in less compliant lungs.

⊗ **Learning point** Invasive pressure monitors

Central venous pressure (CVP)

Left ventricular end-diastolic volume (LVEDV) is an ideal marker of volume status but cannot be measured routinely. Pulmonary artery occlusion pressure (PAOP) is used as a substitute for LVEDV, but its measurement requires a PAC. Right atrial pressure (i.e. CVP) may be used as a surrogate of PAOP. However, the non-linear relationship between CVP and LVEDV means that static measurements of CVP do not provide an accurate indication of volume status, or of fluid responsiveness [16].

Dynamic interpretation of CVP may be beneficial. Titrating fluid boluses to a CVP increase of >3 mmHg 15 min after the bolus has been shown to improve outcome when compared to routine care in the perioperative care of patients with fractured neck of femur [17]. Central venous catheter placement also allows the administration of potent vasoactive medications.

Invasive arterial blood pressure

Whereas isolated arterial pressure monitoring gives limited information on intravascular volume status, arterial access allows frequent blood gas monitoring, rapid recognition of haemodynamic instability and facilitates use of pulse pressure/pulse contour cardiac output monitors (see Learning point, Cardiac output monitors).

> ✪ **Learning point** Cardiac output monitors
>
> ### Pulmonary artery catheter (PAC) (Figure 2.2)
>
> Considered by many to be a gold standard monitor due to the multitude of information provided, historical use within GDT trials, and because they predate many other monitors currently in clinical practice. However, the measurements provided by the pulmonary artery catheter (PAC) are not 100% reliable. Cardiac output is typically derived using a temperature (cold) dilution curve analysis, a technique now also used to calibrate less invasive pulse contour-based devices. PAC use has declined significantly in UK practice, following studies that showed an increase in mortality associated with use of the PAC, especially in lower risk patients. Some part of this may be attributed to over-zealous use of PACs and substandard practice in terms of interpretation of derived data and clinical decisions made as a consequence.
>
>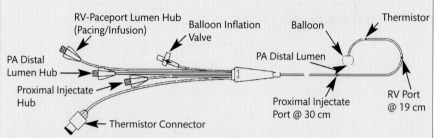
>
> **Figure 2.2** Swan–Ganz thermodilution catheter. Reproduced with permission of Edwards Lifesciences LLC, Irvine, CA, USA. Paceport and Swan–Ganz are trademarks of Edwards Lifesciences Corporation.
>
> ### Oesophageal Doppler monitor (ODM) (Figures 2.3–2.5)
>
> A Doppler probe is placed in the oesophagus at the level of T5/T6 (mid-lower oesophagus) and manipulated to obtain the optimal signal from the descending aorta. The Doppler probe measures the aortic red cell velocity and the period of flow (flow time). Based on assumptions about the cross-sectional diameter of the descending aorta this can be converted into an estimate of blood flow and hence SV.
>
> SV estimates assume a constant cross-sectional area and proportion of cardiac output reaching the descending aorta. Although these assumptions may lead to inaccuracy in the absolute value of SV displayed, trends are not affected and responses to dynamic (fluid) challenges such as an increase in cardiac output are well mapped. It has a short learning curve for the operator to generate reproducible measurements. Peak velocity (PV) is a surrogate measure of left ventricular contractility (Figure 2.4 and Table 2.3).
>
> Corrected flow time (FTc) is the time spent in systole normalized for heart rate. It can be used to identify changes in afterload and preload. Values <330 ms typically indicate hypovolaemia or high systemic vascular resistance, whereas values >360 ms suggest the opposite. The user may enter values of central venous and arterial pressures to obtain an estimate of systemic vascular resistance, thus differentiating causes of low FTc. Postoperative monitoring, after extubation, is not practical. Nasal probes are available, but still uncomfortable for the awake patient.
>
> Meta-analysis of ODM use, which included 920 patients across nine RCTs, demonstrated that its use reduced complications and length of hospital stay [8]. A further, recent meta-analysis concluded
>
> **Table 2.3 Predominant effects of changes in cardiovascular status upon the oesophageal Doppler monitor waveform**
>
> | State | Peak velocity | Flow time |
> | --- | --- | --- |
> | Preload reduction | – | ↓ |
> | Preload increase | – | ↑ |
> | Afterload increase | ↓ | ↓ |
> | Afterload decrease | ↑ | ↑ |
> | Positive inotropy | ↑ | – |
> | Myocardial depression | ↓ | – |
>
> (continued)

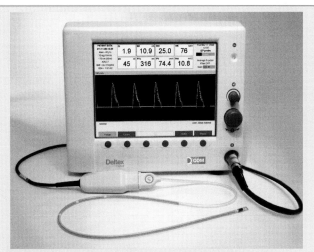

Figure 2.3 Oesophageal Doppler monitor (CardioODM; Deltex Medical). Reproduced with kind permission from Deltex Medical.

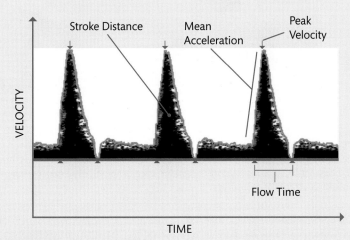

Figure 2.4 The oesophageal Doppler monitor waveform. Reproduced with kind permission from Deltex Medical.

that flow-based cardiac output monitoring may reduce morbidity and mortality (pooled odds ratio (95% confidence interval) of 0.48 (0.33–0.78); p = 0.0002) in high-risk surgical patients. Postoperative complications were reduced overall, although these are difficult to quantify due to differences in classification criteria between the studies [9]. A US government review has described the evidence base for intraoperative use of ODM as 'strong' [18]. NICE supports the use of ODM in high-risk patients and in those in whom the clinician plans to insert invasive monitoring.

Pulse contour analysis

Pulse contour analysis is based upon the physiological principle that pulse pressure, defined as the difference between systolic and diastolic pressure, is proportional to SV. This relationship assumes a constant arterial compliance between repeated measurements. In most commercially available monitors, a calibration step is performed at intervals, using a dilution curve for a known marker (temperature or lithium), to limit drift and account for interpatient variation in arterial compliance. Changes of compliance in between these calibration steps are ignored. After calibration the monitor

(continued)

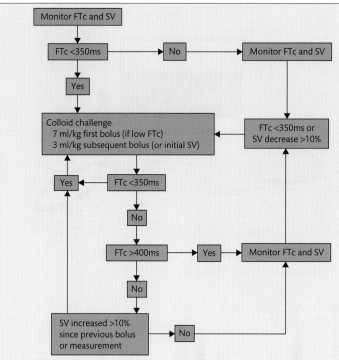

Figure 2.5 A typical goal-directed therapy algorithm. FTc, descending aortic corrected flow time; SV, stroke volume. Reproduced with permission from S. E. Noblett et al., 'Randomized clinical trial assessing the effect of Doppler-optimized fluid management on outcome after elective colorectal resection', *British Journal of Surgery*, 93, 9, pp. 1069–1076. Copyright © 2006 British Journal of Surgery Society Ltd. Published by John Wiley & Sons, Ltd.

continuously analyses the pulse wave (different devices use different algorithms) to provide a continuously displayed cardiac output (or SV). The upward slope of the arterial pressure wave provides a surrogate marker of ventricular contractility.

Stroke volume variation (SVV) is an additional measure, which formalizes the concept of arterial waveform 'swing'. During positive pressure ventilation there is an increase in left ventricular preload during inspiration caused by an increase in pulmonary capillary and venous blood returning to the ventricle: this reverses during expiration. This results in a cyclical change in SV with respiration and the extent of the SVV with the respiratory cycle can be used as a predictor of fluid responsiveness: SVV >12% generally predicts fluid responsiveness and SVV <9% makes it unlikely. SVV relies on a fully ventilated patient, with a tidal volume >8 mL/kg and no arrhythmias. The most recent ODM model also incorporates SVV variables.

The LiDCO® monitor (LiDCO plus system; LiDCO Ltd, Cambridge, UK) is calibrated using lithium dilution administered via a peripheral venous cannula; the only 'invasive' line required is an arterial catheter. It was used as a tool to guide postoperative cardiac output optimization in a study of mostly elective vascular and general surgical patients which demonstrated reduced postoperative morbidity and length of stay in the intervention group [12].

PiCCO® (Philips Healthcare, Guildford, UK) calibrates using warmed or cooled saline injected into a central venous catheter. The temperature change is recorded at a femoral (or brachial) arterial line. The injected bolus must pass through the entire cardiopulmonary unit, and will therefore be in flux with water throughout this volume. The thermodilution curve obtained therefore describes the total intrathoracic thermal volume, and is equal to the sum of global end-diastolic volume (GEDV), pulmonary blood volume (PBV) and extravascular lung water. By comparing the shape of the thermodilution curve with the transit time of the thermal bolus, PiCCO® calculates estimates of these individual volumes. GEDV (or GEDI) is a marker of preload. In a single-centre study, intraoperative use of PiCCO® reduced intensive care stay and vasopressor use [19].

(continued)

Pulse contour devices which do not require calibration are available, they utilize standard arterial lines or estimate pulse volume from the plethysmograph signal. Despite displaying SV, these devices should be considered to record trends alone. Without an index of compliance the derivation of flow from pressure is intrinsically flawed. Some devices include SVV in spontaneously ventilated patients and have the difficult task of accounting for variation in preload with different tidal volumes.

Transthoracic impedance

The NiCOM monitor (Cheetah Medical, Inc., Vancouver, WA, USA) measures thoracic bioimpedance. Changes resulting from cardiac output must be differentiated from those due to ventilation. This is achieved through frequency and phase modulation of an applied voltage.

Echocardiography

This is a specialized skill and echocardiography is not currently in routine use for intraoperative fluid management. Direct visualization of the heart can provide information regarding LVEDV, cardiac contractility, and may identify a range of pathological processes. Transthoracic images of ventilated patients, beyond the substernal view, are notoriously difficult to interpret. Transoesophageal echocardiography (TOE) provides improved images but carries a small risk of oesophageal trauma. TOE requires skill in interpretation. Used most in cardiac surgery, it is also used by a minority for non-cardiac surgery too.

✪ **Learning point** Perfusion monitors

Global perfusion

The use of venous saturations, lactate and base excess to guide fluid therapy is based on perceived underlying physiological principles. There is no strong evidence demonstrating that targeting specific values improves outcomes.

Mixed venous oxygen saturation ($S\bar{v}O_2$), obtained by sampling blood from the pulmonary artery via the distal lumen of the PAC, is considered to be a marker of global oxygen utilization in the acutely ill patient. Central venous sampling from a central venous catheter ($Sc\bar{v}O_2$) may provide a reliable surrogate estimate of $S\bar{v}O_2$. Many studies have demonstrated that the two values are strongly correlated, although not necessarily absolutely predictive; one study found that both measures were poorly correlated with cardiac output [20]. Threshold values for $Sc\bar{v}O_2$ are generally considered to be 70% and 65% for $S\bar{v}O_2$, with lower values implying increased oxygen extraction and hence reduced tissue oxygen delivery. $S\bar{v}O_2$ may be less reliable in established critical illness where the oxygen supply–utilization relationship is disturbed [21], and in situations such as sepsis or anaphylaxis where arteriolar-to-venule shunting may occur.

Tissue hypoperfusion leads to lactate release from anaerobic glucose metabolism, and normalizing lactate levels are routinely used as a target of fluid resuscitation. The phases of surgery and fluid resuscitation are key to lactate interpretation. A rise may represent reperfusion of previously ischaemic or underperfused tissues. Unrelated causes of an elevated lactate include adrenergic medication or ethanol metabolism and poor lactate clearance due to severe liver disease.

Base excess is dependent on many factors. It is incorrect to administer a fluid challenge simply on the basis of a base deficit without full interpretation of the patient's electrolyte and acid/base status, especially in the presence of an elevated chloride.

Individual tissue beds

Measurement of non-essential tissue bed perfusion exploits the body's preference to shut these down first in the context of hypovolaemia. Gut tonometry uses a balloon which rests against gastric mucosa and measures pH, with a fall in pH indicating gut hypoperfusion. In single-centre studies low gastric pH predicts poor outcome in paediatric cardiac surgery [22], and fluid challenges reverse the presence of low gastric pH [23]. These tools are not used routinely outside of research studies.

an appropriate blood pressure—further fluid was not administered. Plasma lactate reached a plateau, and began to fall. The patient's blood glucose rose to 11.3 mmol/L, and an insulin infusion was started.

At 22:30 the patient became hypotensive, with evidence of vasodilation; a further fluid challenge failed to improve SV, and FTc rose from 320 to 400 ms.

An infusion of noradrenaline was started and titrated to the target blood pressure. At 22:45 the patient developed fast atrial fibrillation, with associated hypotension. Magnesium 10 mmol in 100 mL of 0.9% sodium chloride was administered over 10 min. The ODM was switched to average SV spanning 1 min epochs and a further fluid challenge administered. After waiting a further 10 min a repeat dose of magnesium was administered, with successful cardioversion.

In view of significant metabolic derangement and likely worsening inflammatory response overnight, the patient was transferred to the ICU intubated with planned morning extubation. Paracetamol and morphine were prescribed for postoperative analgesia. Non-steroidal anti-inflammatory drugs were omitted. During the course of the procedure the patient's haemoglobin fell to 7.6 g/dL. One unit of blood was transfused. At this time activated partial thromboplastin time (APTT) and prothrombin time (PT) results were fractionally elevated, but a thromboelastogram demonstrated that the patient was hypercoagulable and clotting factors were not replaced.

Discussion

Optimal fluid balance will prevent tissue hypoperfusion and avoid iatrogenic injury through overhydration. It is not possible to directly regulate perfusion to specific tissue beds. Rather, this is achieved through the manipulation of global cardiac output, MAP and attention to the interstitial electrolyte environment. The perceived requirements of individual tissue beds may be in conflict and these individual requirements must be reconciled to provide an overall optimal balance.

Data from goal-directed therapy trials suggest that differences in the volume of fluid, in the order of a few litres, and the timing of administration, can contribute to a diverse range of post-surgical outcomes [8, 9]. The implication is that subclinical tissue hypoperfusion drives the development of complications. This is a plausible mechanism because tissue hypoxia is a powerful inflammatory stimulus [24]. An alternative interpretation is that the fluid has a drug-like effect, interacting with inflammation in a way that is currently unknown. A database analysis of more than 100,000 patients demonstrated that the occurrence of a complication within the first 30 days after surgery was the strongest predictor of survival over 8 years [25], underlining the importance of avoiding early postoperative morbidity.

Underperfusion of the gut and kidney may be the key events as these 'non-essential' tissue beds are subject to early neurohumeral vasoconstriction. Hypoperfusion of the gut may permit endotoxin and bacterial translocation, which are believed to contribute to a range of systemic postoperative complications [26, 27]. Such instances of hypoperfusion may be relatively common; up to 60% in one series of patients undergoing major surgery, when assessed by gut tonometry [26]. Minor increases in postoperative serum creatinine are associated with increased morbidity [28].

Excessive fluid administration may also cause harm. The Starling principle states that the heart is a demand pump. Venoconstriction and the addition of fluid to the vascular space increases preload, and therefore SV. Overzealous resuscitation may impair cardiac function through work-related ischaemia, reduce oxygen delivery through haemodilution and theoretically impair interstitial oxygen diffusion. This is a concern with protocols that challenge cardiac output to maximal values. Oedema threatens the integrity of bowel anastomoses, while intestinal oedema is associated with impaired gastrointestinal function and delayed enteral feeding [29, 30].

An adequate cardiac output is required to maintain oxygen delivery, and an adequate blood pressure is required to maintain tissue perfusion. Anecdotal evidence suggests that a MAP of 60–65 mmHg is sufficient, although a higher pressure may be required in established untreated hypertensive patients. Whereas vasopressors may increase global perfusion pressure, there is potential for inappropriate use of these medications to compound tissue bed hypoperfusion, and contribute to the complications described above

The delivery of anaesthesia interacts with most of the physiological mechanisms involved in fluid homeostasis. High doses of anaesthetic agents obtund autonomic

---

✪ Learning point The evolution of goal-directed therapy (GDT)

GDT specifically describes the evolution of protocols concerning the perioperative manipulation of global oxygen delivery ($\dot{D}O_2$) as a consequence of measurements made with the PAC. In the 1970s Shoemaker demonstrated that survivors of high-risk surgery had a higher haemoglobin, arterial pH, cardiac index, $\dot{D}O_2$ and oxygen consumption ($\dot{V}O_2$) when compared with those who died [32]. An algorithm was developed from these data that was able to predict survivors with high sensitivity and specificity [33]. Survivors' average $\dot{D}O_2$ values were used as targets in a prospective goal-directed study, with $\dot{V}O_2$ expected to improve by association. The mortality in the treatment group was reduced, particularly if $\dot{D}O_2$ was >600 mL/min/m^2 [34]. In the UK, Boyd et al. achieved similar results with their own GDT algorithms [35]; other groups identified critical values of $\dot{D}O_2$, below which lactate formation became dependent on $\dot{D}O_2$ [36, 37]. The findings from these studies were amalgamated into a unified theory, where a defect in $\dot{V}O_2$ may be eliminated by driving $\dot{D}O_2$ to either a set target, or to a level where the relationship with $\dot{V}O_2$ is lost. In this model the degree of perioperative 'oxygen debt' is related to postoperative complications and death, in keeping with current knowledge of the relationship between hypoperfusion, hypoxia and inflammation.

Despite positive trial results, and a plausible pathophysiological mechanism, the use of PAC-directed GDT is now rare in the UK. Possible reasons include the lack of multicentre trials, the declining use of PAC, and a lack of integration between pre-, intra- and postoperative care. There are methodological criticisms. Analysis of the equations used to calculate $\dot{V}O_2$ and $\dot{D}O_2$ in early PAC research reveals that they are mathematically coupled. Second, the capacity to increase $\dot{V}O_2$ through GDT may simply be an indicator of previously unidentified physiological reserve—benefit is revealed, not derived, by GDT. An element of distrust in GDT was partly generated by the large doses of dobutamine which some protocols allowed—doses which are now generally agreed to be harmful.

✪ Learning point Examining the evidence: which fluid?

Evidence-based fluid administration is hampered by a lack of adequately powered randomized studies of fluid composition examining clinically relevant outcomes in a controlled perioperative setting.

Current prescription practices are predominantly influenced by the biophysical properties of the available fluids, and the expected pathophysiological consequences of administration. Many regulatory bodies do not classify fluids as drugs, so new fluids may be released to the market with relatively limited clinical safety data.

(continued)

❝ Expert comment

There is continued debate regarding the advantages of crystalloid over colloid and vice versa. What is clear is that there is no definitive evidence to choose one over the other, but both must be given in the right quantity at the right time. The addition of cardiac output monitoring allows an assessment of flow and is recommended for administering fluids in high-risk surgical patients. It is important to remember that there are significant differences in the way perioperative fluids are administered across Europe and the USA.

Crystalloid or colloid?

Given the large volumes of effectively foreign molecules involved, critics argue that colloid use cannot be justified until robust data demonstrate that they improve clinical outcomes, and do not cause harm. Proponents of colloids respond that the physiological rationale behind their use and the—albeit limited—evidence base available make this extreme view unjustified.

The Saline versus Albumin Fluid Evaluation (SAFE) study was a pragmatic, prospective trial comparing albumin with 0.9% saline in a mixed intensive care population. It demonstrated non-inferiority of albumin within this group, and settled concerns raised by previous Cochrane analysis that albumin may be harmful [38]. An interesting second finding of this study was that the ratio of crystalloid to albumin required to achieve particular goal-directed targets of volume status was 1.4:1 rather than 3:1 as previously taught.

The semi-synthetic colloids are heterogeneous products; each has distinct properties. Manufacturers of dextrans and starches provide maximum dose levels with their products. All semi-synthetic colloids may affect blood coagulation. Gelatins are the most widely used, but have been associated with renal impairment within a critical care population [39].

In 2008 the Efficacy of Volume Substitution and Insulin Therapy in Severe Sepsis (VISEP) study suggested that hydroethyl starch (HES) resuscitation in severe sepsis increased the risk of renal failure, and possibly death [40]. Criticism of study methodology prevented widespread acceptance of VISEP's findings, and provided the catalyst for further investigation. The recapitulation of these findings by the 6S trial in 2011 prompted an immediate review of the literature by the European Society of Intensive Care Medicine (ESICM) [41]. The ESICM issued a consensus statement in March 2012 cautioning against the use of HES in severe sepsis or in those at risk of renal failure [42]. In June 2013 the MHRA suspended the use of starch solutions to treat critically ill patients and those undergoing surgery, with widespread support from professional bodies.

Balanced or unbalanced?

Fluids with an ionic composition and osmolality similar to plasma are termed 'balanced'. It seems intuitive to use balanced solutions, but due to the multitude of anions present in plasma, no fluid is truly balanced. Bicarbonate is the predominant plasma anion subject to metabolism, but making up the entire anion gap with bicarbonate in fluids would be unphysiological.

Bicarbonate readily degrades to carbon dioxide, which diffuses through the majority of plastics used to store fluids. Carbon dioxide-resistant bags containing bicarbonate are available outside the UK, but are more expensive.

'Balanced fluids' therefore strike a compromise. First, they are slightly hypotonic, which reduces the amount of substituted anion required. Second, they substitute an alternative anion that may be metabolized, such as lactate or, more recently, acetate. Even this may be unphysiological; compound sodium lactate (Hartmann's solution) contains racemic lactate. Human metabolic processes have evolved to metabolize L-lactate. Concerns have been raised concerning the metabolism and effects of D-lactate.

The archetypal unbalanced fluid is 0.9% saline and its use is associated with a hyperchloraemia, and consequently acidosis [43]. The relationship between chloride and acidosis may be explained by Stewart's approach to acid/base disturbances, and to an extent by the 'anion gap' principle [44]. Hyperchloraemia is associated with renal artery vasoconstriction [45] and with gut hypoperfusion [43]. The associated acidosis may also lead to clinical confusion, and the incorrect diagnosis of acidosis secondary to hypovolaemia.

❝ Expert comment
Author's opinion: which fluid?

The deliberate expansion of the vascular space with the intention of increasing cardiac output must be distinguished from replacement of intraoperative fluid losses. A pragmatic approach would include a mixture of balanced crystalloids for water and electrolyte, 5% dextrose for evaporative losses and gelatin boluses targeted to an appropriate index of vascular filling.

reflexes. Positive intrathoracic pressure impairs right heart filling, and high volume ventilation triggers pulmonary and systemic inflammation which may contribute to capillary leak. During critical illness the regulatory systems themselves may become dysfunctional: inotropic and vasomotor reflexes respond unpredictably to fluid and drug challenges [31].

A Final Word from the Expert

Intraoperative fluid balance can be a difficult subject, but the availability of advanced monitoring technology has helped significantly.

Elderly patients presenting with abdominal catastrophes and multiple comorbidities are numerous and represent an extremely high-risk group of surgical patients. The important points to remember here are:

1. It is extremely important to recognize these patients early as being at high risk of a poor perioperative outcome; their immediate care should be planned before theatre and intraoperatively, and likewise their postoperative care, which for the majority of these patients should be done in an ICU.
2. The scientific evidence to support the use of one type of fluid over another is not strong, but fluid must be used appropriately and is probably best administered in a goal-directed fashion against a cardiac output monitor.
3. In reality the use of a central venous line, arterial line, and a cardiac output monitor represent best care for these patients. The best evidence for improving outcome is from using GDT such as the challenging of SV with fluid boluses. There is also evidence for lactate clearance as a surrogate target for resuscitation. Central access may be needed for the administration of vasopressors, but this also allows measurement of central venous oxygen saturations. Clinicians have to be able to assimilate this complex information at all stages of the patient's care, and recognize where best evidence exists to guide their practice.

References

1. Powell-Tuck J, Gosling P, *et al. British Consensus Guidelines on Intravenous Fluid Therapy for Adult Surgical Patients* (GIFTASUP); 2009. < http://www.bapen.org.uk/pdfs/bapen_pubs/giftasup.pdf >
2. National Institute for Health and Care Excellence. *CardioQ-ODM oesophageal Doppler monitor*; 2011 < http://guidance.nice.org.uk/MTG3/Guidance/pdf/English >
3. Prytherch D, Whiteley M, Higgins B, Weaver P, Prout W, Powell S. POSSUM and Portsmouth POSSUM for predicting mortality. *Br J Surg* 1998;85:1217–20.
4. Copeland GP, Jones D, Walters M. POSSUM: a scoring system for surgical audit. *Br J Surg* 1991;78:355–60.
5. Wei S, Tian J, Song X, Chen Y. Association of perioperative fluid balance and adverse surgical outcomes in esophageal cancer and esophagogastric junction cancer. *Ann Thoracic Surg* 2008;86:266–72.
6. Tandon S, Batchelor A, Bullock R, *et al.* Peri-operative risk factors for acute lung injury after elective oesophagectomy. *Br J Anaesth* 2001;86:633–8.
7. Jones RM, Moulton CE, Hardy KJ. Central venous pressure and its effect on blood loss during liver resection. *Br J Surg* 1998;85:1058–60.
8. Phan TD, Ismail H, Heriot AG, Ho KM. Improving perioperative outcomes: fluid optimization with the esophageal Doppler monitor, a metaanalysis and review. *J Am Coll Surg* 2008;207:935–41.
9. Hamilton MA, Cecconi M, Rhodes A. A systematic review and meta-analysis on the use of preemptive hemodynamic intervention to improve postoperative outcomes in moderate and high-risk surgical patients. *Anesth Analg* 2011;112:1392–1402.
10. Noblett SE, Snowden CP, Shenton BK, Horgan AF. Randomized clinical trial assessing the effect of Doppler-optimized fluid management on outcome after elective colorectal resection. *Br J Surg* 2006;93:1069–76.

11. Shoemaker W, Appel P, Waxman K, Schwartz S, Chang P. Clinical trial of survivors' cardiorespiratory patterns as therapeutic goals in critically ill postoperative patients. *Crit Care Med* 1982;10:398–403.

12. Pearse R, Dawson D, Fawcett J, Rhodes A, Grounds RM, Bennett ED. Early goal-directed therapy after major surgery reduces complications and duration of hospital stay. A randomised, controlled trial. *Crit Care* 2005;9:R687–93.

13. Marik PE, Corwin HL. Efficacy of red blood cell transfusion in the critically ill: a systematic review of the literature. *Crit Care* 2008;36:2667–74.

14. Pettilä V, Westbrook AJ, Nichol AD, *et al*. Age of red blood cells and mortality in the critically ill. *Crit Care* 2011;15:R116.

15. De Montmollin E, Aboab J, Mansart A, Annane D. Bench-to-bedside review: beta-adrenergic modulation in sepsis. *Crit Care* 2009;13:230.

16. Osman D, Ridel C, Ray P, *et al*. Cardiac filling pressures are not appropriate to predict hemodynamic response to volume challenge. *Crit Care Med* 2007;35:64–8.

17. Venn R, Steele A, Richardson P, Poloniecki J, Grounds M, Newman P. Randomized controlled trial to investigate influence of the fluid challenge on duration of hospital stay and perioperative morbidity in patients with hip fractures. *Br J Anaesth* 2002;88:65–71.

18. Agency for Healthcare Research and Quality. Esophageal Doppler ultrasound-based cardiac output monitoring for real-time therapeutic management of hospitalized patients; 2007. < https://www.ecri.org/Documents/EPC/Esophageal_Doppler_Ultrasound-Based_Cardiac_Output_Monitoring.pdf >

19. Goepfert M, Reuter A, Akyol D, Lamm P, Kilger E, Goetz A. Goal-directed fluid management reduces vasopressor and catecholamine use in cardiac surgery patients. *Intens Care Med* 2007;33:96–103.

20. el-Masry A, Mukhtar AM, el-Sherbeny AM, Fathy M, el-Meteini M. Comparison of central venous oxygen saturation and mixed venous oxygen saturation during liver transplantation. *Anaesthesia* 2009;64:378–82.

21. Protti A, Singer M. Bench-to-bedside review: potential strategies to protect or reverse mitochondrial dysfunction in sepsis-induced organ failure. *Crit Care* 2006;10:228.

22. Bichel T, Kalangos A, Rouge JC. Can gastric intramucosal pH (pHi) predict outcome of paediatric cardiac surgery? *Paediatric Anaesthesia* 1999;9:129–34.

23. Mythen M, Webb A. Perioperative plasma volume expansion reduces the incidence of gut mucosal hypoperfusion during cardiac surgery. *Arch Surg* 1995;130:423–29.

24. Eltzschig HK, Carmeliet P. Hypoxia and inflammation. *N Engl J Med* 2011;364:656–65.

25. Khuri SF, Henderson WG, DePalma RG, Mosca C, Healey NA, Kumbhani DJ. Determinants of long-term survival after major surgery and the adverse effect of postoperative complications. *Ann Surg* 2005;242:326–43.

26. Mythen M, Barclay G, Purdy G, *et al*. The role of endotoxin immunity, neutrophil degranulation and contact activation in the pathogenesis of post-operative organ dysfunction. *Blood Coagul Fibrinolysis* 1993;4:999–1005.

27. Baker J, Deitch E, Li M, Berg R, Specian R. Hemorrhagic shock induces bacterial translocation from the gut. *J Trauma* 1988;28:896–906.

28. Lassnigg A, Schmid ER, Hiesmayr M, *et al*. Impact of minimal increases in serum creatinine on outcome in patients after cardiothoracic surgery: do we have to revise current definitions of acute renal failure? *Crit Care Med* 2008;36:1129–37.

29. Falk J. Fluid resuscitation and colloid–crystalloid controversy: new thoughts on an old debate. *Crit Care Med* 1991;19:451–53.

30. Moss G. Plasma albumin and post operative ileus. *Surg Forum* 1967;18:333–6.

31. Goldstein B, Fiser DH, Kelly MM, Mickelsen D, Ruttimann U, Pollack MM. Decomplexification in critical illness and injury: relationship between heart rate variability, severity of illness, and outcome. *Crit Care Med* 1998;26:352–7.

32. Shoemaker W, Montgomery ES, Kaplan E, Elwyn DH. Physiological patterns in surviving and nonsurviving shock patients. *Arch Surg* 1973;106:630–6.

33. Shoemaker W, Appel P, Bland R, Hopkins J, Chang P. Clinical trial of an algorithim for outcome prediction in acute circulatory failure. *Crit Care Med* 1982;10:398–403.

34. Shoemaker W, Appel P, Kram H, Waxman K, Lee T. Prospective trial of supranormal values of survivors as therapeutic goals in high-risk surgical patients. *Chest* 1988;94:1176–86.

35. Boyd O, Grounds RM, Bennett ED. A randomized clinical trial of the effect of deliberate perioperative increase of oxygen delivery on mortality in high-risk surgical patients. *JAMA* 1993;270:2699–707.

36. Cain S. Appearance of excess lactate in anaesthetised dogs during anemic and hypoxic hypoxia. *Am J Physiol* 1965;209:604–10.

37. Shibutani K, Komatsu T, Kubal K, Sanchala V, Kumar V, Bizzari D. Critical level of oxygen delivery in anaesthetised man. *Crit Care Med* 1983;11:640–3.

38. Finfer S, McEvoy S, Bellomo R, McArthur C, Myburgh J, Norton R. Impact of albumin compared to saline on organ function and mortality of patients with severe sepsis. *Intens Care Med* 2011;37:86–96.

39. Bayer O, Reinhart K, Sakr Y, *et al*. Renal effects of synthetic colloids and crystalloids in patients with severe sepsis: a prospective sequential comparison. *Crit Care Med* 2011;39:1335–42.

40. Brunkhorst FM, Engel C, Bloos F, *et al*. Intensive insulin therapy and pentastarch resuscitation in severe sepsis. *N Engl J Med* 2008;358:125–39.

41. Perner A, Haase N, Wetterslev J, *et al*. Comparing the effect of hydroxyethyl starch 130/0.4 with balanced crystalloid solution on mortality and kidney failure in patients with severe sepsis (6S—Scandinavian Starch for Severe Sepsis/Septic Shock trial): study protocol, design and rationale for a double-blinded randomised clinical trial. *Trials* 2011;12:24.

42. Reinhart K, Perner A, Sprung CL, *et al*. Consensus statement of the ESICM task force on colloid volume therapy in critically ill patients. *Intens Care Med* 2012;38:368–83.

43. Wilkes NJ, Woolf R, Mutch M, *et al*. The effects of balanced versus saline-based hetastarch and crystalloid solutions on acid–base and electrolyte status and gastric mucosal perfusion in elderly surgical patients. *Anesth Analg* 2001;93:811–16.

44. Badr A, Nightingale P. An alternative approach to acid–base abnormalities in critically ill patients. *Cont Educ Anaesth Crit Care Pain* 2007;7:107–11.

45. Gazitùa S, Scott J, Swindal LB, Haddy F. Resistance responses to local changes in plasma osmolality in three vascular beds. *Am J Physiol* 1971;220:384–91.

2.2 Accidental awareness during general anaesthesia

Nikki Freeman

Expert Commentary Paul Myles

CPD Matrix Code: 1A03, 2A03, 2A04

Case history

Mrs C is a 58-year-old woman who has been referred for an elective total abdominal hysterectomy following diagnosis of endometrial carcinoma. While undergoing an emergency caesarean section more than 30 years ago, she experienced an episode of awareness. She reports that, at the time, her experiences were dismissed by the surgical and anaesthetic teams involved. Since then she has suffered from anxiety, has experienced recurrent nightmares, and has had problems socializing. She had not discussed her experiences with anyone, including her husband, until she confided in her general practitioner after the prospect of an operation was raised. She understands that it is important for her to undergo surgery but is terrified at the prospect of being awake during anaesthesia. Her general practitioner made an early referral to the anaesthetic department at her local hospital as he was concerned that her understandable fear would deter her from going through with surgery.

⭐ **Learning point** Awareness in anaesthesia; definitions, incidence and risk factors

Accidental awareness during general anaesthesia (AAGA) is an iatrogenic complication, which many patients are understandably very worried about. As a result of coverage in the press, and horror films such as *Awake*, the topic has a high public profile. Concern about AAGA is often raised by patients preoperatively and may increase preoperative anxiety. AAGA is ranked the second highest outcome to avoid by patients (after postoperative nausea and vomiting) and by anaesthetists (after death). Patients who are unexpectedly awake during their operation may experience pain, an inability to move or breathe, as well as a sense of intense fear, and complete helplessness.

Two forms of AAGA must be distinguished. During implicit awareness, a period of wakefulness takes place but the patient does not recall it afterwards, although behaviour or performance may be altered. Implicit awareness requires intraoperative techniques for its detection. In explicit awareness the patient experiences a period of wakefulness and is able to recall and report these events afterwards [1]. The psychological sequelae of AAGA are frequent with 50% of those experiencing awareness reporting some form of psychological distress afterwards. The most significant manifestation is post-traumatic stress disorder (PTSD) [2].

There have been several large multicentre studies attempting to quantify the incidence of accidental awareness during general anaesthesia (AAGA). These studies vary in their methodology and in the timing and structure of the postoperative assessment, and they fail to study a consistent anaesthetic

(continued)

Expert comment

It is believed that most cases of awareness go undetected. Patients may be too distressed to express their experience or are worried that they will not be believed. Reliable detection can include open-ended enquiry but this should be followed by a structured questionnaire early after recovery from anaesthesia, and repeated on at least one further occasion at around one week later.

technique; however, collectively they suggest an incidence of explicit AAGA of ~1 in 600 [3–5]. This equates to >1 case per UK anaesthetic consultant every 2 years. Only Pollard's study using retrospective analysis of quality control data (which included a modified Brice questionnaire) reported a much lower incidence of ~1 in 14,000 [6]. Historically patient groups who are high risk for awareness, due to the use of lower doses of anaesthetic agent, include major trauma (11–43%), cardiac surgery (1–1.5%), and obstetric emergency caesarean section (0.4%) [7]. Many of these studies are at least a decade old. Studies reflecting AAGA risk in routine patients during modern anaesthetic practice are limited.

✪ **Learning point** The Brice protocol

The Brice interview is a post-anaesthesia questionnaire used by anaesthetists to detect awareness which comprises five questions. The questions are based on the study by Brice *et al.* in 1970 and are:

1. What was the last thing you remember before going to sleep?
2. What is the first thing you remember on waking up?
3. Can you remember anything in between?
4. Did you dream during the procedure?
5. What was the worst thing about your operation?

In most research projects the Brice protocol (or a variant) is administered on three occasions (on waking, in the following 24–48 h, and after 2–3 weeks) to identify all cases. Cases suggestive of awareness in clinical research generally require ratification by an external independent panel [8].

Reproduced from Brice DD, 'A simple study of awareness and dreaming during anaesthesia', *British Journal of Anaesthesia*, 1970, 42, 6, pp. 535–542, by permission of The Board of Management and Trustees of the British Journal of Anaesthesia and Oxford University Press.

✪ **Learning point** Classification of AAGA

In an attempt to define the broad range of experiences and to provide a tool for research, a simple classification system called the Michigan Awareness Classification Instrument was developed (Table 2.4) [2]. This classification is used by the American Society of Anesthesiologists' Anesthesia Awareness Registry and several large, prospective, randomized controlled trials relating to the prevention of intra-operative awareness [9, 10]. An alternative classification of grades of awareness has been recently devised by Wang *et al.* (Table 2.5). Their classification explores not only the intraoperative state but also the psychological sequelae [11]. Not all cases fit into even this classification.

Table 2.4 Michigan Awareness Classification Instrument

Class 1	Isolated auditory perceptions
Class 2	Tactile perceptions, e.g. surgical manipulation, endotracheal tube
Class 3	Pain
Class 4	Paralysis, e.g. a feeling that one cannot move, speak or breathe.
Class 5	Paralysis and pain
D	Associated distress, e.g. reports of fear, anxiety, suffocation, a sense of doom or of impending death

Reproduced from Reproduced from G Mashour et al., 'A novel classification instrument for intraoperative awareness events', *Anesthesia and Analgesia*, 110, 3, pp. 813–815, copyright 2010 with permission from the International Anesthesia Research Society.

Table 2.5 Grades of awareness

	Intraoperative state		Immediate postoperative state		
	Consciousness	Signs	Recall	Sequelae	Wakefulness
0	Unconscious	No signs	No recall		
1	Conscious	Signs/+IFT[a]	No recall	No recall or sequelae	Intraoperative wakefulness with obliterated explicit and implicit memory
2	Conscious; word stimuli presented	Signs/+IFT[a]	No recall	No explicit recall, but implicit memory for word stimuli but no sequelae	Intraoperative wakefulness with subsequent implicit memory
3	Conscious	Signs/+IFT[a]	No recall	PTSD/nightmares/etc. No explicit recall	Intraoperative wakefulness with implicit emotional memory
4	Conscious	Signs/+IFT[a]	Explicit recall with or without pain	Explicit recall but no sequelae	Awareness but resilient patient
5	Conscious	Signs/+IFT[a]	Explicit recall with distress and/or pain	Explicit recall and PTSD/nightmares	Awareness with sequelae

[a] Positive isolated forearm technique (+IFT).

Reproduced from M Wang et al., 'The topography of awareness: a classification of intra-operative cognitive states', *Anaesthesia*, 67, 11, pp. 1197–1201, Wiley, © 2012 The Association of Anaesthetists of Great Britain and Ireland, with permission.

○ **Learning point** Risk factors for awareness

Defining risk factors associated with awareness is challenging, as data have been obtained from small, unrelated studies, reported over many decades. It is however clear, that the single most important cause of awareness remains underdosing of anaesthesia relative to a specific patient's requirements. Table 2.6 lists the wide range of factors described as increasing risk of AAGA. This may occur because of equipment failure, a deliberate low-dose anaesthetic technique, drug error, or where an individual's anaesthetic requirements are higher than expected (e.g. due to concurrent drug use). Of particular importance is the use of neuromuscular blocking agents (NMBA) which double the incidence of awareness and increase the likelihood of painful awareness and subsequent PTSD [12, 13].

Table 2.6 Potential risk factors for accidental awareness during anaesthesia

Surgical factors	Cardiac surgery
	Cardiopulmonary bypass
	Emergency surgery (including trauma)
	Obstetric surgery
Patient factors	Severe aortic stenosis
	Pulmonary hypertension
	ASA 4 or 5 status
	Cardiac ejection fraction <40%
	Marginal exercise tolerance
	Long-term use of opiates, benzodiazepines, anticonvulsants, cocaine
	Daily alcohol consumption
	Protease inhibitor use
	End-stage lung disease
	Paediatrics
	Previous AAGA
Anaesthetic factors	Use of muscle relaxants
	Difficult intubation or prolonged airway management
	Non-propofol, non-volatile-based anaesthetic techniques

ASA, American Society of Anesthesiologists; AAGA, accidental awareness during general anaesthesia.

Learning point Obstetric anaesthesia past and present

In the 1970s when Mrs C underwent her caesarean section it was not unusual for low doses of anaesthetic agent to be used in an attempt to provide safety for mother and child. As a result many women experienced AAGA. Awareness and its repercussions were not widely appreciated and counselling services and psychological support were not commonplace. Many women were left to deal with the traumatic consequences of awareness on their own [14]. During the 1990s, higher standards of monitoring and safety within anaesthesia, combined with improved access to neonatal resuscitation resulted in the use of higher doses of anaesthetic agent being used. Subsequently, the incidence of AAGA for caesarean section fell to 0.26% [15]. Today, the use of regional anaesthesia for caesarean section, including rapid sequence spinal for emergencies, has made an important contribution to avoiding the need for general anaesthesia with a consequent reduction in AAGA [16].

Learning point Post-traumatic stress disorder following AAGA

Experience of awareness can vary; however, mental distress is reported in up to 50% of those who experience awareness, with the most extreme psychological outcome being PTSD [17]. Diagnosing post-awareness PTSD can be difficult. Patients who have experienced AAGA are often resistant to further medical contact and presentation can occur a long time after the event. Moreover, patients who do present with psychological distress are often reluctant to volunteer information about the traumatic event without direct questioning, preferring instead to block out the painful memories. This may affect male patients to a greater extent than females. Patients may be diagnosed with anxiety or depressive illness which subsequently proves resistant to pharmacological treatment. The mainstay of treatment for PTSD is cognitive behavioural therapy. Eye movement desensitization may also be helpful [18]. The American Association of Awareness Anesthesia Awareness Registry collects voluntary data from patients who have experienced AAGA. This and the NAP5 study (see A Final Word from the Expert) offer the opportunity to study a larger cohort of patients who have experienced AAGA and will provide further information on the topic in due course.

Diagnostic criteria for PTSD ICD-10 (*International Classification of Diseases*, 10th revision)

A. Exposure to a stressful event or situation of an exceptionally threatening or catastrophic nature which is likely to cause pervasive distress in almost anyone.
B. Persistent remembering or re-living of the stressor in intrusive flashbacks, vivid memories, recurring dreams, or by experiencing distress when exposed to reminders.
C. Actual or preferred avoidance of reminders of the stressor.
D. Either of the following:
    1. Inability to recall, either partially or completely, some important aspects of the period of exposure to the stressor.
    2. Two or more newly arising persistent symptoms of hyperarousal—difficulty in falling or staying asleep, irritability or outbursts of anger, difficulty in concentrating, hypervigilance, exaggerated startle response.

For diagnosis, criteria B, C and D should all be met within 6 months of the stressful event (delayed onset PTSD can be diagnosed after this time).

Reproduced from 'Diagnostic criteria for research', The ICD-10 Classification of Mental and Behavioural Disorders, http://www.who.int/classifications/icd/en/GRNBOOK.pdf, with permission from the World Health Organization, Geneva, 1993.

Management plan

The approach to Mrs C's anaesthetic required careful consideration and planning. Because her surgery was for endometrial carcinoma, there was limited time for psychological preparation. The first step was to invite Mrs C to meet the anaesthetist. A clinical psychologist was present at the meeting and she began regular sessions with him in the weeks preceding her surgery. Mrs C made an accompanied visit to the anaesthetic room and theatre. The technical aspects of the anaesthetic and the best approach to prevent a second episode of awareness were planned by her anaesthetist and discussed with her in full.

⊗ **Learning point** Neuropharmacology of anaesthesia

In order for awareness with recall to occur there must be consciousness and memory formation. The exact mechanisms by which anaesthetic agents modify consciousness and memory are not clear. Indeed the neuroscience (neuroanatomy and neurophysiology) underlying consciousness is far from understood, which makes studying its alteration and reversal problematic. Study of the normal state of awareness and sleep–wake cycles has helped to elucidate the importance of allosteric modulation of the gamma-aminobutyric acid receptor type A ($GABA_A$) in hypnosis [19], with the α_5-subunit containing $GABA_A$ receptors strongly implicated in learning and memory [20]. However, the study of sleep mechanisms is limited in its relevance to AAGA, as anaesthesia is a distinct entity, being physiologically more akin to coma than sleep [21].

It is increasingly clear that anaesthetic agents have a diverse and complex action on the brain. Despite a clear role for the GABA receptor, it is by no means the only molecular target for the modulation of consciousness and memory. Recent scientific advances have shown that halothane anaesthesia is associated with a reduction of cholinergic transmission in parts of the reticular activating system, which regulate arousal and sleep–wake transitions [22], whereas propofol and isoflurane may cause hypnosis by inhibiting or interrupting histaminergic transmission from the tuberomammillary nucleus in the hypothalamus [23]. Furthermore, no single anatomical centre for consciousness has been identified. Consciousness instead appears to be mediated by the co-ordinated activity of higher-order cortical areas with both inhalational and intravenous general anaesthetics selectively suppressing feedback activity in these areas [24]. Greater understanding of the neuroscience of consciousness and of the effects of anaesthesia on consciousness and memory formation are required before strategies to prevent AAGA can be progressed in a genuinely scientific manner.

⊗ **Learning point** Depth of anaesthesia monitoring

Physiological variables

Typically, depth of anaesthesia is assessed by monitoring the patient's response to surgery, i.e. movement and/or changes in physiological variables. Movement responses under anaesthesia are primarily reflexes mediated in the spinal cord, as opposed to cortical pathways in the brain. As a result, movement under anaesthesia does not usually correlate with recollection after anaesthesia; equally, absence of movement (even in an unparalysed patient) does not assure lack of awareness.

Depth of anaesthesia assessment using physiological responses relies on signs of autonomic stimulation: lacrimation, tachycardia, bradycardia, hypertension, tachypnoea, sweating, and dilated pupils. However, the use of such physiological signs is unreliable. Hypovolaemia, sepsis, beta-blockade, the use of antimuscarinic agents or anaesthetic agents themselves can all interfere with the interpretation of heart rate and blood pressure measurements. Additionally, sympathetic activation may occur in the presence of adequate anaesthesia or be obtunded by neuraxial or regional anaesthetic techniques [25].

Isolated forearm technique

The isolated forearm technique has been used as a clinical and experimental technique. A tourniquet is applied to the forearm and inflated above systolic blood pressure. The tourniquet acts to separate the forearm from the systemic circulation, so that any muscle relaxant subsequently administered is unable to perfuse beyond the tourniquet and paralyse the distal muscles of the arm. Therefore, an anaesthetized and otherwise paralysed patient is able to squeeze a hand on command to show if they are awake [26]. This technique has highlighted some of the difficulties of understanding awareness and the limitations of our understanding of the mechanisms of sedation, anaesthesia and memory formation. When used in a study of patients under an intentionally light plane of propofol, without surgical stimulus, two-thirds were able to move their arm in response to command. Of these, only one in four had explicit recall of the event postoperatively [27]. The ability to follow commands under sedation is therefore not necessarily connected to memory formation and recall. This may be because anaesthetic agents prevent memory formation at doses considerably lower than those required for loss of consciousness and immobility [28]. For example, the concentration of isoflurane needed to suppress learning and memory of verbal cues is approximately one-quarter of the dose required to

(continued)

achieve an unconscious state [29]. Furthermore, drugs such as propofol and midazolam cause greater memory inhibition than thiopental at equisedative doses [30].

The unreliability of physiological observations and variation of memory formation under different anaesthetic agents has led to the development of more sophisticated methods which attempt to assess anaesthetic depth. Exhaled anaesthetic gas concentrations, minimum alveolar concentration (MAC) and brain function monitoring are discussed.

Volatile anaesthetic agents: end-tidal anaesthetic concentration

The end-tidal anaesthetic agent concentration (ETAC) can be measured using infra-red absorbance techniques, and its monitoring, during anaesthesia, is considered standard in current UK practice. ETAC monitoring allows real-time dose adjustment of the agent. End-tidal monitoring is used to estimate alveolar gas partial pressure and extrapolate, at equilibrium, plasma and therefore end-organ volatile partial pressure. From these measurements the concept of MAC was developed. MAC is the partial pressure of vapour in the alveoli, at 1 atmosphere, which will prevent 50% of subjects from responding to a standard surgical groin incision, by visibly moving (i.e. an ED_{50}). Different inhalational agents can therefore be compared using MAC: the MAC of isoflurane is approximately 1.2% whilst the MAC of desflurane is 6% (isoflurane is more potent than desflurane because it achieves the same effect at a lower concentration). Due to the accuracy of modern gas analysers and the clear end-point (movement or no movement), MAC studies are precise, and have demonstrated low biological variability [31]. An exhaled concentration of anaesthetic agent >0.7 MAC has been proposed as an appropriate threshold to prevent awareness, as it may suppress the formation of emotionally charged memories [28], and has been used as the lower alarm limit in large awareness studies such as B-Unaware [32] and BAG-RECALL [10] (see Landmark trials). However, from these studies it can be seen that hypnosis and amnesia will not always be achieved at this concentration [10, 32, 33]. It is therefore important for the anaesthetist to understand how MAC can be altered due to co-administration of other drugs and by patient factors (Table 2.7), and maintain vigilance to the possibilities of awareness.

Table 2.7 Factors affecting minimum alveolar concentration (MAC)

Factors that increase MAC	Factors that decrease MAC
Hyperthermia	Hypothermia
Chronic alcohol use	Hypotension
Chronic opiate use	Hypoxia
Chronic benzodiazepine use	Acidosis
Hyponatraemia	Sedative drugs: benzodiazepines, opiates, α_2-agonists
L-DOPA	Regional anaesthesia
Thyrotoxicosis	Neonates
Paediatric patients	Increasing old age
	Hypothyroidism
	Pregnancy

L-DOPA, L-3,4-dihydroxyphenylalanine.

Total intravenous anaesthesia (TIVA) involves the delivery of an anaesthetic agent (usually propofol with or without opioids) by continuous intravenous infusion to a patient. The anaesthetic is delivered via pumps preprogrammed with pharmacokinetic algorithms based on experimental data. These data are used to calculate the amount of drug required to produce a preselected plasma or target organ concentration. However, the algorithms used are based on population studies and are not specific for an individual: the actual dose of intravenous anaesthetic agent needed to render a patient unaware varies widely [34]. These factors may explain some reports of a higher incidence of awareness when this technique is used. Devices for monitoring plasma propofol concentration in clinical practice are in early development and not widely available. Newer techniques may allow prediction of propofol concentrations in serum by determination of propofol concentration in exhaled gases; however, these methods are still highly experimental [35]. As plasma propofol concentrations cannot be measured routinely, the use of brain function monitoring has been advocated while using TIVA. This is especially so when TIVA is used in conjunction with muscle relaxation (see Learning point, NICE recommendations).

(continued)

Brain function monitoring

The electrical activity of cortical cells can be recorded by scalp electrodes. Two main types of electrical signals can be observed: spontaneous activity in the form of an electroencephalogram (EEG) or stimulus-evoked activity detected as evoked potentials (EPs). By contrast with an EEG, which contains information from superficial layers of the cerebral cortex, EPs reflect the pathway of stimulus perception from deeper brain regions.

Full EEG

The EEG measures the spontaneous electrical activity of the outer cortical layers of the brain through the use of scalp electrodes. The recorded signal has a very low amplitude of <200 μV and therefore requires strong amplification. The frequencies of classical EEG bands range from 0.5–30 to >70 Hz (Table 2.8).

Table 2.8 EEG band frequencies

EEG band	Frequency range (Hz)
Gamma	>30
Beta	13–30
Alpha	8–13
Theta	4–8
Delta	0.5–4

The gamma band reflects neuronal signal transmission, in particular cortico-cortical communications. In awake subjects, the main activity is the alpha band. There is a shift towards beta activity if the subject's eyes are closed or during induction of anaesthesia. Increasing sedative and anaesthetic agents leads to signal slowing that reflects increasing activity in the delta band. High doses of anaesthetic induce burst suppression: an EEG 'flat line' [36]. Overall increasing depth of anaesthesia leads to a general slowing (left shift) of the EEG activity.

EEG recordings only reflect the activity of superficial cortical layers and it has not yet been determined whether anaesthetic agents induce unconsciousness by cortical or subcortical mechanisms. It is therefore unclear whether EEG monitoring truly analyses the central nervous system structures or functions essential for unconsciousness and anaesthetic depth [36]. In practical terms this technique has further limitations during use in a theatre setting as multiple electrodes need to be glued to the scalp. This can be time-consuming and technically challenging. Furthermore, the waveforms recorded require expert analysis. Processed EEG has to some extent overcome many of the technical difficulties of full EEG monitoring. However, both methods remain prone to interference artefacts from external electrical activity such as diathermy, or electromyogram activity from facial muscles [37].

Processed EEG

In an attempt to simplify the measurement of electrical brain activity a number of commercially available devices have been studied and developed. They involve rapid analysis of the EEG waveforms with proprietary mathematical manipulation and modelling which generates a power frequency spectrum (i.e. an analysis of the degree to which different frequency waveforms contribute to the electrical energy of the EEG). There are several processed EEG monitors on the market, including the Bispectral Index System monitor (Covidien), E-Entropy monitor (GE Healthcare) and Narcotrend-Compact M monitor (MT MonitorTechnik). All use proprietary (and commercially protected) algorithms and analyses.

Bispectral Index System (BIS)

This uses an electrode sensor strip which is attached via adhesive to the patient's forehead. Electrical activity in the brain is processed using a rapid Fourier analysis algorithm to calculate a dimensionless number between 0 (absence of brain electrical activity) and 100 (fully awake). The BIS score is designed to provide a direct measure of the patient's response to the hypnotic component of anaesthetic drugs (Table 2.9). The target range of BIS values during general anaesthesia is recommended to be 40–60; this range indicates a low probability of awareness with recall. To reliably eliminate AAGA, a lower target range is likely to be necessary. The manufacturers recommend that when BIS is used clinical signs should also be considered in judging the likelihood of adequate anaesthesia.

(continued)

Table 2.9 Relationship of Bispectral Index System (BIS) value with brain activity

BIS number	Brain activity
100	Awake—responds to normal voice
80	Light/moderate sedation—may respond to loud commands or mild prodding/shaking
60	General anaesthesia—low probability of explicit recall. Unresponsive to verbal stimulus
40	Deep hypnotic state
20	Burst suppression
0	Flat line EEG

Reproduced with permission from Kelley SD, *Monitoring consciousness. Using the bispectral index during anesthesia. A pocket guide for clinicians.* Covidien. 2010. <http://www.covidien.com/imageServer.aspx/doc252087.pdf?contentID=32980&contenttype=application/pdf>. Accessed 12/12/13.

Narcotrend-Compact M

The Narcotrend-Compact M monitor is different from BIS in the manner in which the EEG data are processed. Spectral analysis is used to convert raw EEG data into several variables, to which multivariate statistical methods (using proprietary pattern recognition algorithms, developed from the visual classification of EEGs), are then applied. The EEG classification scale is from stage A (awake) to stage F (very deep hypnosis), with stage E indicating the appropriate depth of anaesthesia for surgery. As a refinement to the A–F scale, an EEG index (100 = awake, 0 = very deep hypnosis) is also calculated.

E-Entropy

The E-Entropy monitor measures irregularity in both spontaneous brain (EEG) and facial muscular activity (facial electromyography). It again uses a proprietary algorithm to process these data to produce two values: response entropy (RE) and state entropy (SE). Highly irregular signals with variation of wavelength and amplitude over time produce high values of entropy, whereas more ordered signals with less variation in wavelength and amplitude produce low or zero entropy values. Therefore, the RE scale ranges from 0 (no brain activity) to 100 (fully awake) and the SE scale ranges from 0 (no brain activity) to 91 (fully awake). The recommended target range for entropy values during anaesthesia is 40–60 for RE with SE values near 40.

All of these monitors have calibration limitations as they were all tested on healthy adult volunteers, and extrapolations cannot necessarily be made to other patient populations [38, 39]. There is also concern that current brain monitors are unable to discriminate reliably between consciousness and anaesthesia because of variability in patients' dose responses and EEG responses [40]. As the monitors have delays of between 30 s and 2 min before they indicate a change in the level of anaesthesia, brief periods of wakefulness could occur before any change in monitor output [41].

Several large studies have taken place to assess whether the use of BIS, in combination with an anaesthetic dosing protocol, can reduce the incidence of intraoperative awareness (see Landmark trials). Some authors advocate the use of BIS to prevent anaesthetic overdose and enable downward titration of anaesthetic dose during anaesthesia. However, this may be hazardous due to time lag and the possibility of a narrow range of drug concentration over which the brain undergoes transition states from unconsciousness to wakefulness [42].

Evoked potentials (auditory)

Auditory evoked responses (AERs) represent the passage of electrical activity from the cochlea to the cortex in response to auditory stimuli of 6–10 Hz. The recorded electrical activity consists of an early brainstem response followed by early and late cortical responses. EEG analysis of the early cortical (middle latency) activity reveals characteristic waveforms whose latency increases and amplitude decreases with the onset of anaesthesia [43]. AER monitoring can correlate with the transition from the awake to the asleep state, but it is a poor predictor of movement in response to painful stimuli [44]. It has not yet gained wide popularity as a depth of anaesthesia monitor due to problems with signal interference and wide variation in awake values, with overlap between the awake and asleep state [45]. However, it has been reported to have detected intraoperative awareness successfully, and may emerge as a more useful tool in the future.

❝ Expert comment

BIS, like most anaesthetic monitors, is prone to artefact. BIS can be misleading (about 5% of the time). Greater clinical utility will be achieved if there is integration of the patient's characteristics, anaesthetic drug delivery (including recovery of neuromuscular block), surgical stimulation and visual inspection of the raw EEG trace.

> **Landmark trials** Debate on the usefulness of BIS monitoring
>
> The B-Aware trial [33], published in 2004, studied 2463 patients in high-risk groups for AAGA and demonstrated that titration of anaesthesia to maintain a target BIS range, compared with standard anaesthetic practice, decreased the incidence of intraoperative awareness (two cases in the BIS-guided group compared with 11 cases in the standard group, an absolute risk reduction of 82%, $P = 0.022$).
>
> The 2008 B-Unaware study compared a BIS-guided protocol with an ETAC-guided protocol in 2000 patients at high risk of AAGA [32]. The authors found no statistically significant differences in the incidence of AAGA or anaesthetic delivery between the two groups. However, both protocols in the trial resulted in a lower incidence of AAGA than predicted (0.2% vs 1.0%) which led some to conclude that the use of some form of depth-of-anaesthesia monitoring, whether BIS or ETAC, to guide anaesthetic dose administration combined with an overall increase in vigilance by anaesthetists could contribute to reduced incidence of awareness [32, 46].
>
> In support of these studies, a 2010 Cochrane database meta-analysis of 31 randomized control trials concluded that BIS-guided anaesthesia could reduce the risk of intraoperative recall in surgical patients with high risk of awareness compared with using standard anaesthetic practice. However, when compared with an ETAC protocol, BIS-guided anaesthesia was not superior in the prevention of awareness [47].
>
> The BIS or Anaesthetic Gas to Reduce Explicit Recall (BAG-RECALL) trial (2009) [10] was designed to investigate whether BIS-guided anaesthesia was superior to ETAC-guided anaesthesia in decreasing the incidence of intraoperative awareness among high-risk patients. The international, three-centred, randomized, controlled study included a total of 5713 patients. Of these, 49 patients reported having memories of the period between 'going to sleep' and 'waking up' at the end of surgery. Experts determined that 27 patients (0.47%) met the criteria for 'possible awareness'. Of these, 9 (0.16%) were identified to have experienced definite intraoperative awareness. There was no statistically significant difference in the incidence of awareness between groups (ETAC group 2 versus BIS group 7), $P = 0.98$. This study therefore failed to demonstrate superiority of BIS-guided anaesthesia over ETAC-guided anaesthesia in the reduction of intraoperative awareness.
>
> This topic remains controversial. Currently underway is the Michigan Awareness Control Study [14], the largest prospective trial of awareness prevention. The trial aims to compare BIS monitoring with a non-electroencephalographic gauge of anaesthetic depth. They aim to recruit 30,000 patients at both low and high risk of awareness. The anaesthesia providers will receive a warning via a pager during the anaesthetic to tell them if the BIS is >60 or the ETAC is <0.5. Results are awaited with interest.
>
> To date, the methodology of all trials has been to target a BIS value of between 40 and 60 to indicate adequate depth of anaesthesia with a low probability of awareness. No research group has yet used a lower BIS value of, say, 30–50 or even 20–40 as a target which would logically reduce the incidence of AAGA further. There is concern that anaesthesia which is 'too deep' can lead to prolonged recovery, and increase the incidence of complications (stroke, myocardial infarction, death), or long-term cognitive decline in susceptible individuals [48]. There is limited evidence to support these concerns, and this area, like so many associated with AAGA, remains controversial and in need of further research.

> **Clinical tip** Checklist for preventing awareness
>
> **Preoperative and on induction**
>
> - Evaluate risk factors for awareness. If specific risk factors are identified, consider increasing administered anaesthetic dose.
> - Consider administering a benzodiazepine as an amnesic premedication.
> - Check all equipment, drugs, and dosages; ensure that drugs are clearly labelled and that infusions are running into veins.
> - Re-dose intravenous anaesthesia when delivery of inhalation anaesthesia is difficult, such as during a long intubation attempt or during rigid bronchoscopy.
>
> **Intraoperative**
>
> - Avoid the administration of muscle relaxants wherever possible. If muscle relaxants are required, use the minimum dose necessary, monitor paralysis with a peripheral nerve stimulator to avoid excessive dosing and assess adequacy of reversal.
> - Administer at least 0.7 MAC of the inhalation agent and set an alarm for a low anaesthetic gas concentration.
> - Ensure adequate dose of antinociceptive agents.
> - If using TIVA, ensure that the intravenous cannula is patent, connected, and visible whenever possible. Be familiar with the equipment, drugs and algorithms you are using. Consider use of depth-of-anaesthesia monitoring.

Expert comment

Midazolam has amnestic properties, but these are dose-related and unlikely to provide protection against awareness throughout the duration of surgery. Propofol almost certainly has comparable amnestic properties at equipotent hypnotic doses.

⊗ Learning point NICE recommendations

The National Institute for Health and Care Excellence (NICE) has recently issued guidance for the use of processed EEG monitoring during anaesthesia. Recommendations are based on a health technology assessment and a cost-benefit analysis. They recommend that BIS, E-Entropy or Narcomed should be 'considered' as depth of anaesthesia monitors for the reduction of adverse outcome from anaesthesia in patients at increased risk of AAGA. Groups highlighted include those receiving TIVA and those at high risk of unintended awareness, cognitive dysfunction or the adverse physiological effects of deep anaesthesia. These recommendations were made despite the Health Technology Report failing to find robust evidence for reducing rates of AAGA by depth of anaesthesia monitoring. E-Entropy and Narcotrend monitors have very limited evidence to support their use but NICE gave these monitors the same levels of support [48]. The NICE recommendations are controversial.

Expert comment

Many doctors won't acknowledge that an adverse incident occurred because of perceived litigation risk, as well as professional pride and denial of having caused patient distress. This is best expressed to the patient and/or the patient's family as regret, for this has far fewer connotations of fault or blame, and this, if anything, is likely to reduce ongoing distress as well as litigation risk.

⊕ Clinical tip In the event of a suspected episode of awareness

It is of some surprise that there are no clear guidelines on how a report of AAGA should be managed. Pragmatically, if awareness is suspected during an operation, it is essential that this possibility is explored postoperatively and that patients are treated in a supportive manner. Reassure and talk to the patient in recovery. Visit the patient on the ward accompanied by a senior anaesthetist with an interest in AAGA. Listen to the patient's account of events and validate every aspect, putting the events into context. Where an episode of AAGA appears probable or is clear-cut, it is important to tell patients that you believe them. Be frank, open, and apologize. Try to explain the cause of the awareness. Where the episode is not clear-cut, it is still important to be open and supportive, and to explore further. Make an immediate referral to a mental health expert with relevant expertise. Maintain contact with the patient during their hospital stay and beyond if necessary. It is also important that surgeons and general practitioners are able to recognize post-awareness PTSD, as the psychological effects can present some time after surgery [49].

Primarily, the prevention of awareness involves the correct administration of an adequate dose of anaesthesia. To achieve this, the anaesthetist must have a full understanding and experience of the drugs which are being used. All anaesthetic equipment must be maintained, serviced regularly and checked before use. The patient should be monitored appropriately. Furthermore, it is essential that the anaesthetist is vigilant to the possibility of awareness (see Clinical tip, Checklist for preventing awareness).

Mrs C's operation

It took a great deal of courage for Mrs C to confide in her GP and anaesthetist that she had previously been aware under anaesthesia. She was surprised and reassured that she was at last believed. Steps were put in place to support Mrs C through her cancer surgery. Gentle reassurance and an honest explanation of each step of the anaesthetic helped Mrs C go through with her surgery. She was anaesthetized by an experienced anaesthetist. She received a midazolam pre-med and an intravenous induction. Maintenance was with sevoflurane and MAC of 1.0 was maintained throughout. Her operation was changed to a vaginal hysterectomy, and intubation avoided by use of a ProSeal™ LMA. A remifentanil infusion was used throughout and muscle relaxants were not administered. BIS monitoring was used, maintaining the BIS score of 40–50. She was delighted that she did not experience intraoperative awareness on this occasion. She continued to see the counsellor postoperatively and is no longer experiencing flashbacks. She has stopped using temazepam to help her sleep at night and has become a patient expert helping others who have experienced AAGA come to terms with their experience.

Discussion

AAGA is a potentially avoidable but devastating iatrogenic complication. By far the best approach is its prevention, through safe, vigilant practice and monitoring administered drug concentration and brain function. Simplistically, increasing dosage of anaesthetic drugs reduces the risk of AAGA, but patient variability and the potential for complications of excessive anaesthetic drug doses means that a balance must be achieved. For AAGA to be eradicated completely, a better knowledge of the underlying neurobiology is required to influence clinical practice. To achieve this there must be a greater understanding of consciousness, as well as of the mechanisms underlying anaesthesia. For example, it is known that induction of, and emergence from, anaesthesia are a hysteresis, occurring at different drug concentrations. However, at present, there are several contradictory theories on how these processes truly work. The information integration theory of consciousness predicts a graded return to consciousness [50]; the flip-flop theory of binary sleep–wake transition predicts a discrete shift from unconsciousness to consciousness [51]; whereas non-linear analysis of anaesthesia emergence suggests both multiple and discrete phase transitions leading to consciousness [42]. It is hoped that clarity of understanding may help identify more reliable methods of dosing, delivering and monitoring intravenous anaesthetics, and the development of new drugs that target consciousness and memory, while minimizing adverse effects on the cardiovascular system that can constrain anaesthetic dosing.

Audit of practice

The Royal College of Anaesthetists recommends that all anaesthetic departments should audit the incidence of definite or probable awareness. The ideal standard is that no patient undergoing general anaesthesia should have awareness. However, in line with published data the following targets have been recommended [52].

For general surgical cases: $n < 0.2\%$ should have intraoperative awareness.
For obstetric anaesthesia: $n < 0.4\%$ of women should have intraoperative awareness.
For cardiac anaesthesia: $n < 1\%$ should have intraoperative awareness.

A Final Word from the Expert

The 5th National Audit Project of the Royal College of Anaesthetists and the Association of Anaesthetists of Great Britain and Ireland (NAP5) is currently studying the topic of AAGA. This project will potentially identify the largest ever cohort of patients who report AAGA with the potential to learn both quantitatively and qualitatively from the data and the patient experiences. The results of this project and subsequent recommendations are awaited with interest.

References

1. Chortkoff BS, Bennett HL, Eger EI. Subanesthetic concentrations of isoflurane suppress learning as defined by the category-example task. *Anaesthesiology* 1993;79:16–22.
2. Mashour GA, Esaki RK, Tremper KK, Glick DB, O'Connor M, Avidan MS. A novel classification instrument for intraoperative awareness events. *Anesth Analg* 2009;110:813–815.
3. Ghoneim MM, Block RI, Haffarnan M, Mathews MJ. Awareness during anesthesia: risk factors, causes and sequelae: a review of reported cases in the literature. *Anesth Analg* 2009;108:527–535.
4. Sebel PS. The incidence of awareness during anesthesia: a multicenter United States study. *Anesth Analg* 2004;99:833–9.
5. Sandin R, Enlaund G, Samuelson P, Lennmarken C. Awareness during anaesthesia: a prospective case study. *Lancet* 2000;355:707–11.
6. Pollard RJ, Coyle JP, Gilbert RL, Beck JE. Intraoperative awareness in a regional medical system: a review of 3 years' data. *Anaesthesiology* 2007;106:269–74.
7. Mashour GA. Posttraumatic stress disorder after intraoperative awareness and high-risk surgery. *Anesth Analg* 2010;110:668–70.
8. Brice D, Hetherington RR, Utting JE. A simple study of awareness and dreaming during anaesthesia. *Br J Anaesth* 1970;42:535–42.
9. Mashour G, Tremper K, Avidan M. Protocol for the "Michigan Awareness Control Study": a prospective, randomized, controlled trial comparing electronic alerts based on bispectral index monitoring or minimum alveolar concentration for the prevention of intraoperative awareness. *BMC Anesthesiol* 2009;9:7.
10. Avidan M, Palanca B, Glick D, *et al.* Protocol for the BAG-RECALL clinical trial: a prospective, multi-center, randomized, controlled trial to determine whether a bispectral index-guided protocol is superior to an anesthesia gas-guided protocol in reducing intraoperative awareness with explicit recall in high risk surgical patients. *BMC Anesthesiol* 2009;9:8.
11. Wang M, Messina AG, Russell IF. The topography of awareness: a classification of intra-operative cognitive states. *Anaesthesia* 2012;67:1197–1201.
12. Paech MJ, Scott KL, Clavisi O, Chua S, McDonnell N. The ANZCA Trials Group. A prospective study of awareness and recall associated with general anaesthesia for caesarean section. *Int J Obstet Anesth* 2008;17:298–303.
13. Sneyd JR, Mathews DM. Memory and awareness during anaesthesia. *Br J Anaesth* 2008;100:742–44.
14. Crawford JS. Awareness during operative obstetrics under general anaesthesia. *Br J Anaesth* 1971;43:179–82.
15. Lyons G, Macdonald R. Awareness during caesarean section. *Anaesthesia* 1991;46:62–4.
16. Kinsella SM, Girgirah K, Scrutton MJL. Rapid sequence spinal anaesthesia for category-1 urgency caesarean section: a case series. *Anaesthesia* 2010;65:664–9.
17. Bruchas RR, Kent CD, Wilson HD, Domino KB. Anaesthesia awareness. Narrative review of psychological sequalae, treatment and incidence. *J Clin Psychol Med Settings* 2011;18:257–67.
18. Reed R. Easily missed? Post-traumatic stress disorder. *Br Med J* 2012;344:44.
19. Caraiscos VB, Elliott EM, You-Ten KE, *et al.* Tonic inhibition in mouse hippocampal CA1 pyramidal neurons is mediated by alpha5 subunit-containing gamma-aminobutyric acid type A receptors. *Proc Natl Acad Sci USA* 2004;101:3662–7.
20. Cheng VY, Martin LJ, Elliott EM, *et al.* a5GABAA receptors mediate the amnestic but not sedative–hypnotic effects of the general anesthetic etomidate. *J Neurosci* 2006;26:3713–20.
21. Franks NP, Lieb WR. What is the molecular nature of general anaesthetic target sites? *Trends Pharmacol Sci* 1987;8:169–74.
22. Keifer JC, Baghdoyan HA, Lydic R. Pontine cholinergic mechanisms modulate the cortical electroencephalographic spindles of halothane anesthesia. *Anaesthesiology* 1996;84:945–4.

23. Luo T, Leung LS. Basal forebrain histaminergic transmission modulates electroencephalographic activity and emergence from isoflurane anesthesia. *Anaesthesiology* 2009;111:725–33.

24. Imas OA, Ropella KM, Ward BD, Wood JD, Hudetz AG. Volatile anesthetics disrupt frontal–posterior recurrent information transfer at gamma frequencies in rat. *Neurosci Lett* 2005;387:145–50.

25. Russell IF. Conscious awareness during general anaesthesia: relevance of autonomic signs and isolated arm movements as guides to depth of anaesthesia. *Baillière's Clin Anaesthesiol* 1989;3:511–32.

26. Russell IF. Intraoperative awareness and the isolated forearm technique. *Br J Anaesth* 1995;75:819–21.

27. Russell IF, Wang M. Absence of memory for intraoperative information during surgery with total intravenous anaesthesia. *Br J Anaesth* 2001;86:196–202.

28. Chortkoff BS, Gonsowski CT, Bennett HL, *et al*. Subanesthetic concentrations of desflurane and propofol suppress recall of emotionally charged information. *Anesth Analg* 1995;81:728–36.

29. Eger EI, Koblin DD, Harris RA, *et al*. Hypothesis: inhaled anesthetics produce immobility and amnesia by different mechanisms at different sites. *Anesth Analg* 1997;84:915–18.

30. Veselis RA, Reinsel RA, Feshchenko VA, Wronski M. The comparative amnestic effects of midazolam, propofol, thiopental, and fentanyl at equisedative concentrations. *Anaesthesiology* 1997;87:749–64.

31. Eger EI, Saidman LJ, Brandstater B. Minimum alveolar anesthetic concentration: a standard of anesthetic potency. *Anesthesiology* 1965;26:756–63.

32. Avidian M. Anaesthesia awareness and bispectral index. *N Engl J Med* 2008;358:1097–1107.

33. Myles PS, Leslie K, McNeil J, Forbes A, Chan MT. Bispectral index monitoring to prevent awareness during anaesthesia: the B-Aware randomised controlled trial. *Lancet* 2004;363:1757–63.

34. Newton DE, Thornton C, Konieczko K, *et al*. Levels of consciousness in volunteers. *Anesthesiology* 2011;114:1218–33.

35. Takita A, Masui K, Kazama T. On-line monitoring of end-tidal propofol concentration in anesthetized patients. *Anesthesiology* 2007;106:659–64.

36. Kortelainen J, Koskinen M, Mustola S, Seppanen T. EEG frequency progression during induction of anesthesia: from start of infusion to onset of burst suppression pattern. *Conf Proc IEEE Engng Med Biol Soc* 2007;1570–3.

37 Castro A, Amorim P, Nunes CS. Modeling state entropy of the EEG and auditory evoked potentials: hypnotic and analgesic interactions. *Conf Proc IEEE Engng Med Biol Soc* 2007;1949–52.

38. Dahaba AA. Different conditions that could result in the bispectral index indicating an incorrect hypnotic state. *Anesth Analg* 2005;101:765–73.

39. Niedhart DJ, Kaiser HA, Jacobsohn E, Hantler CB, Evers AS, Avidan MS. Intrapatient reproducibility of the BISxp monitor. *Anaesthesiology* 2006;104:242–8.

40. Dutton RC, Smith WD, Smith NT. Brief wakeful response to command indicates wakefulness with suppression of memory formation during surgical anesthesia. *J Clin Monit* 1995;11:41– 6.

41. Zanner R, Pilge S, Kochs EF, Kreuzer M, Schneider G. Time delay of electroencephalogram index calculation: analysis of cerebral state, bispectral, and Narcotrend indices using perioperatively recorded electroencephalographic signals. *Br J Anaesth* 2009;103:394–9.

42. Walling PT, Hicks KN. Nonlinear changes in brain dynamics during emergence from sevoflurane anesthesia: preliminary exploration using new software. *Anaesthesiology* 2006;105:927–35.

43. Plourde G. Auditory evoked potentials. *Best Pract Res Clin Anaesthesiol* 2006;20:129–39.

44. Kumar A, Anand S, Yaddanapudi LN. Comparison of auditory evoked potential parameters for predicting clinically anaesthetized state. *Acta Anaesthesiol Scand* 2006;50:1139–44.

45. Scheller B, Schneider G, Daunderer M, Kochs EF, Zwissler B. High-frequency components of auditory evoked potentials are detected in responsive but not in unconscious patients. *Anaesthesiology* 2005;103:944–50.

46. Kertai MD, Pal N, Palanca BJ, *et al.* Association of perioperative risk factors and cumulative duration of low bispectral index with intermediate-term mortality after cardiac surgery in the B-Unaware trial. *Anesthesiology* 2010;112:1116–27.

47. Punjasawadwong Y, Bunchungmonkol N, Phongchiewboon A. Bispectral index for improving anaesthetic delivery and postoperative recovery. *Cochrane Database Syst Rev* 2010;CD003843.

48. National Institute for Health and Care Excellence. *Depth of anaesthesia monitors (E-Entropy, BIS and Narcotrend): diagnostics consultation document.* London: NICE; June 2012.

49. Kertai MD, Palanca BJ, Pal N, *et al.* Bispectral index monitoring, duration of bispectral index below 45, patient risk factors, and intermediate-term mortality after noncardiac surgery in the B-Unaware trial. *Anesthesiology* 2011;114:545–56.

50. Tononi G. An information integration theory of consciousness. *BMC Neurosci* 2004;5:42.

51. Lu J, Sherman D, Devor M, Saper CB. A putative flip-flop switch for control of REM sleep. *Nature* 2006;441:589–94.

52. Girgirah K, Kinsella M. Awareness and general anaesthesia. In: Colvin JR, Peden CJ editors. *Raising the standard: a compendium of audit recipes for continuous quality improvement,* 3rd ed. London: Royal College of Anaesthetists; 2011. p. 106–7. < http://www.rcoa.ac.uk/system/files/CSQ-ARB-2012.pdf >

Further reading

Mashour GA editor. *Consciousness, awareness, and anesthesia.* New York: Cambridge University Press.

2.3

Cardiopulmonary exercise testing: utility in major surgery

Steve Tolchard

ⓒ Expert Commentary Paul Older

CPD Matrix Code: *2A03, 3A03, 3A05*

Case history

A 74-year-old male under surveillance for a 5 cm abdominal aortic aneurysm (AAA) was referred for preoperative assessment following an expansion of the aneurysm of 1.8 cm during the previous 2 years. He weighed 79 kg and was 165 cm tall (BMI: 29 kg/m²). The aneurysm was associated with bilateral common iliac stenoses and therefore was not suitable for endovascular aneurysm repair (EVAR) (Figure 2.6). The patient had a past history of hypertension and hypercholesterolaemia (treated with candesartan and atorvastatin), and curative surgery for a renal cell carcinoma. He also took aspirin daily. He was an ex-smoker of 20 pack-years. His exercise was limited by claudication at 40 yards without development of any symptoms attributable to his cardiovascular system.

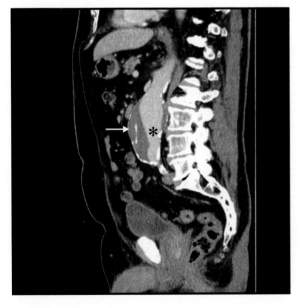

Figure 2.6 CT angiogram of abdominal aortic aneurysm (arrow) demonstrating presence of thrombus surrounding central luminal flow (*).

➕ **Clinical tip** Associated
conditions

AAA is associated with, among
other conditions, coronary
artery disease, hypertension
and peripheral vascular disease.
Careful preoperative investigation
for cardiac ischaemia and renal
impairment combined with
assessment of functional capacity is
essential in these patients [4–7].

⭐ **Learning point** Timing of aneurysm surgery

The law of Laplace means that as aneurysmal diameter increases so does wall tension: this increases
the risk of rupture. This patient's risk with a 6 cm aneurysm is 10–20% per year [1, 2]. Emergency repair
of a leaking aneurysm carries a mortality of nearly 50%, and is higher still following rupture [3]. Current
guidelines suggest that surveillance should continue until the aneurysm reaches ≥5.5 cm, or expands
≥1 cm per year, at which point surgery is considered [1].

Clinical examination was unremarkable. Baseline observations included oxygen
saturations of 99% on room air, blood pressure of 160/70 mmHg and heart rate of
68 beats/min. Blood test results included a haemoglobin concentration of 14.7 g/dL
and evidence of moderate chronic kidney disease (CKD 3: estimated glomerular filtration rate: 53 mL/min/1.73 m^2; creatinine: 114 μmol/L). His chest X-ray was unremarkable and his ECG showed sinus rhythm with no evidence of ventricular hypertrophy,
cardiac ischaemia, prior infarct or conduction abnormality. In view of his reported
exercise tolerance, the nature of the surgery, and in order to better evaluate his perioperative risk, a cardiopulmonary exercise test (CPET) was requested to provide an
objective dynamic assessment of his functional capacity.

🔵 **Expert comment**

As is often the case, clinical
examination was unrewarding. In view
of the history and the type of surgery
this patient should definitely have
a CPET. The joint American College
of Cardiology and American Heart
Association (ACC/AHA) guidelines
for perioperative cardiovascular
evaluation for non-cardiac surgery
describe a group of patients with
'surgery specific risk' [8]. These patients
are deemed at risk due to the extent
of the surgery and the likely fluid shifts
associated with that surgery. Aortic
surgery is included in these guidelines.
All such patients should be admitted
to an ICU following major surgery
regardless of their aerobic capacity.
The CPET should be performed to
help assess the surgical risk and the
necessity for prolonged invasive
monitoring. It will also identify
cardiopulmonary problems such
as pulmonary artery hypertension,
inducible cardiac ischaemia and poor
ventilatory function.

⭐ **Learning point** Cardiopulmonary exercise testing

Cardiopulmonary exercise testing (CPET) is a means of objectively measuring a patient's
cardiopulmonary reserve. The test involves a limited exercise programme on a cycle ergometer while
performing continuous gas exchange analysis with a metabolic cart (Figure 2.7). Patients are seated on a
cycle ergometer connected to a 12-lead ECG and continuous non-invasive blood pressure monitoring.
Respiratory gas exchange is measured via side-stream analysis from a tight-fitting facemask. During the
initial 2 min period baseline data are collected at rest followed by a 1–2 min period of unloaded cycling.
A ramp protocol is then applied and the patient is instructed to continue cycling at a constant cadence
(leg rotational speed) of 60 revolutions per minute (rpm) for as long as possible. Tests are terminated if
patients indicate that they cannot continue, if cadence falls below 55 rpm due to fatigue or dyspnoea,
or if they develop signs or symptoms suggestive of cardiac ischaemia or arrhythmia. Patients are then
continually monitored during a recovery period of 2 min unloaded cycling prior to disconnection from
the test equipment.

The CPET test is standardized except for the 'ramp' which can be varied based on the calculations
below. The ramp (expressed in W/min) is the rate at which the resistance to cycling is increased, which
is proportional to the work the patient has to do to maintain the same cadence. During loaded cycling,
the work of cycling is increased by the calculated ramp and the patient continues cycling until maximum
effort. At this point the ramp is switched back to unloaded cycling for a 2 min recovery period.

Estimated work ramp for a CPET test can be calculated as:

Ramp (W/min) = peak-unloaded $\dot{V}O_2$/100

Peak $\dot{V}O_2$ (mL/min) = (height-age) × 20

Unloaded $\dot{V}O_2$ (mL/min) = 150 + (weight (kg) × 6)

During each test more than 5000 individual measurements are taken and from analysis of gas
exchange and ECG data a nine-panel plot is constructed (the Wasserman nine-panel plot; Figure 2.8).
From this plot it is possible to derive measurements such as anaerobic threshold (AT) (Figure 2.9),
ventilatory equivalents for carbon dioxide and oxygen ($\dot{V}E/\dot{V}CO_2$ and $\dot{V}E/\dot{V}O_2$) and peak oxygen uptake
($\dot{V}O_2$ peak) (see Figure 2.8 for definitions). These measurements, either alone or combined, have
been shown to be predictive of postoperative morbidity and mortality, and provide useful additional
information which can be used to guide preoperative discussion about risk and in determining
perioperative levels of care.

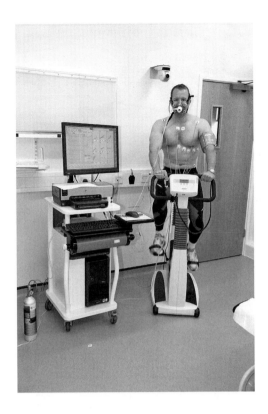

Figure 2.7 Volunteer undergoing cardiopulmonary exercise test (CPET) on cycle ergometer demonstrating side-stream analysis of respiratory gas exchange by metabolic cart.

The CPET was organized 2 weeks preoperatively (Figure 2.8). An incremental work ramp of 10 W/min was applied and the patient stopped at 82 W. He reached a peak oxygen uptake ($\dot{V}O_2$) of 14 mL/kg/min, and a maximum heart rate of 115 bpm (Figure 2.7). There were no exercise-induced ECG changes and he remained asymptomatic throughout. V-Slope analysis (Figure 2.9) revealed an AT of 10 mL/kg/min. With this AT the patient was considered high risk for his surgery. Following a discussion with the patient and explanation of risks he was booked for an open AAA repair with postoperative ICU care. Perioperative beta-blockers were not prescribed.

The patient was prepared for anaesthesia by insertion of two large-bore intravenous cannulae, a thoracic epidural at interspace $T_{8/9}$, and invasive arterial and central venous monitoring. The patient was induced with a target controlled infusion (TCI) of propofol (4 µg/mL; Marsh model) and a bolus of 5 µg/kg fentanyl. Intubation was facilitated by atracurium and followed by maintenance anaesthesia using propofol TCI, combined with epidural boluses of bupivacaine (0.25%). The aortic aneurysm was cross-clamped, excised and repaired using a bifurcated aortic graft to the common iliac arteries via a mid-line laparotomy. Cross-clamp time was 120 min and prior to release of the clamp the patient received 1500 mL sodium lactate solution (Hartmann's, Baxter, UK) effecting a CVP rise of 5 mmHg. Total fluid input was 4000 mL crystalloid. The decrease in systemic vascular resistance secondary to clamp removal was reversed with an infusion of 0.45 µg/kg/min metaraminol (an α_1-agonist). Blood loss was minimal at 400 mL. At the end of surgery the patient was extubated and transferred to the HDU. On the HDU he received intensive nursing and invasive monitoring was continued. Fluid management, epidural analgesia and oxygen delivery were optimized while avoiding hypotension to maintain renal and cardiac function. Epidural analgesia was

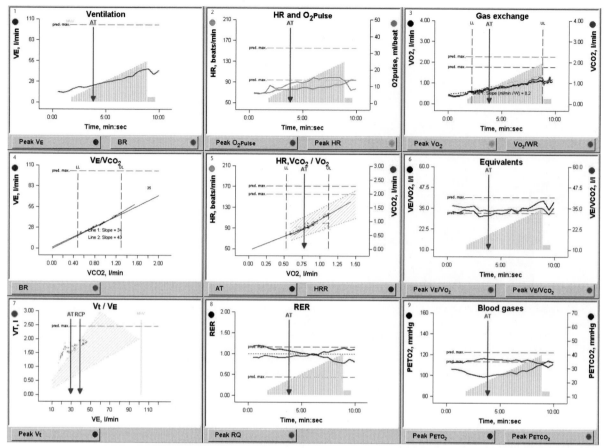

Figure 2.8 The Wasserman nine-panel plot derived from a cardiopulmonary exercise test (CPET). (Plots are numbered 1–9 from top left to bottom right, respectively.) Definitions:

- Oxygen pulse is $\dot{V}O_2$/heart rate and reflects SV (panel 2).
- AT is the $\dot{V}O_2$ at which aerobic metabolism is supplemented by anaerobic metabolism; a value of <11 mL/kg/min is considered to indicate high risk (all panels).
- $\dot{V}O_2$ peak is the highest value of $\dot{V}O_2$ obtained during the test (panel 5).
- Ventilatory equivalents ($\dot{V}E/\dot{V}CO_2$ and $\dot{V}E/\dot{V}O_2$) are markers of ventilation:perfusion matching and reflect lung efficiency (panels 4 and 6).
- RER is the respiratory exchange ratio (panel 8).

Plots 1, 4, 6 and 7 examine ventilatory effort and efficiency.

Plot 2 reflects the cardiac output.

Plot 3 shows the exercise $\dot{V}O_2$ and $\dot{V}CO_2$ relationships.

Plot 5 is a plot of $\dot{V}O_2/\dot{V}CO_2$: the V-plot (see Figure 2.9).

Plots 8 and 9 show the changes in RER and end-tidal gas exchange, respectively.

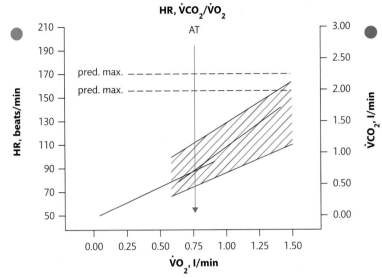

Figure 2.9 The V-slope demonstrating the derivation of the anaerobic threshold (AT). Below the AT the patient respires aerobically during exercise and $\dot{V}O_2$ and $\dot{V}CO_2$ are matched. Above the AT, aerobic metabolism is maximal and ATP production is supplemented by anaerobic metabolism, so the ratio of CO_2 produced to O_2 used increases. The AT is indicated by the inflection point on the V-slope. In the majority of tests the inflection is obvious and the AT is identified automatically by CPET software. In a few cases the inflection point is not clear and the AT is derived manually, usually by two independent experts interpreting the V-slope in relation to the RER and $\dot{V}E/\dot{V}O_2$ and $\dot{V}E/\dot{V}CO_2$ curves in Wasserman plots 6 and 8. HR, heart rate.

> **❝ Expert comment**
>
> Claudication is a difficult situation for the clinician reporting the CPET. This patient is reporting moderate claudication symptoms and thus one might expect a poor result with CPET. Interpretation of the CPET is not easy in such patients as it may be a challenge to differentiate the cause of a poor AT. Is it primarily a cardiac problem or a peripheral vascular problem?
>
> If the cause of a lower AT is the peripheral vasculature then the heart rate response will be less than expected as the central cardiac performance is not challenged as much as the poor AT might suggest. In addition there will be abnormalities in the $\dot{V}O_2$/work rate and $\dot{V}CO_2$/work rate relationships. Not only would there be a slow rise in the $\dot{V}O_2$ due to the poor blood supply to the limbs but the rate of rise in $\dot{V}CO_2$ would also be slow for the same reason [9].
>
> In this patient the nine-panel plot tends to support these observations with a low maximum heart rate (~115 bpm; predicted 146 bpm, i.e. 220 – age). The $\dot{V}O_2$/work rate slope is low at 8 mL/min/watt and the $\dot{V}CO_2$/ work rate slope rises very slowly. This may be an expression of diffuse lower peripheral vascular disease and one would have to query whether the poor AT was in part due to poor vascular supply to the legs.

> **❝ Expert comment**
>
> The AT of just higher than 760 mL (~10 mL/min/watt) determined by the V-slope method (Figure 2.9) indicates moderate cardiac failure by the Weber and Janicki definition [10]. Quoting an AT in decimal places is not recommended as it suggests a degree of precision that could not be justified. In addition to the poor ventricular performance, the ventilatory efficiency of 34 from panel 4 is poor. The ventilatory efficiency slope can only be used up to the respiratory compensation point. Hence ventilatory efficiency is 34 and not 43. The ventilatory equivalents support this with values of around 35. It is quite possible that this man will have some respiratory problems immediately post surgery. These numbers do not suggest pulmonary artery hypertension.

➕ **Clinical tip** Type of surgery

Open AAA surgery may be indicated for cases which are not suitable for treatment by EVAR due to anatomical issues relating to stent placement (such as bilateral iliac stenosis, as in this case). These anatomical issues may have implications for open surgery; longitudinal incisions may be chosen over transverse incisions to optimize surgical access. Clear communication between surgeon and anaesthetist is required to ensure consensus on management to minimize perioperative risk.

❝ Expert comment

I quote: 'Perioperative beta-blockers were not prescribed'. There can be no argument with this decision. In the PeriOperative ISchemic Evaluation (POISE) study [11] (which showed that starting perioperative beta-blockers soon before surgery in patients with an underlying high cardiovascular risk, increased overall mortality) involving more than 8,000 patients the following statement was made: 'Our results highlight the risk in assuming a perioperative beta-blocker regimen has benefit without substantial harm, and the importance and need for large randomized trials in the perioperative setting. Patients are unlikely to accept the risks associated with perioperative extended-release metoprolol.'

In the opinion of this reviewer there is no doubt that most beta-adrenergic blocking drugs are not only negative chronotropes but also negative inotropes. Given the increase in oxygen demand after surgery, there is inevitably a need for an increase in cardiac output. What exactly is one going to achieve in potentially preventing this essential cardiac response by use of beta-blockade? It was decided not to start the beta-blockade in this patient. The situation may have been different if he was already on beta-blockers (which should then have been maintained) and had poor ventricular function as well. With an AT of perhaps only 8 mL/min/watt, it might be an idea to reduce the dose if there were no signs of myocardial ischaemia, but that is another story!

➕ **Clinical tip** Cardiac output monitoring

The use of cardiac output monitoring to guide fluid administration should be considered during anaesthesia for open AAA surgery, though supporting evidence for this specific patient group is lacking. Various devices are available which estimate cardiac output from arterial flow or pressure measurements; all are based on algorithms which make assumptions about vascular compliance. Absolute values may therefore prove inaccurate during aortic cross-clamping; the displayed values must be interpreted carefully before acting upon them.

administered by infusion of 0.1% bupivacaine with 2 μg/mL fentanyl. The patient left HDU after 48 h, and following an unremarkable recovery was discharged and returned home 5 days later.

Discussion

Major surgery places a severe stress on a patient's cardiopulmonary reserve, increasing oxygen demand by 40–50% [12]. Preoperative assessment strategies are designed to identify patients with poor cardiopulmonary reserve who are at increased risk of perioperative complications and death as a result of surgery. Assessment is designed to enable adequate counselling, discussion of treatment options and risk in order to assist patients in making informed decisions. Preoperative assessment ideally serves to direct interventions to reduce perioperative risk and improve outcome. Traditionally tests designed to assess cardiac structure and function, or the presence of cardiac ischaemia, have been employed. These include echocardiography, stress electrocardiography, dobutamine stress tests, and ventriculography, although none has been validated as risk predictive preoperative screening tests [4, 13]. Whereas the presence of cardiac ischaemia is undoubtedly important, evidence [14] suggests that the presence of heart failure is a considerably greater risk factor for perioperative death in major non-cardiac surgery. The focus on heart failure has led to the use of new technologies such as CPET in perioperative risk evaluation.

There is little doubt that exercise capacity is related to perioperative risk and there is an increasing number of guidelines suggesting the preoperative assessment of exercise capacity as a risk assessment tool [6, 15, 16]. The ACC/AHA [16] and European Society for Cardiology [6] guidelines for cardiac assessment in non-cardiac surgery highlight the importance of functional capacity estimation in assessing perioperative risk. The Royal College of Surgeons and Department of Health Report on the Perioperative Care of the General Surgical Patient [17] endorsed this view by recommending the objective assessment of perioperative risk by a range of risk scores and exercise testing. Furthermore the Vascular Society of Great Britain and Ireland [3] have recommended preoperative CPET testing in their Framework for Improvement of AAA Repair.

CPET provides a dynamic assessment of a patient's cardiac and respiratory capacity which has powerful diagnostic utility and prognostic value [9, 12, 18–21]. It is a non-invasive test which objectively determines cardiopulmonary performance under stress [9, 20]. It is safe, cost-effective, and easy to perform in most patients. It yields physiological data which can be used to detect cardiac ischaemia, pulmonary hypertension, chronic obstructive airways disease and, in particular, diagnose the presence, degree and progression of heart failure [9, 19, 22]. CPET has the ability to risk-stratify patients presenting for major non-cardiac surgery through calculation of the AT, peak $\dot{V}O_2$, $\dot{V}E/\dot{V}O_2$ and $\dot{V}E/\dot{V}CO_2$ [5, 18–20]. Elderly patients (> 60 years) with AT < 11 mL/kg/min are at higher risk of cardiopulmonary death compared to those with higher AT. The coexistence of ECG evidence of cardiac ischaemia further elevates that risk [5–12, 20]. Death and postoperative cardiopulmonary morbidity can result from patients with low AT being unable to meet the 40–50% increase in oxygen demand in the postoperative period [16]. In patients presenting for aortic aneurysm repair, AT, $\dot{V}O_2$ peak, $\dot{V}E/\dot{V}O_2$ and, in particular, $\dot{V}E/\dot{V}CO_2$ are all predictive of short- and mid-term survival [18]. AT has been used to risk-stratify surgical patients, direct perioperative care, and reduce their cardiopulmonary mortality [20].

With the possible exception of lung resection surgery [15], in the UK there is currently no consensus on which patients require CPET. This is not surprising considering that risk stratification using this technology is relatively new and only around 17% of National Health Service trusts possess this technology as of 2010 [23]. Those trusts with CPET use a combination of age, type of surgery and/or presence of comorbidities as criteria for testing and a majority use CPET parameters of AT < 11 mL/kg/min and $\dot{V}E/\dot{V}CO_2$ ≥34 to define high risk. Considering the utility of CPET in risk stratification, which both facilitates frank discussion of perioperative risk with patients and the planning of perioperative care, there is a strong argument that all patients undergoing major non-cardiac surgery should be tested. However, it is apparent that agreed, definitive pathways with defined test criteria and perioperative care pathways for those at high risk do not currently exist [23]. The ACC/AHA guidelines recommend the use of the Duke Activity Scale Index (DASI) to estimate physiological reserve. However, the DASI and the incremental shuttle walk test, while showing good correlation with each other, fail to discriminate between potentially high- and low-risk patients [24].

AAA is a progressive condition associated with cardiovascular disease and carries significant risk of mortality when aneurysm size exceeds a diameter of 5.5 cm [1]. Historically, elective open aneurysm repair has a variably reported perioperative mortality of between 1% and 10%; however, recently the national UK mortality has been 2.4% [1–3]. Mortality for aneurysm repair depends on numerous factors such as the type and quality of the surgery and the local perioperative care facilities. A reduction in mortality is seen in centres with high activity. However, patient factors are also very important. In this case an AT of < 11 mL/kg/min increased this patient's likelihood of developing perioperative morbidity or mortality [5, 12, 21]. However, he was discharged after 48 h from HDU and only stayed a further 5 days in hospital. Despite his risk profile, this is not an unusual finding as it will be the natural course in 80% of patients with an AT < 11 mL/kg/min presenting for major non-cardiac surgery [20]. For fitter patients undergoing this type of surgery with AT > 11 mL/kg/min, studies performed by Older et al. [5, 12, 20, 21] and Swart and Carlisle [18] suggest similar outcomes whether cared for postoperatively on a general ward or in the ICU. However, as AT falls, mortality increases, in particular in patients with coexisting cardiac ischaemia; these patients have better outcomes if cared for in a high-dependency environment [5]. Thus, in the future, preoperative assessment of functional capacity using CPET is likely not just to inform discussions regarding perioperative risk, but may also determine the patient pathway and level of care provided postoperatively.

A Final Word from the Expert

The important point made in the discussion comes at the very end. CPET is designed to ensure that the patient is looked after in the best possible area, e.g. in an ICU. It is not designed to offer a reason to cancel surgery. I believe that the issue to be targeted in order to improve perioperative mortality of AAA surgery is postoperative care. In fact I believe that all patients for AAA surgery should be admitted to ICU; not only because of issues such as nursing ratios but also because the most experienced clinicians in postoperative management are to be found in ICU.

Finally all that has been said implies that cardiac failure, not myocardial ischaemia, is the predominant cause of cardiac mortality following major surgery [14].

The outcome here was first-rate with no increase in duration of stay and in my view excellent use of hospital facilities.

References

1. Ashton HA, Buxton MJ, Day NE, *et al.* The Multicentre Aneurysm Screening Study (MASS) into the effect of abdominal aortic aneurysm screening on mortality in men: a randomised controlled trial. *Lancet* 2002;360(9345):1531–9.
2. Brewster DC, Cronenwett JL, Hallett JW, Johnston KW, Krupski WC, Matsumura JS. Guidelines for the treatment of abdominal aortic aneurysms. Report of a subcommittee of the Joint Council of the American Association for Vascular Surgery and Society for Vascular Surgery. *J Vasc Surg* 2003;37:1106–17.
3. Vascular Society of Great Britain and Ireland. *Outcomes after elective repair of infra-renal abdominal aortic aneurysm*. National Abdominal Aortic Aneurysm Quality Improvement Programme Report; 2012 [online].
4. Dunselman PH, Kuntze CE, van Bruggen A, *et al.* Value of New York Heart Association classification, radionuclide ventriculography, and cardiopulmonary exercise tests for selection of patients for congestive heart failure studies. *Am Heart J* 1988;116:1475–82.
5. Older P, Smith R, Courtney P, Hone R. Preoperative evaluation of cardiac failure and ischaemia in elderly patients by cardiopulmonary exercise testing. *Chest* 1993;104:701–4.
6. Poldermans D, Bax JJ, Boersma E, *et al.* Guidelines for preoperative risk assessment and perioperative cardiac management in non-cardiac surgery: the Task Force for Preoperative Cardiac Risk Assessment and Perioperative Cardiac Risk Management in Non-Cardiac Surgery of the European Society of Cardiology. *Eur Heart J* 2009;30:2769–812.
7. Swart M, Carlisle JB. Prospective randomised controlled trial of high dependency care. *Br J Anaesth* 2007;99:273–6.
8. Fleisher LA. Evaluation of the patient with cardiac disease undergoing noncardiac surgery: an update on the original AHA/ACC guidelines. *Int Anesthesiol Clin* 2002;40:109–20.
9. Wasserman K, Hansen JE, Sue DY, *et al. Principles of exercise testing and interpretation*. 5th edn. Philadelphia: Wolters Kluwer/Lippincott Williams & Wilkins; 2012.
10. Weber KT, Janicki JS. Cardiopulmonary exercise testing for evaluation of chronic cardiac failure. *Am J Cardiol* 1985;55:22A–31A.
11. Devereaux PJ, Yang H, Yusuf S, *et al.* Effects of extended-release metoprolol succinate in patients undergoing non-cardiac surgery (POISE trial): a randomised controlled trial. *Lancet* 2008;371:1839–47.

12. Older P, Smith R. Experience with preoperative invasive measurement of haemodynamic, respiratory and renal function in 100 elderly patients scheduled for major abdominal surgery. *Anaesth Intensive* Care 1988;16:389–95.

13. Halm EA, Browner WS, Tubau JF, Tateo IM, Mangano DT. Echocardiography for assessing cardiac risk in patients having non-cardiac surgery. Study of Peri-operative Ischaemia Research Group. *Ann Intern Med* 1996;125:433–41.

14. Hernandes AF, Whellan DJ, Stroud S, Sun JL, O'Connor M, Jollis JG. Outcomes in heart failure after major non-cardiac surgery. *J Am Coll Cardiol* 2004;44:1446–53.

15. Colice GL, Shafazand S, Griffin JP, Keenan R, Bolliger CT. Physiologic evaluation of the patient with lung cancer being considered for resectional surgery: ACCP evidence based clinical practice guidelines. *Chest* 2007;132:161–77.

16. Eagle KA, Berger PB, Calkins H, *et al*. American College of Cardiology; American Heart Association. ACC/AHA guideline update for perioperative cardiovascular evaluation for noncardiac surgery—executive summary: a report of the American College of Cardiology/ American Heart Association Task Force on Practice Guidelines (Committee to Update the 1996 Guidelines on Perioperative Cardiovascular Evaluation for Noncardiac Surgery). *J Am Coll Cardiol* 2002;39:542–53.

17. Royal College of Surgeons of England and The Department of Health. *The higher risk general surgical patient: towards improved care for a forgotten group*; 2011 [online].. Available from: < http://www.rcseng.ac.uk/publications/docs/higher-risk-surgical-patient/@@ download/pdffile/higher_risk_surgical_patient_2011_web.pdf >

18. Carlisle J, Swart M. Mid-term survival after abdominal aortic aneurysm surgery predicted by cardiopulmonary exercise testing. *Br J Surg* 2007;94:966–9.

19. Gitt AK, Wasserman K, Kilkowski C, *et al*. Exercise anaerobic threshold and ventilatory efficiency identify heart failure patients for high risk of early death. *Circulation* 2002;106:3079–84.

20. Older P, Hall A, Hader R. Cardiopulmonary exercise testing as a screening test for peri-operative management of major surgery in the elderly. *Chest* 1999;116:355–62.

21. Older P, Hall A. Clinical review: How to identify high risk surgical patients. *Crit Care* 2004;8:369–72.

22. Mancini D. Predicting survival in heart failure: exercise based prognosticating algorithms. In: Wasserman K editor. *Cardiopulmonary exercise testing and cardiovascular health*, 1st ed. Austin, TX: Futura Publishing; 2002. p. 165.

23. Simpson JC, Sutton H, Grocott MPW. Cardiopulmonary exercise testing—a survey of current use in England. *J Intens Care Soc* 2010;10:275–8.

24. Struthers R, Erasmus P, Holmes K, Warman P, Collingwood A, Sneyd JR. Assessing fitness for surgery: a comparison of questionnaire, incremental shuttle walk and cardiopulmonary exercise testing in general surgical patients. *Br J Anaesth* 2008;101:774–80.

CHAPTER 3

Laparoscopic and bariatric surgery

3.1 Prolonged laparoscopic surgery

Alex Middleditch and Vassilis Athanassoglou

ⓘ **Expert Commentary** Timothy E. Miller
CPD Matrix Code: *1A01, 3A03*

Case history

A 75-year-old female presented to her general practitioner with a short history of rectal bleeding, preceded by a longer history of altered bowel habit with a tendency to constipation. A referral to a colorectal surgeon was made, and in clinic a rigid sigmoidoscopy revealed a mass in the distal sigmoid. Biopsies taken from this showed a moderately differentiated adenocarcinoma. A colonoscopy confirmed the presence of a solitary, non-obstructing sigmoid tumour, and a staging CT scan showed no evidence of metastatic spread. The patient was subsequently listed for an anterior resection. Routine preoperative assessment elicited a history of chronic obstructive pulmonary disease, hypertension, and well-controlled type 2 diabetes mellitus. Past surgical history was remarkable only for a previous lower segment caesarean section. Medications included aspirin, candesartan, fluticasone/salmeterol, gliclazide, metformin, and tiotropium. The patient was noted to be obese (BMI: 34 kg/m^2), but was normotensive with resting oxygen saturations of 95% on room air. The results of blood tests taken are shown in Table 3.1.

Due to a limited exercise tolerance of around 2–3 metabolic equivalents (METs) she underwent CPET. This showed an anaerobic threshold of 14 mL/kg/min, which placed her in the low-risk group for postoperative cardiovascular complications. P-POSSUM gave a preoperative predicted mortality risk of 1.6%.

Table 3.1 Blood tests at preoperative assessment

Haematology	Haemoglobin: 12.0 g/dL
	White cell count: 6.5 × 10^9/L
	Platelets: 214 × 10^9/L
Biochemistry	Creatinine: 138 µmol/L
	Urea: 7.1 mmol/L
	Na: 136 mmol/L
	K: 4.7 mmol/L
	HbA1c: 58 mmol/mol (equivalent to 7.5%)

> **⊗ Learning point** Metabolic equivalents
>
> The metabolic equivalent of task (MET), or metabolic equivalent, is a measure of energy expenditure. Exact definitions vary—but there is consensus that one MET is the resting metabolic rate, i.e. the energy utilization or oxygen consumption, of an individual sitting at rest in a chair. This has previously been quoted at 3.5 mL oxygen per kg body weight per minute, and elsewhere 1 kcal per kg body weight per hour—though there is significant variability between individuals, and for most individuals this value is an overestimate [1]. This resting metabolic rate is used as a reference to give a ratio of energy expenditure for different physical activities. Thus sleeping equates to 0.9 METs; walking up stairs at a steady pace 4 METs; and running at a rapid pace 18 METs or more. This simple tool allows the anaesthetist to estimate the ability of an individual to cope with the increased energy requirements associated with the postoperative period. Less than 4 METs maximum capacity may help predict higher risk of perioperative complications, especially in the presence of other risk factors [2].

In view of potential postoperative pulmonary complications the decision was made by the surgical team that it was in the patient's best interests to attempt surgery laparoscopically. Following consultation with the anaesthetic team she was felt to be a suitable candidate and was enlisted in an 'enhanced recovery after surgery' programme.

> **⊗ Learning point** Laparoscopy—what and why?
>
> Laparoscopy in its current form was first described in 1901, when Kelling used a cystoscope to examine the abdominal viscera of dogs. It took nearly a century for the technique to gain popularity among all groups of surgeons, but this minimally invasive type of approach now plays a significant role in many modern forms of surgery. Laparoscopy involves insufflation of a gas into the abdominal cavity to expand the potential space, enabling visualization of structures and insertion of surgical instruments. Other related techniques may involve extra- or retroperitoneal approaches depending on the site of surgical interest. Entry to the abdomen for insufflation is achieved via a number of possible methods—the open surgical 'Hasson' technique, the Veress needle trocar, direct trocar insertion, and optical, shielded and radially expanding trocars. Gas insufflation on modern systems is electronically controlled, achieving a chosen pressure rapidly, and maintaining it reliably. Most laparoscopic systems generate intra-abdominal pressures of between 5 and 20 mmHg, with modern users avoiding the higher pressures. This gives an increase in intra-abdominal volume of between 2 and 5 L [3]. Various different gases have been used including: air, helium, nitrous oxide and carbon dioxide, the last of which has been most popular due to its high solubility in blood resulting in reduced risk of clinically significant gas embolism [4, 5].
>
> The increase in laparoscopic surgery followed shortly after the advent of enhanced recovery or fast track surgical programmes and has enabled this philosophy of approach to be widely expanded. These programmes first came into existence in the early 1990s—using a multimodal approach in an attempt to speed the recovery, discharge, and resumption of normal activities of patients following elective surgery. The multimodal approach includes changes in patient preparation and education, surgical technique, anaesthetic management and ward culture. The anaesthetist as a true perioperative physician has a central role in the enhanced recovery team: medically optimizing the patient preoperatively, limiting the adverse physiological impact of the surgery intraoperatively, and facilitating early recovery and preventing complications in the postoperative phase.
>
> Laparoscopic surgery is associated with a reduced surgical stress response and can offer the following benefits:
>
> - less surgical tissue trauma and potentially reduced intraoperative blood loss
> - less catabolism
> - less intense and shorter duration of postoperative pain
> - shorter postoperative ileus
> - improved postoperative pulmonary function
> - lower rates of wound infection
> - improved short-term quality of life
> - shorter hospital stay [6, 7]
>
> (continued)

> **❝ Expert comment**
>
> Laparoscopic colectomy within an enhanced recovery programme provides the best short-term clinical outcomes for patients with resectable colorectal cancer. Many centres now have a median length of stay of 3–4 days. Patients can return to their usual activities as early as a week after discharge from hospital and less than 2 weeks from surgery, whereas patients undergoing open surgery often take 8 weeks or more to recover.

When combined as part of an enhanced recovery programme, these benefits may be improved further [8].

In spite of these advantages, laparoscopic surgery is associated with increased operative time and has not been shown to improve mortality or oncological outcome. In addition, these factors are dependent on the experience of the surgeon and the institution, and some have suggested that for several of these the effect of an enhanced recovery programme is more important than the use of a laparoscopic technique [9, 10].

✪ **Learning point**   Contraindications to laparoscopy

With increasing use and experience with laparoscopy, the list of contraindications is shrinking.

Absolute
- Unrestricted ventriculoperitoneal shunt
- Right-to-left intracardiac shunt

Relative
- Raised intracranial pressure (ICP)
- Cardiac disease:
  - poor ventricular function
  - significant valvular disease
  - significant coronary artery disease
  - patent foramen ovale
- Hypovolaemia
- Previous extensive abdominal surgery

⊕ **Clinical tip** Airway management for laparoscopy

The use of a laryngeal mask for procedures of long duration and some laparoscopic surgery is accepted and supported by evidence of safety, particularly in gynaecological laparoscopic surgery [11]. The ProSeal LMA has potential benefits and an evidence base (in terms of performance characteristics) that suggests it might be suitable for simple abdominal laparoscopic surgery [12]. It has been used for laparoscopic cholecystectomy [13]. However, the use of supraglottic devices in prolonged laparoscopic surgery with extremes of positioning has not been sufficiently well studied to be recommended.

The patient was admitted on the morning of surgery having been fasted for a period of 6 h, but having been encouraged to take clear fluids including a carbohydrate-rich drink until 2 h prior to theatre. Anaesthesia was induced with propofol and fentanyl, and an intubating dose of atracurium facilitated tracheal intubation. At the time of intubation a nasogastric tube was passed to decompress the stomach—decreasing the risk of gastric perforation on trocar placement. Maintenance was undertaken by pressure-controlled ventilation with a mixture of oxygen, air, and desflurane in combination with a remifentanil infusion. For monitoring purposes a radial artery catheter and an oesophageal Doppler probe were sited. A urinary catheter was also sited to allow improved pelvic access and monitoring of urine output.

❝ **Expert comment**

An arterial line should be considered in all patients with cardiac disease undergoing prolonged laparoscopic surgery. In severe cardiac disease TOE, where available, may also be helpful to assess whether the patient is going to tolerate the pneumoperitoneum, and to monitor cardiac status intraoperatively. Non-invasive cardiac output monitoring is a more readily available alternative.

✪ **Learning point**   Anaesthetic technique for prolonged laparoscopy

Laparoscopic surgery has been performed under local, regional (both with and without sedation), general anaesthesia and numerous combinations. For prolonged surgery, general anaesthesia is the usual primary technique but there is a relatively small evidence base. There is little strong evidence of a superior anaesthetic technique for prolonged laparoscopy. Balanced anaesthesia using short-acting agents with low emetic potential in association with good, multimodal postoperative analgesia that may include local and regional techniques should be the intention.

The patient was positioned on the operating table in Lloyd-Davies position on a non-slip mattress. The arms were placed in a neutral position by the patient's sides. Padded supports were placed to keep them in position with particular care paid to the padding of the elbows. Shoulder braces were placed over the coracoid processes to prevent intraoperative cephalad movement of the patient during steep head-down tilt—these were intermittently checked intraoperatively to ensure that they had not moved medially to overlie the soft tissue superficial to the path of the brachial plexus.

❝ **Expert comment**

All prolonged laparoscopic surgeries should be considered at least moderate risk for postoperative nausea and vomiting (PONV), and therefore receive two prophylactic antiemetic agents. Any patients with additional risk factors should be treated as high risk. Therapeutic options in these patients include multimodal treatment with two to four antiemetic agents from different classes, as well as total intravenous anaesthesia (TIVA).

✪ **Learning point** Positioning

Positioning patients for prolonged surgery requires meticulous attention to body position, pressure areas and other potential sources of injury resulting from extended immobility. Modern materials used for operating table mattresses show excellent pressure distribution properties. In spite of this, prolonged time on the operating table has been shown to be independently associated with the development of pressure sores [14]. Rhabdomyolysis has also been reported following long-duration surgery [15]. There is also a well-recognized complication associated with prolonged lithotomy or Lloyd-Davies position or steep Trendelenburg—termed 'well-leg compartment syndrome'. Intraoperative ischaemia and reperfusion injury results in compartment syndrome with threat to limb, and potential renal injury [16]. Some would advocate peripheral oximetry to monitor the pulsatility of flow, and regular breaks in position to improve perfusion intermittently.

One of the major concerns regarding prolonged immobilization during surgery is the potential for peripheral nerve damage. A large series (380,000 patients from a single centre in various surgical specialties) estimated the risk of perioperative nerve injury at 0.03%, although many would contend that this is likely a significant underestimate [17, 18]. This is of particular interest, in that subsequent litigation claims involving perioperative nerve damage may identify the anaesthetist as the responsible party, especially where positioning is involved. Risk appears to be increased in patients with diabetes mellitus, hypertension and in smokers. The majority (60%) are upper limb – with the ulnar and radial nerves and the brachial plexus commonly injured. Lower limb nerves at risk include the femoral, sciatic and superficial peroneal. Nerve damage may occur via direct compression, extreme stretch and ischaemia [19]. Thus during prolonged surgery it is important to ensure that excessive extension, flexion, abduction, adduction, or rotation of joints is avoided, and that there are no points of pressure exerted over areas where nerves are known to overlie bony structures (e.g. ulnar nerve over the medial epicondyle of the elbow, superficial peroneal nerve over the fibular head).

❝ **Expert comment**

Rhabdomyolysis due to ischaemia from excessive compression can occur in prolonged procedures in the lateral decubitus and lithotomy positions. Male sex and elevated BMI are additional risk factors. To reduce the risk vacuum, 'bean bags' or cushioning pads should be used, and use of the kidney rest and high lithotomy position minimized. As well as adequate intravascular volume, higher perfusion pressures should be maintained in high-risk patients [20, 21].

Intravenous fluids were started, and blood sugar was checked. As this was within the normal range, an insulin sliding scale was not started at this stage. There was no significant change in monitored variables at the start of surgery. Pneumoperitoneum was instituted via an optical trocar and intra-abdominal pressure was increased at moderate gas flow rates to 12 mmHg. This was associated with an initial increase, followed by a steady decrease in stroke volume measured by oesophageal Doppler to 20% below baseline levels. Blood pressure remained stable. There was a significant decrease in tidal volume, necessitating increase in ventilator inspiratory pressure.

➕ **Clinical tip** Ventilation: volume control or pressure control?

Many clinicians have a preferred ventilatory strategy and often provide justification for their choice. During laparoscopic surgery volume-controlled ventilation has the advantage of being unaffected by changes in compliance, thus may require less manipulation to control elevation in end-tidal CO_2. Conversely pressure-controlled ventilation gives lower peak and plateau inspiratory airway pressures [22, 23], which in the morbidly obese or steep Trendelenburg position may help decrease the risk of barotrauma. A potential compromise strategy is the use of pressure-controlled volume-guaranteed ventilation; however, this is not currently widely available. Limited data suggest that improved oxygenation is associated with the use of pressure-controlled ventilation during laparoscopic surgery in obese patients, but this is insufficient to warrant firm recommendation [24, 25]. Thus the ventilation strategy chosen should be based on patient comorbidities and an understanding of positioning during surgery. Different modalities may be appropriate at different stages of surgery.

✪ **Learning point** Physiological effects of pneumoperitoneum (Table 3.2)

Pneumoperitoneum, or more correctly capnoperitoneum, involves insufflation of carbon dioxide into the peritoneal cavity under pressure. The normal intra-abdominal pressure is ≤5 mmHg, excepting morbidly obese patients where it may be elevated to 9–10 mmHg [26]. An acute increase in

(continued)

intra-abdominal pressure causes a number of significant physiological changes that impact on all major organ systems. As a result there have been attempts to avoid this: the use of low-pressure systems, and gasless laparoscopy with abdominal-wall lift methods using a fan-like retractor within the abdomen have been described and used; the physiological manifestations of these less conventional techniques are not well described but may be less pronounced than standard techniques [27, 28].

Cardiovascular

The cardiovascular effects of pneumoperitoneum have been extensively studied in both animal models and human subjects. They result from the direct pressure effect of intra-abdominal gas, absorption of carbon dioxide, and the activation of both sympathetic and parasympathetic nervous systems. These changes may be either potentiated or attenuated during laparoscopic surgery by the extreme positioning sometimes used to improve or achieve surgical access.

In general, the following cardiovascular changes may be seen with pneumoperitoneum [29, 30]:

- minor increase in heart rate
- increased systemic vascular resistance (SVR) and pulmonary vascular resistance (PVR)
- increased mean arterial pressure (MAP)
- decreased cardiac output (CO)
- increased central venous pressure (CVP)

The aetiology of these alterations is complex and multifactorial. The increase in SVR may be caused by direct compression of the abdominal aorta, as well as elevations in plasma levels of noradrenaline, vasopressin, renin, and aldosterone observed during pneumoperitoneum [31–33]. These may result from direct effects of absorbed carbon dioxide, or by central activation of the sympathetic nervous system. The biphasic change sometimes seen in cardiac output may be secondary to an initial increase in venous return from abdominal organs on institution of pneumoperitoneum, followed by a combination of increased afterload and reduced venous return due to compression of the abdominal inferior vena cava [29, 34]. A high partial pressure of carbon dioxide that may result from both transperitoneal absorption, and impairment of ventilation, has direct myocardial depressant and arrythmogenic effects. These effects may be more pronounced in otherwise healthy morbidly obese patients—who show a similar cardiovascular profile, in terms of echocardiographic changes, to that observed in patients with significant cardiac disease [35]. Peritoneal stretch can also cause a well-documented vagally induced bradycardia.

There is, however, significant discordance between the findings of studies looking at the haemodynamic effects of pneumoperitoneum. Some studies on healthy subjects using low intra-abdominal pressure have shown a persisting increase in cardiac output—possibly due to increased venous return [29], whereas others have shown little effect [36, 37]. Others have shown the effect to be relatively short-lived—with cardiac output returning to baseline within 20 min of insufflation [30]. All of the studies have small sample sizes and use a multitude of methods in order to quantify the effects—this variability in conditions makes it difficult to compare findings. However, knowledge of the following variables may allow greater predictability of clinical manifestations:

- Surgical factors
  - o abdominal insufflation pressure and initial flow rate
  - o surgical technique
- Anaesthetic factors
  - o anaesthetic technique
  - o ventilatory strategy and carbon dioxide absorption and level
- Patient factors
  - o patient positioning
  - o patient volaemic status
  - o patient cardiac function
  - o obesity [31, 38]

Administration of intravenous fluids to maintain normovolaemia, and the use of remifentanil, may significantly reduce the cardiovascular sequelae of pneumoperitoneum in healthy individuals [37]. In addition the increase in SVR will be at least partially offset by the use of vasodilatory anaesthetic agents. Thus in a healthy, normovolaemic individual with normal cardiac function undergoing a laparoscopic

(continued)

procedure with insufflation pressures limited to <12 mmHg, there may be little clinically significant change in haemodynamic variables [36].

Respiratory

During pneumoperitoneum, the increase in intra-abdominal pressure displaces the diaphragm cephalad which increases intrathoracic pressure [30, 39]. This causes a marked decrease in chest wall and lung compliance [40], leading to atelectasis [39], decreased functional residual capacity [41] and changes in ventilation/perfusion ratios [42]. These all result clinically in an increased airway pressure for a given tidal volume, and an increased risk of hypoxaemia. The increased airway pressure is not usefully reduced by neuromuscular blockade [43]. The negative effects on gas exchange can be significantly improved by the application of positive end-expiratory pressure (PEEP), although this may also cause haemodynamic impairment [44].

An increase in arterial carbon dioxide ($PaCO_2$) results from impaired ventilation—at least in part as a result of increased physiological dead space [45], but mainly due to absorption of carbon dioxide from the peritoneal cavity. The extent of this absorption is limited by compression of local blood vessels, and thus $PaCO_2$ should reach a plateau level by 30 min from insufflation [46]. It is important to increase minute ventilation to avoid significant acid–base disturbance. Even in healthy patients this may require an increase in minute volume of anywhere between 12% and 54% [47, 48]. In addition, the relationship between end-tidal carbon dioxide and $PaCO_2$ levels is complex—and may vary both between individuals and over time in the same individual during pneumoperitoneum [48, 49], therefore both exact values and trends may be misleading. This phenomenon may be exaggerated in those patients with cardiopulmonary disease and during prolonged pneumoperitoneum, leading to an increased risk of both significant acidaemia and hypercarbia [45, 50]. Arterial blood gas analysis may therefore be useful during prolonged laparoscopy. Transcutaneous CO_2 monitoring, where available, may also provide a more accurate estimation of $PaCO_2$ during pneumoperitoneum [51].

During pneumoperitoneum, a significant quantity of carbon dioxide is absorbed and buffered by the body; following cessation of pneumoperitoneum elimination of carbon dioxide may continue for a significant period [47]. This leads to an increase in work of breathing postoperatively which may be compounded by impairment in postoperative respiratory function present after laparoscopic surgery. This impairment is less marked than after open abdominal surgery, but occurs with both upper and (to a lesser extent) lower abdominal procedures [52]. It is sufficient to cause significant postoperative hypoxia, even after short laparoscopic procedures in healthy individuals [53].

Renal + splanchnic

During pneumoperitoneum, there is a decrease in renal blood flow, impairment of renal function, and decreased urine output. The mechanism of this is not fully understood, but the degree of impairment may be associated with preoperative renal function, volaemic status, raised intra-abdominal pressure, positioning, and duration of pneumoperitoneum [54]. As a result, intraoperative clearance of renally excreted drugs may be impaired. This effect appears to be short-lived, and reverses even after prolonged (>4 h) surgery in patients with pre-existing renal impairment [55]. In spite of this, it is prudent to avoid nephrotoxic drugs where possible, especially in patients with renal impairment.

The effects of pneumoperitoneum on hepatic and intestinal blood flow vary between models. Splanchnic blood flow may fall, leading to an increase in biochemical markers of oxidative stress, which is related to duration and level of intra-abdominal pressure [56]. The clinical significance of this is unclear, although evidence from one study showing impaired indocyanine green clearance by the liver during pneumoperitoneum suggests that effects on drug metabolism are plausible [57]. Conversely recent evidence shows that with increasing duration of abdominal insufflation, hepatic blood flow and metabolism may adapt and paradoxically improve [58].

Cerebral

An increase in ICP has been noted in experimental models with pneumoperitoneum – even after correction of $PaCO_2$ [59]. The presumed mechanism for this is an increase in intrathoracic pressure, leading to raised CVP, transmitted to the sagittal sinus where it impairs resorption of cerebrospinal fluid. It is possible that raised ICP may be responsible for some of the cardiovascular sequelae of

(continued)

pneumoperitoneum [60]. Diagnostic laparoscopy in a patient with a closed head injury caused a spectacular elevation in ICP following pneumoperitoneum; thus laparoscopy should be avoided in any patient with possible raised ICP [61]. Prolonged laparoscopic surgery with the patient in head-down (Trendelenburg) position has also been associated with development of cerebral oedema affecting emergence from anaesthesia [62]. The mechanism for this is unclear, but it appears to be transient in nature, and resolves with head-up positioning.

Haematological and immunological

During pneumoperitoneum the compression of the abdominal veins results in venous stasis of the lower limbs, which in combination with the hypercoagulability associated with surgical trauma, and a prolonged operating time, increases the risk of venous thrombosis. Venous stasis can be partially overcome by sequential calf compression devices [63] but these may not be appropriate for some patients (e.g. Lloyd-Davis or lithotomy position), so adequate pharmacological thromboprophylaxis should be the norm in this group of patients.

Laparoscopic surgery results in a less marked stress response when compared with open surgery, as assessed via numerous surrogate biochemical markers [6]. There is also evidence of less suppression of cell-mediated immune function [64, 65]. This may lead to less risk of postoperative complications, both infective and oncological, although the latter is not supported by current evidence. Despite this there is evidence for a direct effect of carbon dioxide pneumoperitoneum on local immune function—with some models showing that it impairs the function of peritoneal macrophages [65]. Theoretically, this could adversely affect the ability of these cells to deal with microscopic deposits of tumour in the early postoperative period.

Hypothermia

During laparoscopy there is a steady flow of gas into the abdomen to replace that absorbed, and more significantly that which leaks from around port sites. Over a period of time the continual escape of warm, moist gas can equate to large volumes—and can result in significant loss of heat and therefore fall in body temperature. A reduction in heat loss (and indeed postoperative pain) may be achieved by heating and humidifying the insufflated gas—although this is the subject of debate [66, 67]. Thus adequate warming facilities must be available for prolonged laparoscopy, and temperature should be monitored throughout.

Table 3.2 Summary of physiological changes of pneumoperitoneum

Cardiovascular	
Heart rate	↑/↔
Cardiac output	↓
Systemic vascular resistance	↑
Mean arterial pressure	↑
Pulmonary vascular resistance	↑

Respiratory	
Compliance	↓
Atelectasis	↑
Functional residual capacity	↓
PaO_2	↔/↓
$PaCO_2$	↑ (without increased minute ventilation)
Airway pressure	↑

Other	
Renal blood flow	↓
Renal clearance	↓
Urine output	↓
Hepatic blood flow	?↓
Hepatic clearance	↓
Intestinal blood flow	?↓
Intracranial pressure	↑

🔆 Expert comment

There have been major concerns about the effect of impaired venous outflow from the brain on cerebral perfusion during prolonged laparoscopic surgery in the steep Trendelenburg position. However, a recent study using transcranial Doppler flow velocity to assess cerebral blood flow in robotic prostatectomies found that cerebral perfusion was not compromised. As expected the investigators found that care must be taken to avoid hyperventilation with consequent hypocapnia and reduced cerebral blood flow [68].

✪ **Learning point** Complications of pneumoperitoneum (Table 3.3)

Table 3.3 Complications of pneumoperitoneum

Trauma	Caused by trocar/Verres needle insertion
	• Results in haemorrhage, injury to solid organs, perforation of bladder/intestine
Incorrect gas placement	Pneumo(capno)thorax (uni/bilateral)
	Pneumomediastinum
	Pneumopericardium
	Subcutaneous emphysema
	• Insufflation of gas under pressure will dissect into any possible tissue plane. This includes both normal and abnormal planes, and embryonic remnants.
	Gas embolism
Respiratory	Bronchial intubation
	• Caused by cephalad movement of the diaphragm moving the bronchial tree
	Pneumothorax
	• From barotrauma caused by high inspiratory pressures

❝ **Expert comment**

Venous gas embolism is a rare but potentially lethal complication of laparoscopic surgery. Carbon dioxide enters the bloodstream during insufflation through a tear in a vessel in the abdominal wall or peritoneum and obstructs the right ventricular outflow tract causing sudden cardiovascular collapse. The risk decreases after completion of the pneumoperitoneum as the increased abdominal pressure causes the injured vessel to collapse. Treatment includes immediate desufflation of the pneumoperitoneum, ventilation with 100% oxygen, and positioning in steep head-down and left-lateral decubitus position.

❝ **Expert comment**

Subcutaneous emphysema occurs when insufflated carbon dioxide dissects from the peritoneal cavity to the subcutaneous tissues. This may occur at the trocar site or via a defect in the diaphragm. The carbon dioxide bubbles under the skin and is annoying for the patient, although it is usually harmless and settles in a day or two. Intra-abdominal pressure of carbon dioxide should be monitored, since high pressures are associated with a higher incidence of subcutaneous emphysema.

⊕ **Clinical tip** Anaesthetic management of pneumoperitoneum (Table 3.4)

Table 3.4 Measures to reduce the physiological effects of pneumoperitoneum

Adequate preload	A bolus of fluid prior to commencement partially compensates for decreased venous return
Adequate anaesthesia	Reduces sympathetic nervous system activation, limiting increases in SVR
Gradual insufflation	Allows time for adaptation to changes
Limiting intra-abdominal pressure	Using the minimum level of intra-abdominal pressure that provides adequate and safe surgical access
Gradual changes in position	Allows time for adaptation to changes.
Cautious increase in PEEP	Reduces atelectasis or ventilation/perfusion mismatch and improves functional residual capacity to improve oxygenation

If there are difficulties tolerating pneumoperitoneum in spite of these measures, and reversible complications have been excluded, the decision must be made as to whether the procedure should be performed open or abandoned completely. An inability to tolerate pneumoperitoneum may represent previously unrecognized severe cardiorespiratory disease that may significantly affect the postoperative course.

Following pneumoperitoneum the patient was tilted into Trendelenburg position at 15% to allow better surgical access. This resulted in some improvement in cardiac output, but a further significant decrease in tidal volumes, requiring increased inspiratory airway pressure. Several minutes after this the pulse oximeter alarm indicated that the oxygen saturations had fallen from 97% to < 90%.

⊕ Clinical tip Pathophysiological causes of acute hypoxia during laparoscopy (Table 3.5)

Table 3.5 Pathophysiological causes of acute hypoxia during laparoscopy

Cause	Associated features	Management
Bronchial intubation	Reduced air entry (usually) left side Raised inspiratory pressures/decreased tidal volume Usually occurs following pneumoperitoneum/change in position. Little initial increase in end-tidal CO_2 (Note: can be bilateral)	Partial withdrawal of tracheal tube
Pneumothorax/ capnothorax	Reduced air entry on relevant side Chest asymmetry Hyper-resonance Raised inspiratory pressures Increase in end-tidal CO_2	Release pneumoperitoneum Cautious application of PEEP[a] (capnothorax—not pneumothorax) Pleural drain
Impaired perfusion	Decreased peripheral perfusion/ cardiac output	Exclude: • significant haemorrhage/hypovolaemia • tension pneumothorax • gas embolism • myocardial impairment Treat as appropriate
Pulmonary shunt Ventilation/perfusion mismatch	Air entry reduced at bases/unchanged	Increase FiO_2 Apply PEEP Increase mean airway pressure Improve position—head up Release/reduce pneumoperitoneum Alveolar recruitment measures

[a] Application of positive end-expiratory pressure (PEEP) has been successfully used in the management of capnothorax, but may cause significant worsening of cardiovascular parameters so should be used with caution [69, 70].

❻ Expert comment

Cardiovascular changes and significant respiratory acidosis have been observed in otherwise healthy patients during prolonged laparoscopic surgery. The cardiovascular compromise can be caused by mechanical factors directly related to increased intra-abdominal pressure affecting ventilation and venous return, as well as to absorption of carbon dioxide into the circulation, leading to acidosis and further cardiopulmonary depression.

✪ Learning point Effect of positioning

In order to provide good surgical access and view of the operative site, patients undergoing laparoscopic procedures are occasionally subject to steep and unnatural positions. This creates difficulty for the anaesthetist in several forms.

Trendelenburg (head down)

This position reduces the effects of abdominal compression on lower limb venous stasis. This results in a marked increase in CVP—up to 3-fold [71], but also offsets some of the impairment induced by pneumoperitoneum—improving stroke volume and cardiac output in healthy patients [72]. A doubling in mean pulmonary artery pressure and pulmonary capillary wedge pressure caused no cardiac impairment in American Society of Anasthesiologists status I–II radical prostatectomy patients, but may have significant adverse effects in the presence of impaired cardiac function [71].

Trendelenburg position potentiates the effect of pneumoperitoneum on respiratory mechanics, increasing diaphragmatic incursion on the thorax, decreasing lung compliance and increasing physiological dead space. This impairment is well tolerated in healthy individuals [73], but increased in obese patients [74]. Effects increase with greater degrees of tilt [75].

Increases in intraocular pressure have been observed in patients in Trendelenburg position [76]. Caution should therefore be exercised in patients with pre-existing visual problems, especially glaucoma.

Following prolonged head-down laparoscopic surgery position, patients frequently have facial oedema. This is an indication of a potentially dangerous anaesthetic complication as it is likely to be associated with a degree of laryngeal oedema. As such a tracheal cuff leak test should be performed prior to extubation of

(continued)

these patients [77]. The risk of this complication can be reduced by judicious intraoperative intravenous fluid administration, limiting degree of head-down tilt, and upright positioning following surgery for a period prior to extubation [78].

Reverse Trendelenburg

The head-up position exacerbates impaired venous return from the lower body, which may further reduce the cardiac output in conjunction with pneumoperitoneum [81]. This has potentially profound effects on major organ blood supply—including brain, heart and kidneys. The effects on respiratory function are less marked, with little discernible change [82].

Following withdrawal of the tracheal tube by 1.5 cm, breath sounds improved on the left side of the chest, tidal volumes increased markedly, and the oxygen saturation improved. Surgery continued with minimal blood loss, but was complicated by adhesions presumed to be secondary to her previous obstetric surgery. This increased the time required to mobilize the large bowel, although did not necessitate conversion to open surgery given the patient's stable physiological state. Fluid therapy was administered as guided by oesophageal Doppler readings. Despite this, oliguria was noted—but this was not associated with elevation of blood lactate levels that might indicate impaired global tissue perfusion. Clonidine was given to a dose of 1 µg/kg for analgesic purposes and to limit the potential catecholamine effect of pneumoperitoneum. Once resection was complete and the anastomosis underway, intravenous paracetamol was given and morphine was gradually titrated in. A serotonin (5HT$_3$) antagonist was administered for antiemesis. On release of pneumoperitoneum cardiac output increased significantly. Following completion of surgery bilateral transversus abdominis plane (TAP) blocks were placed under ultrasound guidance. The patient was then woken, extubated and transferred to the recovery unit. Following further doses of intravenous morphine, intravenous fluids were discontinued and she was transferred to a general surgical ward with ongoing oxygen therapy. Urine output improved over the next few hours.

Postoperative analgesia included regular oral paracetamol, with oral tramadol and oral morphine as required. An NSAID was not used in view of preoperative renal impairment. Thromboprophylaxis was prescribed in the form of compression stockings and a low-molecular-weight heparin.

Learning point Analgesia for laparoscopic surgery

Laparoscopic surgery usually involves less tissue trauma than open surgery, and therefore postoperative pain and analgesia requirements are generally lower in intensity and duration. However, significant pain, particularly immediately postoperatively, is still a frequent complaint of patients undergoing laparoscopy [83]—and there remains significant ongoing research into optimal analgesic techniques. In addition, the degree of surgical trauma varies depending on the procedure: some laparoscopy-assisted procedures still involve large incisions (e.g. for removal of resected tumour). The mechanisms and pattern of pain following laparoscopy are complicated. Pain results from trocar insertion points, surgical visceral trauma, and the stretch of the peritoneal nerves and vessels induced by pneumoperitoneum [84]. Use of low intra-abdominal pressure may therefore decrease postoperative pain [85]. Also, excitation of the phrenic nerve can result in right shoulder-tip pain that may last for up to 3 days [84]. This pain is associated with the continued radiological presence of a subdiaphragmatic gas bubble. Active removal of gas at the end of the procedure decreases postoperative pain [86], and ongoing drainage may be helpful [87], but does not universally result in resolution of symptoms [88].

Oral

The use of simple analgesics, such as paracetamol and NSAID, is a routine part of any analgesic ladder. The effect of NSAIDs on pain after laparoscopy is variably reported. They may be especially helpful

(continued)

in treating the classical shoulder-tip pain [84]. The use of oral opioids is widespread, although is associated with PONV.

Intravenous opiates

These are the mainstay of rescue analgesia in the immediate post-anaesthetic phase, and are widely effective. In addition they are still used beyond this early period in the form of patient-controlled analgesia (PCA) for the more painful laparoscopic procedures. However, they have multiple side-effects, including increasing the risk of PONV, impaired gastrointestinal motility/prolongation of ileus and respiratory depression. This offsets some of the intended benefits of laparoscopy so their use should be avoided where possible.

Local anaesthesia infiltration

Local anaesthetic techniques potentially play a useful role in post operative pain control. The use of intraperitoneal local anaesthetic has shown mixed promise [89], whereas infiltration at port sites has demonstrated analgesic benefit [90].

Regional anaesthesia

The use of rectus sheath [91], paravertebral [92], and more recently TAP blocks [93] have all been successfully demonstrated to reduce postoperative analgesia requirement, in particular systemic opiates, after laparoscopy.

Central neuraxial blockade

Central neuraxial techniques have been used as the sole anaesthetic technique for laparoscopic surgery. However, for prolonged laparoscopic surgery with potentially extreme positioning, this is not appropriate. They can, however, be used in conjunction with general anaesthesia.

Epidural anaesthesia is accepted to provide optimal analgesia after open abdominal surgery. Spinal (subarachnoid) anaesthesia with an opiate can increase the duration of analgesia without some of the undesirable associations of continuous epidural anaesthesia, such as restrictions on mobility and hypotension. The use of epidurals in laparoscopic surgery is being challenged in the context of increased use of enhanced recovery programmes. The evidence base is very limited, but a recent single-centre trial comparing thoracic epidural, spinal anaesthesia with opiate (diamorphine) and morphine PCA in patients undergoing laparoscopic colorectal surgery found that the epidural group had longer hospital stay and longer postoperative ileus [94]. The group receiving spinal anaesthesia reported better analgesia than the PCA group. A further (unblinded) observational trial comparing spinal and epidural anaesthesia in this setting reported increased duration of stay and slower mobilization associated with thoracic epidural anaesthesia and perhaps surprisingly also reported better analgesia in the spinal group [95]. Caudal epidural anaesthesia may be a useful adjunctive technique for laparoscopic pelvic surgery [91].

A combination of effective analgesic techniques is essential for maximizing the potential benefits that result from a minimally invasive approach to the abdomen.

That evening she was able to take small amounts of oral diet, limited by mild nausea which was treated with an antiemetic. Pain was treated with an evening dose of tramadol. Due to an increased blood glucose an insulin sliding scale was commenced overnight. This was discontinued the following morning as she was tolerating normal diet, and was able to restart her normal diabetic medications. Postoperative blood tests showed minimal changes from preoperative. Her urinary catheter was removed, and she was able to mobilize to a chair on the first postoperative day. Bowel function had returned to normal by day 2 postoperatively, and on day 3 she was discharged home.

Discussion

This case highlights the impact of the increasing complexity of surgical techniques on anaesthetic management decisions. The advent of enhanced recovery surgery with its benefits to patients and improved cost-effectiveness places additional responsibility on anaesthetists to consider the implications of their chosen anaesthetic technique on patient outcomes, including length of stay. The anaesthetist plays a key role as perioperative physician in the management of patients undergoing prolonged laparoscopic surgery. From the preoperative preparation and optimization, to limiting the operative physiological insult, through to ensuring rapid postoperative recovery, high-quality evidence-based management can have a significant impact on patient outcome.

A Final Word from the Expert

The last 10 years have seen huge advances in laparoscopic surgery, so that in the near future some predict that the majority of operations will be minimally invasive. The increase in complexity of cases performed laparoscopically and the steep learning curve needed to attain the necessary skills will inevitably lead to a greater number of prolonged laparoscopic surgeries.

Anaesthetists need to be aware of the specific problems and challenges that can occur with prolonged laparoscopic surgery so that patients can experience the benefits that they expect from this new era in surgical care.

References

1. Byrne NM, Hills AP, Hunter GR, Weinsier RL, Schutz Y. Metabolic equivalent: one size does not fit all. *J Appl Physiol* 2005;99:1112–19.
2. Fleisher LA, Beckman JA, Brown KA, *et al.* ACC/AHA 2007 guidelines on perioperative cardiovascular evaluation and care for noncardiac surgery: a report of the American College of Cardiology/American Heart Association Task Force on Practice Guidelines (Writing Committee to Revise the 2002 Guidelines on Perioperative Cardiovascular Evaluation for Noncardiac Surgery). *Circulation* 2007;116:e418–99.
3. Mulier JP, Dillemans B, Van Cauwenberge S. Impact of the patient's body position on the intraabdominal workspace during laparoscopic surgery. *Surg Endosc* 2010;24:1398–1402.
4. Yau P, Watson DI, Lafullarde T, Jamieson GG. Experimental study of effect of embolism of different laparoscopy insufflation gases. *J Laparoendosc Adv Surg Tech A* 2000;10:211–16.
5. Roberts MW, Mathiesen KA, Ho HS, Wolfe BM. Cardiopulmonary responses to intravenous infusion of soluble and relatively insoluble gases. *Surg Endosc* 1997;11:341–6.
6. Luo K, Li JS, Li LT, Wang KH, Shun JM. Operative stress response and energy metabolism after laparoscopic cholecystectomy compared to open surgery. *World J Gastroenterol* 2003;9:847–50.
7. Schwenk W, Haase O, Neudecker J, Müller JM. Short term benefits for laparoscopic colorectal resection. *Cochrane Database Syst Rev* 2005;20(3):CD003145.
8. Vlug MS, Wind J, Hollmann MW, *et al.* LAFA study group. Laparoscopy in combination with fast track multimodal management is the best perioperative strategy in patients undergoing colonic surgery: a randomized clinical trial (LAFA-study). *Ann Surg* 2011;254:868–75.
9. Abraham N, Albayati S. Enhanced recovery after surgery programs hasten recovery after colorectal resections. *World J Gastrointest Surg* 2011;27:1–6.
10. Khan S, Gatt M, MacFie J. Enhanced recovery programmes and colorectal surgery: does the laparoscope confer additional advantages? *Colorectal Dis* 2009;11:902–8.
11. Verghese C, Brimacombe JR. Survey of laryngeal mask airway usage in 11,910 patients: safety and efficacy for conventional and nonconventional usage. *Anesth Analg* 1996;82:129–33.

12. Cook TM, Lee G, Nolan JP. The ProSeal laryngeal mask airway: a review of the literature. *Can J Anaesth* 2005;52:739–60.

13. Maltby JR, Beriault MT, Watson NC, Liepert D, Fick GH. The LMA-ProSeal is an effective alternative to tracheal intubation for laparoscopic cholecystectomy. *Can J Anaesth* 2002;49:857–62.

14. Kemp MG, Keithley JK, Smith DW, Morreale, B. Factors that contribute to pressure sores in surgical patients. *Res Nurs Health* 1990;13:293–301.

15. Alterman I, Sidi A, Azamfirei L, Copotoiu S, Ezri T. Rhabdomyolysis: another complication after prolonged surgery. *J Clin Anesth* 2007;19:64–6.

16. Beraldo S, Dodds SR. Lower limb acute compartment syndrome after colorectal surgery in prolonged lithotomy position. *Dis Colon Rectum* 2006;49:1772–80.

17. Welch MB, Brummett CM, WelchTD. Perioperative peripheral nerve injuries. A retrospective study of 380,680 cases during a 10-yr period at a single institution. *Anesthesiology* 2009;111:490–7.

18. Prielipp RC, Warner MA. Perioperative nerve injury: a silent scream? *Anesthesiology* 2009;111:464–6.

19. Sawyer RJ, Richmond MN, Hickey JD, Jarrratt JA. Peripheral nerve injuries associated with anaesthesia. *Anaesthesia* 2000;55:980–91.

20. Glassman DT, Merriam WG, Trabulsi EJ, *et al.* Rhabdomyolysis after laparoscopic nephrectomy. *J Soc Laparoendosc Surgeons* 2007:11;432–7.

21. Slater MS, Mullins RJ. Rhabdomyolysis and myoglobinuric renal failure in trauma and surgical patients: a review. *J Am Coll Surg* 1998:186;693–716.

22. Choi EM, Na S, Choi SH, An J, Rha KH, Oh YJ. Comparison of volume-controlled and pressure-controlled ventilation in steep Trendelenburg position for robot-assisted laparoscopic radical prostatectomy. *J Clin Anesth* 2011:23:183–8.

23. Oğurlu M, Küçük M, Bilgin F, *et al.* Pressure-controlled vs volume-controlled ventilation during laparoscopic gynecologic surgery. *J Minim Invasive Gynecol* 2010;17:295–300.

24. Cadi P, Guenoun T, Journois D, Chevallier JM, Diehl JL, Safran D. Pressure-controlled ventilation improves oxygenation during laparoscopic obesity surgery compared with volume-controlled ventilation. *Br J Anaesth* 2008;100:709–716.

25. De Baerdemaeker LE, Van der Herten C, Gillardin JM, Pattyn P, Mortier EP, Szegedi LL. Comparison of volume-controlled and pressure-controlled ventilation during laparoscopic gastric banding in morbidly obese patients. *Obes Surg* 2008;18:680–5.

26. Sanchez NC, Tenofsky PL, Dort JM, *et al.* What is normal intraabdominal pressure? *Am Surg* 2001;67:243–8.

27. Nguyen NT, Lee SL, Anderson JT, *et al.* Evaluation of intraabdominal pressure after open and laparoscopic gastric bypass. *Obes Surg* 2001;11:40–5.

28. Andersson L, Lindberg G, Bringman S, Ramel S, Anderberg B, Odeberg-Wernerman S. Pneumoperitoneum versus abdominal wall lift: effects on central haemodynamics and intrathoracic pressure during laparoscopic cholecystectomy. *Acta Anaesthesiol Scand* 2003;47:838–46.

29. Kelman GR, Swapp GH,Smith I, Benzie RJ, Gordon NL. Cardiac output and arterial blood–gas tension during laparoscopy. *Br J Anaesth* 1972;44:1155–62.

30. Joris JL, Noirot DP, Legrand MJ, *et al.* Hemodynamic changes during laparoscopic cholecystectomy. *Anesth Analg* 1993;76:1067–71.

31. O'Leary E, Hubbard K, Tormey W, Cunningham AJ. Laparoscopic cholecystectomy: haemodynamic and neuroendocrine responses after pneumoperitoneum and changes in position. *Br J Anaesth* 1996;76:640–4.

32. Walder AD, Aitkenhead AR. Role of vasopressin in the haemodynamic response to laparoscopic cholecystectomy. *Br J Anaesth* 1997;78:264–6.

33. Joris J, Lamy M. Neuroendocrine changes during pneumoperitoneum for laparoscopic cholecystectomy. *Clin Circuln* 1992;A33.

34. Kashtan J, Green JF, Parsons EQ, Holcroft JW. Hemodynamic effect of increased abdominal pressure. *J Surg Res* 1981;30:249–55.

35. Popescu WM, Bell R, Duffy AJ, Katz KH, Perrino AC Jr. A pilot study of patients with clinically severe obesity undergoing laparoscopic surgery: evidence for impaired cardiac performance. *J Cardiothorac Vasc Anesth* 2011;25:943–9.

36. Andersson L, Wallin CJ, Sollevi A, Odeberg-Wernerman S. Pneumoperitoneum in healthy humans does not affect central blood volume or cardiac output. *Acta Anaesthesiol Scand* 1999;43:809–14.

37. Lentschener C, Axler O, Fernandez H, *et al.* Haemodynamic changes and vasopressin release are not consistently associated with carbon dioxide pneumoperitoneum in humans. *Acta Anaesthesiol Scand* 2001;45:527–35.

38. Cunningham AJ, Brull SJ. Laparoscopic cholecystectomy: anesthetic implications. *Anesth Analg* 1993;76:1120–33.

39. Andersson LE, Bååth M, Thörne A, Aspelin P, Odeberg-Wernerman S. Effect of carbon dioxide pneumoperitoneum on development of atelectasis during anesthesia, examined by spiral computed tomography. *Anesthesiology* 2005;102:293–9.

40. Fahy BG, Barnas GM, Flowers JL, Nagle SE, Njoku MJ. The effects of increased abdominal pressure on lung and chest wall mechanics during laparoscopic surgery. *Anesth Analg* 1995;81:744–50.

41. Mutoh T, Lamm WJ, Embree LJ, Hildebrandt J, Albert RK. Volume infusion produces abdominal distension, lung compression, and chest wall stiffening in pigs. *J Appl Physiol* 1992;72:575–82.

42. Mutoh T, Lamm WJ, Embree LJ, Hildebrandt J, Albert RK. Abdominal distension alters regional pleural pressures and chest wall mechanics in pigs in vivo. *J Appl Physiol* 1991;70:2611–18.

43. Chassard D, Berrada K, Tournadre J, Boulétreau P. The effects of neuromuscular block on peak airway pressure and abdominal elastance during pneumoperitoneum. *Anesth Analg* 1996;82:525–7.

44. Loeckinger A, Kleinsasser A, Hoermann C, Gassner M, Keller C, Lindner KH. Inert gas exchange during pneumoperitoneum at incremental values of positive end-expiratory pressure. *Anesth Analg* 2000;90:466–71.

45. Monk TG, Weldon BC, Lemon D. Alterations in pulmonary function during laparoscopic surgery. *Anesth Analg* 1993;76:S274.

46. Baraka A, Jabbour S, Hammoud R, *et al.* End-tidal carbon dioxide tension during laparoscopic cholecystectomy. Correlation with the baseline value prior to carbon dioxide insufflation. *Anaesthesia* 1994;49:304–6.

47. Kazama T, Ikeda K, Kato T, Kikura M. Carbon dioxide output in laparoscopic cholecystectomy. *Br J Anaesth* 1996;76:530–5.

48. Wahba RW, Mamazza J. Ventilatory requirements during laparoscopic cholecystectomy. *Can J Anaesth* 1993;40:206–10.

49. Klopfenstein CE, Schiffer E, Pastor CM, *et al.* Laparoscopic colon surgery: unreliability of end-tidal CO_2 monitoring. *Acta Anaesthesiol Scand* 2008;52:700–7.

50. Wittgen CM, Andrus CH, Fitzgerald SD, Baudendistel LJ, Dahms TE, Kaminski DL. Analysis of the hemodynamic and ventilatory effects of laparoscopic cholecystectomy. *Arch Surg* 1991;126:997–1000.

51. Xue Q, Wu X, Jin J, Yu B, Zheng M. Transcutaneous carbon dioxide monitoring accurately predicts arterial carbon dioxide partial pressure in patients undergoing prolonged laparoscopic surgery. *Anesth Analg* 2010;111:417–20.

52. Joris J, Kaba A, Lamy M. Postoperative spirometry after laparoscopy for lower abdominal or upper abdominal surgical procedures. *Br J Anaesth* 1997;79:422–6.

53. Vegfors M, Cederholm I, Lennmarken C, Löfström JB. Should oxygen be administered after laparoscopy in healthy patients? *Acta Anaesthesiol Scand* 1988;32:350–2.

54. Demyttenaere S, Feldman LS, Fried GM. Effect of pneumoperitoneum on renal perfusion and function: a systematic review. *Surg Endosc* 2007;21:152–60.

55. Ahn JH, Lim CH, Chung HI, Choi SU, Youn SZ, Lim HJ. Postoperative renal function in patients is unaltered after robotic-assisted radical prostatectomy. *Korean J Anesthesiol* 2011;60:192–7.

56. Sammour T, Mittal A, Loveday BP, *et al*. Systematic review of oxidative stress associated with pneumoperitoneum. *Br J Surg* 2009;96:836–50.

57. Tuñón MJ, González P, Jorquera F, Llorente A, Gonzalo-Orden M, González-Gallego J. Liver blood flow changes during laparoscopic surgery in pigs. A study of hepatic indocyanine green removal. *Surg Endosc* 1999;13:668–72.

58. Hoekstra LT, Ruys AT, Milstein DM, *et al*. Effects of prolonged pneumoperitoneum on hepatic perfusion during laparoscopy. *Ann Surg* 2013;257:302–7.

59. Rosenthal RJ, Friedman RL, Chidambaram A, *et al*. Effects of hyperventilation and hypoventilation on $PaCO_2$ and intracranial pressure during acute elevations of intraabdominal pressure with CO_2 pneumoperitoneum: large animal observations. *J Am Coll Surg* 1998;187:32–8.

60. Rosin D, Rosenthal RJ. Adverse hemodynamic effects of intraabdominal pressure—is it all in the head? *Int J Surg Invest* 2001;2:335–45.

61. Mobbs RJ, Yang MO. The dangers of diagnostic laparoscopy in the head injured patient. *J Clin Neurosci* 2002;9:592–3.

62. Pandey R, Garg R, Darlong V, Punj J, Chandralekha, Kumar A. Unpredicted neurological complications after robotic laparoscopic radical cystectomy and ileal conduit formation in steep trendelenburg position: two case reports. *Acta Anaesth Belg* 2010;61:163–6.

63. Jorgensen JO, Lalak NJ, North L, Hanel K, Hunt DR, Morris DL. Venous stasis during laparoscopic cholecystectomy. *Surg Laparosc Endosc* 1994;4:128–33.

64. Carter JJ, Whelan RL. The immunologic consequences of laparoscopy in oncology. *Surg Oncol Clin North Am* 2001;10:655–77.

65. Goldfarb M, Brower S, Schwaitzberg SD. Minimally invasive surgery and cancer: controversies. Part 1. *Surg Endosc* 2010;24:304–34.

66. Sajid MS, Mallick AS, Rimpel J, Bokari SA, Cheek E, Baig MK. Effect of heated and humidified carbon dioxide on patients after laparoscopic procedures: a meta-analysis. *Surg Laparosc Endosc Percutan Tech* 2008;18:539–46.

67. Birch DW, Manouchehri N, Shi X, Hadi G, Karmali S. Heated CO(2) with or without humidification for minimally invasive abdominal surgery. *Cochrane Database Syst Rev* 2011;(1):CD007821.

68. Kalmar AF, Dewaele F, Foubert L, *et al*. Cerebral hemodynamic physiology during steep Trendelenburg position and CO_2 pneumoperitoneum. *Br J Anaesth* 2012;108:478–84.

69. Cunningham AJ. Anesthetic implications of laparoscopic surgery. *Yale J Biol Med* 1998;71:551–78.

70. Wahba RW, Tessler MJ, Kleiman SJ. Acute ventilatory complications during laparoscopic upper abdominal surgery. *Can J Anaesth* 1996;43:77–83.

71. Lestar M, Gunnarsson L, Lagerstrand L, Wiklund P, Odeberg-Wernerman S. Hemodynamic perturbations during robot-assisted laparoscopic radical prostatectomy in 45° Trendelenburg position. *Anesth Analg* 2011;113:1069–75.

72. Russo A, Marana E, Viviani D, *et al*. Diastolic function: the influence of pneumoperitoneum and Trendelenburg positioning during laparoscopic hysterectomy. *Eur J Anaesthesiol* 2009;26:923–7.

73. Schrijvers D, Mottrie A, Traen K, *et al*. Pulmonary gas exchange is well preserved during robot assisted surgery in steep Trendelenburg position. *Acta Anaesthesiol Belg* 2009;60:229–33.

74. Meininger D, Zwissler B, Byhahn C, Probst M, Westphal K, Bremerich DH. Impact of overweight and pneumoperitoneum on hemodynamics and oxygenation during prolonged laparoscopic surgery. *World J Surg* 2006;30:520–6.

75. Salihoglu Z, Demiroluk S, Cakmakkaya S, Gorgun E, Kose Y. Influence of the patient positioning on respiratory mechanics during pneumoperitoneum. *Middle East J Anesthesiol* 2002;16:521–8.

76. Awad H, Santilli S, Ohr M, *et al*. The effects of steep trendelenburg positioning on intraocular pressure during robotic radical prostatectomy. *Anesth Analg* 2009;109:473–8.

77. Gainsburg DM. Anesthetic concerns for robotic-assisted laparoscopic radical prostatectomy. *Minerva Anestesiol* 2012;78:596–604.

78. Danic MJ, Chow M, Alexander G, Bhandari A, Menon M, Brown M. Anesthesia considerations for robotic-assisted laparoscopic prostatectomy: a review of 1,500 cases. *J Robotic Surg* 2007;1:119–23.

79. Pinkney TD, King AJ, Walter C, Wilson TR, Maxwell-Armstrong C, Acheson AG. Raised intraocular pressure (IOP) and perioperative visual loss in laparoscopic colorectal surgery: a catastrophe waiting to happen? A systematic review of evidence from other surgical specialities. *Tech Coloproctol* 2012;16:331–5.

80. Wilcox S, Vandam LD. Alas poor Trendelenburg and his position! A critique of its uses and effectiveness. *Anesth Analg* 1998;67;574–8.

81. Hirvonen EA, Poikolainen EO, Pääkkönen ME, Nuutinen LS. The adverse hemodynamic effects of anesthesia, head-up tilt, and carbon dioxide pneumoperitoneum during laparoscopic cholecystectomy. *Surg Endosc* 2000;14:272–7.

82. Fahy BG, Barnas GM, Nagle SE, Flowers JL, Njoku MJ, Agarwal M. Effects of Trendelenburg and reverse Trendelenburg postures on lung and chest wall mechanics. *J Clin Anesth* 1996;8:236–44.

83. Ure BM, Troidl H, Spangenberger W, Dietrich A, Lefering R, Neugebauer E. Pain after laparoscopic cholecystectomy. Intensity and localization of pain and analysis of predictors in preoperative symptoms and intraoperative events. *Surg Endosc* 1994;8:90–6.

84. Alexander JI. Pain after laparoscopy. *Br J Anaesth* 1997;79:369–78.

85. Gurusamy KS, Samraj K, Davidson BR. Low pressure versus standard pressure pneumoperitoneum in laparoscopic cholecystectomy. *Cochrane Database Syst Rev* 2009;(2):CD006930.

86. Phelps P, Cakmakkaya OS, Apfel CC, Radke OC. A simple clinical maneuver to reduce laparoscopy induced shoulder pain: a randomised controlled trial. *Obstet Gynecol* 2008;111:1155–60.

87. Swift G, Healey M, Varol N, Maher P, Hill D. A prospective randomised double blind placebo controlled trial to assess whether gas drains reduce shoulder pain following gynecological laparoscopy. *Aust NZ J Obstet Gynaecol* 2002;42:267–70.

88. Readman E, Maher PJ, Ugoni AM, Gordon S. Intraperitoneal ropivacaine and a gas drain: effects on postoperative pain after laparoscopic surgery. *J Am Assoc Gynecol Laparosc* 2004;11:486–91.

89. Kahokehr A, Sammour T, Soop M, Hill AG. Intraperitoneal use of local anesthetic in laparoscopic cholecystectomy: systematic review and metaanalysis of randomized controlled trials. *J Hepatobiliary Pancreat Sci* 2010;17:637–56.

90. Hasaniya NW, Zayed FF, Faiz H, Severino R. Preinsertion local anesthesia at the trocar site improves perioperative pain and decreases costs of laparoscopic cholecystectomy. *Surg Endosc* 2001;15:962–4.

91. Collins LM, Vaghadia H. Regional anesthesia for laparoscopy. *Anesthesiol Clin North America* 2001;19:43–55.

92. Naja MZ, Ziade MF, Lonnqvist PA. General anaesthesia combined with bilateral paravertebral blockade (T5–6) vs. general anaesthesia for laparoscopic cholecystectomy: a prospective, randomized clinical trial. *Eur J Anaesthesiol* 2004;21:489–95.

93. Conaghan P, Maxwell-Armstrong C, Bedforth N, *et al.* Efficacy of transversus abdominis plane blocks in laparoscopic colorectal resections. *Surg Endosc* 2010;24:2480–4.

94. Levy BF, Scott MJ, Fawcett W, Fry C, Rockall TA. Randomized clinical trial of epidural, spinal or patient-controlled analgesia for patients undergoing laparoscopic colorectal surgery. *Br J Surg* 2011;98:1068–1107.

95. Virlos I, Clements D, Beynon J, Ratnalikar V, Khot U. Short-term outcomes with intrathecal versus epidural analgesia in laparoscopic colorectal surgery. *Br J Surg* 2010;97:1401–6.

3.2 Anaesthesia for bariatric surgery

Louise Savic

Expert Commentary Mark C. Bellamy

CPD Matrix Code: *1A01, 1C01, 2A07, 3A13*

Case history

A 41-year-old woman presented for bariatric surgery. She gave a history of being over-weight from the age of 10 years and had a family history of obesity; both her parents and her sister were morbidly obese. Her sister had undergone bariatric surgery the previous year with a good result.

She described previous successful weight loss through dieting clubs, but each time had rapidly regained this, plus additional, weight. She had a sedentary lifestyle, working as a school secretary.

She was a smoker, with a history of asthma, which was well controlled with salbutamol inhalers and montelukast. She suffered occasional palpitations and was hypertensive, on treatment with an angiotensin-converting enzyme inhibitor (ACEI). She also had a history of gastroesophageal reflux disease, well controlled with a proton pump inhibitor. She had been put on a 10-day diet to reduce liver steatosis, and had been advised to stop smoking.

Following a multi-disciplinary meeting involving a bariatric nurse specialist, surgeon, anaesthetist, psychologist, and respiratory physician she was listed for a laparoscopic Roux-en-Y gastric bypass procedure.

> **❝ Expert comment**
>
> Hepatic engorgement and fatty infiltration increase perioperative risk and conversion from laparoscopic to open surgery. Use of an insulin-suppressing diet in the immediate preoperative period has been shown to bring about rapid resolution of hepatic steatosis.

> **❝ Expert comment**
>
> Smoking is an important risk factor for thromboembolic disease in this patient group.

> **★ Learning point** Defining obesity
>
> - Body mass index (BMI) is calculated as weight in kilograms divided by the square of height in metres (kg/m^2).
> - Obesity can be defined as BMI >30 kg/m^2.
> - BMI >35 kg/m^2 with associated comorbidity, or >40 kg/m^2 without significant comorbidity, is considered morbid obesity.
> - BMI >55 kg/m^2 is termed super-morbid obesity.
> - The duration of obesity is important, since the risk of cardiorespiratory and other comorbidity increases with the number of 'fat-years' [1].
> - 26% of the UK population aged >16 years were classified as obese in 2010 [2].
> - Obesity results, over time, in significant and potentially life-threatening comorbidities. These include hypertension, coronary artery disease, respiratory complications such as obstructive sleep apnoea (OSA) and asthma, metabolic complications such as diabetes, fatty liver disease which can progress to steatosis and cirrhosis, and degenerative joint disease. Quality of life for the individual is often severely impaired.
> - Following surgery, weight loss usually occurs to a plateau level of around 10–20% above ideal body weight, at which point it tends to 'level off'. More than 50% of excess weight may eventually be lost.
>
> (continued)

Only rarely does weight drop to below ideal body weight; if this does occur (for example following extensive malabsorptive procedures), this will often require surgical intervention [3].
- The effect of successful weight loss surgery can be dramatic. Weight loss of 5–10% of initial weight can improve glucose handling, hypertension, and hyperlipidaemia [4]. Diabetes tends to resolve rapidly, long before significant weight loss; hypertension tends to take much longer to resolve. Fatty infiltration of the airway regresses early, with resolution of OSA and obesity hypoventilation syndrome (OHS) [3]. Macrovesicular fatty liver disease will also regress postoperatively.

⭐ **Learning point**   Bariatric procedures

- Surgical procedures deliberately result in either malabsorptive or restrictive defects, or a combination of both.
- Restrictive procedures include vertical banded gastroplasty and gastric banding (which may be adjustable).
- Roux-en-Y gastric bypass combines restriction with a degree of malabsorption, and is considered the 'gold standard' (Figure 3.1).
- These procedures may all be performed laparoscopically.
- Complications from Roux-en-Y gastric bypass include anastomotic leak, gastric pouch outlet obstruction, bleeding, wound infection, respiratory complications and venous thromboembolism.
- Late complications include: persistent nausea, cholelithiasis, anaemia, and protein-calorie malnutrition.

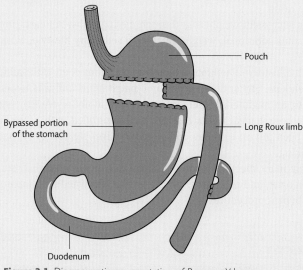

Figure 3.1 Diagrammatic representation of Roux-en-Y bypass.

The patient was 5 feet 9 inches tall (1.75 m), and weighed 186 kg, giving a BMI of 61 kg/m². At the time of her initial referral her BMI had been 55 kg/m², but she had gained 16 kg in the intervening weeks. This is a well-recognized phenomenon in this group, and may result in worsening of cardiac function [5].

She had a blood pressure of 146/78 mmHg, heart rate 69 beats/min and regular, and oxygen saturations of 98% on room air. Her excess adipose tissue was mostly concentrated around her legs, arms and buttocks in a typical gynaecoid distribution.

Airway assessment revealed a Mallampati class 2 view, with good mouth opening and a thyromental distance of >7 cm. Neck extension was normal. There was a single crown on her right central incisor.

> **✪ Learning point Fat distribution**
>
> - Distribution of fat is as important as absolute BMI, in terms of associated comorbidity and risk.
> - The android type of distribution ('apple') is associated with increased fat deposition in the neck and airway, as well as increased risk of cardiovascular and metabolic complications. Intraperitoneal fat can make surgery more complicated. It is defined as a waist-to-hip ratio of >0.8 in women and >1.0 in men.
> - The gynaecoid type of distribution ('pear') is more usually seen in women but may also occur in men. Fat tends to accumulate in the legs, arms and buttocks. Overall morbidity risk is reduced in this group compared with the android type.

> **❝ Expert comment**
>
> The android fat distribution is more commonly associated with the metabolic syndrome, including hyperlipidaemia, diabetes and cardiovascular disease.

> **✚ Clinical tip Airway assessment**
>
> - Mallampati class, mouth opening, neck extension, neck circumference, thyromental distance and sternomental distance should be noted.
> - Obesity and BMI alone are not predictors of difficult intubation. However, a large neck circumference (collar size >17.5 inches) and Mallampati class ≥3 may increase the risk of difficult laryngoscopy and intubation [6, 7].
> - OSA was widely believed to be associated with difficult intubation. A 2009 study sought to determine whether this was in fact an independent risk factor. In 180 morbidly obese patients (122 of whom had OSA) undergoing tracheal intubation for bariatric surgery *in the ramped position*, no relationship between OSA, neck circumference or BMI, and difficult laryngoscopy or intubation was seen. A Mallampati score of 3 or 4 was, however, associated with significant risk of difficult laryngoscopy or intubation [7].
> - Both increased weight (BMI >26 kg/m^2) and snoring are associated with difficult mask ventilation [8]. During airway difficulty (and especially airway obstruction) hypoxia develops considerably more quickly in the obese than in the non-obese patient [9]. The 4th National Audit Project (NAP4) reported a disproportionate number of obese patients who had a major complication of airway management and perhaps an increase in the rate of failure of airway rescue techniques (supraglottic airway placement and emergency surgical airway) [10].
> - Preparations for a difficult laryngoscopy should be made with a clear strategy in case of difficulty decided preoperatively; relevant equipment and personnel should be available.

A more detailed respiratory and cardiovascular history and examination were undertaken, to identify any potential underlying disease in these systems. However, other than the treated hypertension, nothing of any concern was revealed. She had good exercise tolerance, being able to walk for more than one mile and manage stairs without undue breathlessness. She could tolerate lying flat, and gave no history of paroxysmal nocturnal dyspnoea or ankle swelling. There were no clinical signs of heart failure present. The history of asthma was suggestive of mild disease, likely to be weight-related. There was no history of snoring, daytime somnolence, morning headache or poor concentration, suggestive of OSA or OHS. A previous anaesthetic for an appendicectomy as a child had been uneventful.

An ECG was performed, which was unremarkable. A full blood count, urea and electrolytes, and thyroid function tests were taken. All these were in normal range. Neither an echocardiogram nor pulmonary function testing were felt to be indicated in view of her good exercise tolerance.

> **❝ Expert comment**
>
> Asthma is a common comorbidity in morbidly obese subjects (about 30%) and is more common in females than in males. This frequently resolves with weight loss. Its precise aetiology is unclear but may include neuroendocrine factors, microaspiration and chronic inflammation.

> **✪ Learning point Obstructive sleep apnoea (OSA) and obesity hypoventilation syndrome (OHS)**
>
> **Obstructive sleep apnoea**
>
> - OSA is defined as repetitive episodes of upper airway occlusion (pharyngeal collapse) during sleep.
> - >5 episodes per hour or >30 per night is significant.
> - Other features include daytime somnolence, headaches, and poor concentration.
>
> (continued)

- OSA can lead to chronic hypercapnia and hypoxia, associated with polycythaemia, systemic vasoconstriction and/or pulmonary vasoconstriction with resultant right heart failure.
- Obesity is an important risk factor for OSA, with a reported prevalence of 30% in those with BMI >30 kg/m^2 and 40% in BMI >40 kg/m^2 [11]. In particular, an android distribution of fat and large neck circumference ('bull neck') predicts OSA.
- Surgically induced weight loss can significantly improve OSA [12].

Obesity hypoventilation syndrome

- This condition may exist discretely or in combination with OSA, and is characterized by nocturnal hypoventilation leading to daytime hypercapnia and hypoxia ('Pickwickian syndrome'), in patients with BMI >30 kg/m^2.
- Physical factors such as reduced chest wall compliance, as well as blunted central responses to hypercapnia and hypoxia, result in hypoventilation. There is a failure to clear the accumulated carbon dioxide (by contrast with OSA where periods of compensatory hyperventilation prevent carbon dioxide levels rising steadily overnight).
- The condition may result in decompensated respiratory failure, and may be misdiagnosed as chronic obstructive pulmonary disease.

✚ Clinical tip   Preoperative continuous positive airway pressure (CPAP)

- There is evidence that patients found to have OSA benefit from preoperative use of nocturnal CPAP with significant reduction in perioperative complications, including a reduction in postoperative hypoxaemia, cardiac ischaemia, delirium, and unplanned intensive care admissions [13, 14].
- There are thought to be beneficial effects on ventilatory drive, left ventricular ejection fraction, right ventricular function, pulmonary artery pressure, blood pressure, and even tongue size. The ideal length of treatment needed is not known, but patients receiving CPAP should be advised to strictly continue use preoperatively [15].

✪ Learning point   Preassesment scoring tools

- The STOP-BANG assessment tool (Table 3.6) is an 8-point questionnaire covering the salient clinical features of OSA. A score of >5, in combination with other evidence of cardiovascular or respiratory compromise, predicts increased risk and a need for further investigations [16].
- The Epworth Sleepiness Score assesses the extent of daytime somnolence.
- The Obesity Surgery Mortality Risk Score (Table 3.7) is a validated scoring system for patients undergoing all types of bariatric surgery. It allocates one point to each of five preoperative variables and stratifies patients into low, intermediate and high perioperative risk. High-risk patients have a mortality of 7.56% compared to low-risk patients with a risk of 0.3% [17].

Table 3.6 STOP BANG Questionnaire

Do you **S**nore loudly?
Do you often feel **T**ired or sleepy during the daytime?
Has anyone **O**bserved you stop breathing in your sleep?
Do you have high blood **P**ressure?
Is your **B**ody mass index >35 kg/m^2?
Age >50 years?
Neck circumference >40 cm?
Gender male?

Adapted from Chung F *et al*. STOP Questionnaire: a tool to screen obstructive sleep apnea. *Anesthesiology*, 108: 812-821, copyright 2008, with permission from Wolters Kluwer and the American Society of Anesthesiologists; and Chung F et al., 'High STOP-BANG score indicates a high probability of obstructive sleep apnoea', *British Journal of Anaesthesia*, 2012, 108, pp. 768–775, by permission of The Board of Management and Trustees of the British Journal of Anaesthesia and Oxford University Press.

Table 3.7 Obesity Surgery Mortality Score

Risk factor		
Age >45 years		
Male sex		
Risk factors for pulmonary embolus[a]		
Body mass index >50 kg/m^2		
Hypertension		
Class (risk)	Score	Mortality (%)
A (Low)	0–1	0.31
B (Intermediate)	2–3	1.90
C (High)	4–5	7.56

[a] Previous venous thromboembolism, preoperative vena cava filter, pulmonary hypertension, or obesity hypoventilation syndrome.

Each risk factor gives one point.

Reprinted from *Surgery for Obesity and Related Diseases*, 3, 2, DeMaria EJ et al., 'Obesity surgery mortality risk score: proposal for a clinically useful score to predict mortality risk in patients undergoing gastric bypass', pp. 134–140, Copyright 2007, with permission from American Society for Metabolic and Bariatric Surgery (ASMBS), Brazilian Society for Bariatric Surgery, and the Asociacion Latinoamericana de Cirujanos Endoscopistas and Elsevier.

⭐ **Learning point** Respiratory and cardiovascular assessment

- A detailed history is needed, looking for symptoms of heart failure, OSA or OHS. It may be useful to ask specifically about the ability to lie flat; cardiac output and mean pulmonary artery pressure increase when supine and this may be poorly tolerated.
- A preoperative ECG may reveal dysrhythmias, prolonged QT/QTc, signs of right ventricular hypertrophy or strain, P pulmonale indicating right atrial enlargement, or left ventricular hypertrophy.
- Transthoracic echocardiogram can be used to estimate systolic and diastolic function but is usually technically difficult as the fat tissue prevents a good quality image.
- Chest X-ray can be used to assess cardiothoracic ratio and look for evidence of cardiac failure.
- Pulmonary function testing need not be performed routinely in young patients with good exercise tolerance and benign fat distribution [1].
- Oxygen saturations on air are a useful indicator of underlying respiratory disease. Arterial blood gases are indicated where there is evidence or suspicion of hypoxia or hypercapnia.
- Significant cardiovascular dysfunction may be masked by limited mobility. An assessment of functional status may be made simply by asking the patient to walk up a flight of stairs or along the corridor.
- CPET can be considered in patients with unknown exercise tolerance and any significant comorbidity. An increase in serious postoperative complications following laparoscopic Roux-en-Y gastric bypass has been demonstrated in patients with a peak $\dot{V}O_2$<15.8 mL/kg/min [18].
- A history of amphetamine-based appetite suppressant use should be sought, as these increase the risk of perioperative cardiac complications [1].

⭐ **Learning point** Cardiovascular complications of obesity

- In order to meet the metabolic demands of the adipose tissue, cardiac output, blood volume, and arterial pressure are all increased. This can lead to left ventricle dilatation and hypertrophy resulting in diastolic dysfunction (Figure 3.2).
- Systolic dysfunction ('obesity cardiomyopathy') occurs when wall dilatation is not matched by hypertrophy.
- Obesity is associated with a 10-fold increase in systemic hypertension and an increased risk of ischaemic heart disease.
- Ischaemic heart disease in this group is caused by hypertension, hypercholesterolaemia, reduced high-density lipoprotein levels, diabetes and physical inactivity.

(continued)

❝ **Expert comment**

Screening tests such as STOP BANG and the Epworth Sleepiness Score are helpful as reminders but are of low predictive value. The gold standard for diagnosis of sleep apnoea remains polysomnography.

❝ **Expert comment**

The only large study of preoperative dobutamine stress echo in obesity proved inconclusive because of the low event rate and the skewed (female) study population [19]. There may be a role for CPET testing, though as yet this has not been adequately evaluated.

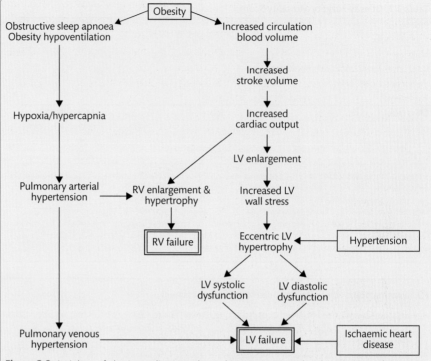

Figure 3.2 Aetiology of obesity cardiomyopathy, and its association with right-sided heart failure, systemic hypertension and ischaemic heart disease. LV, left ventricular; RV, right ventricular.

Reproduced from Adams JP, Murphy PG, 'Obesity in anaesthesia and intensive care', *British Journal of Anaesthesia*, 85, 1, pp. 91–108, copyright 2000, with permission from Oxford University Press and The Board of Management and Trustees of the British Journal of Anaesthesia.

✪ Learning point   Metabolic and other considerations

- Diabetes occurs frequently in this group and random blood glucose testing is a mandatory part of preoperative assessment.
- Obese patients have been shown to have an increased gastric volume with a resultant increased residual volume, although gastric emptying is actually faster than in normal individuals [20]. Other work has demonstrated the resistance gradient between the stomach and the gastro-oesophageal junction to be similar to that in non-obese individuals. However, it is usually considered prudent to routinely protect against acid reflux and aspiration. Agents which have been used include antacids, proton pump inhibitors, histamine H_2 receptor antagonists and prokinetics [21].
- By contrast, there may be an increased risk of pulmonary aspiration in patients who have lost weight following bariatric procedures. The evidence for this comes from a single study demonstrating a significantly increased aspiration risk in this population (6% in the post-bariatric patient versus 0% in non-bariatric patients, $P < 0.05$). This has clear implications for the management of this group presenting for further surgery [22]. Reasons for this phenomenon are not known, but may include reduced lower oesophageal tone and reduced oesophageal–gastric peristalsis.
- Bariatric patients are at high risk of venous thromboembolic disease. One study found that adequate prophylaxis is achieved when calf-length pneumatic compression devices, early ambulation and short operating times were used [23]. However, many units use a blanket anticoagulant policy, continuing anticoagulation (self-injection) after discharge home for two weeks or more. Low-molecular-weight heparin doses need to be adjusted to weight.

On the day of surgery the patient presented fasted, having omitted her ACEI and having taken 30 mL 0.3 M citrate orally on the ward. Venous access was secured in the hand with a 16G cannula. The blood pressure was difficult to measure in the anaesthetic room due to the size of her arms, so an arterial line was sited. She had been warned of the potential need for central venous access.

Prior to induction, the patient was positioned, awake, on the operating table in theatre. She was placed in the 'ramped' position (Figure 3.3).

After preoxygenation, anaesthesia was induced with propofol 350 mg followed by suxamethonium 140 mg. On direct laryngoscopy a Cormack and Lehane grade 2 view was seen and the patient was intubated uneventfully.

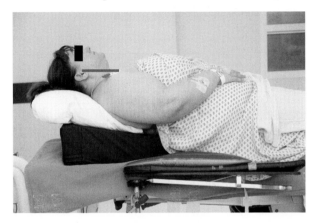

Figure 3.3 Ramped position. Pillows and wedges are used to create a horizontal line between the sternal notch and the external auditory meatus.

⭐ **Learning point** Positioning

- The classical 'sniffing the morning air' position is often difficult to achieve due to soft tissue in the neck and chest wall. The 'ramped' position is ideal for laryngoscopy (Figure 3.3). Pillows or a wedge are used to produce a horizontal line between the sternal notch and the external auditory meatus.
- Obese patients have a reduced functional residual capacity, so the 'oxygen store' following preoxygenation is small. General anaesthesia can reduce chest wall and diaphragmatic tone by up to 50% [24], and there is increased atelectasis and secretion retention. These changes reduce the time it takes for hypoxia to develop; in a study of preoxygenated apnoeic patients, oxygen saturations fell to 90% more than twice as quickly in the morbidly obese group compared with the normal-weight group [25]. Airway management needs to be prompt and reliable. A 25° head-up tilt may slow the desaturation seen when patients are supine [26]. Application of PEEP may also slow the rate of atelectasis and deoxygenation in these patients [27].
- Positioning the patient on the operating table while awake reduces the potential harm to theatre staff involved in moving the patient.
- Rhabdomyolysis has been reported in bariatric surgery, particularly where surgery is prolonged (>240 min), BMI is >50 kg/m^2, and surgery is open. Pressure point protection, careful positioning, and changing patient position during prolonged operations help to reduce risk.
- During laparoscopic Roux-en-Y gastric bypass, the patient will be in a steep head-up position (reverse Trendelenburg). This has cardiovascular and respiratory implications, which are discussed later.

⭐ **Learning point** Drug doses

- Drug effects are unpredictable in obesity. The volume of the central compartment is mostly unchanged, whereas the volume of distribution (V_d) of lipophilic drugs is generally increased in line with increased body mass. However, other factors such as altered tissue binding, increased cardiac output, decreased hepatic blood flow, and increased tubular secretion impact on the pharmacokinetics in a complex manner that can vary from patient to patient.

(continued)

🔵 **Expert comment**

Elective fibreoptic intubation can be reserved for two categories of patient: those with anatomical features suggestive of a difficult intubation independent of their obesity; and those in whom difficulty maintaining oxygenation by bag-and-mask ventilation is anticipated.

Avoidance of sedation may help preserve normal respiratory drive and oxygenation during the procedure. Additionally, supplemental oxygen may be delivered. Awake fibreoptic intubation may be preferably performed orally to minimize discomfort and the risk of epistaxis.

- Drug absorption via oral and intravenous routes is similar to that in non-obese individuals; however, intramuscular and subcutaneous absorption is more variable as a result of poor blood flow to these peripheral sites.
- For calculating drug doses, the total body weight, ideal body weight, or lean body mass may be used (Table 3.8). The use of total body weight or ideal body weight to calculate a dose for the more frequently used drugs is shown in Table 3.9.
- The 'corrected body weight' is sometimes used, which is ideal body weight plus 40% of excess weight [3].

Table 3.8 Definitions of modified body weights used for dose calculation

Ideal body weight (kg) = height (cm) – 100 (male) or 105 (female)
Lean body mass (male) = 1.1 × weight – 128 (weight/height)^2
Lean body mass (female) = 1.07 × weight – 148 (weight/height)^2

Use weight in kg, height in cm.
Reproduced from Bellamy M and Struys M, *Anaesthesia for the Overweight and Obese Patient*, Second Edition, by permission of Oxford University Press.

Table 3.9 Use of total body weight, ideal body weight and lean body mass to calculate drugs doses.

Drug	Dosing
Propofol	IBW for induction, TBW for maintenance
Thiopentone	IBW (at dose of 7.5 mg/kg) [3]
Midazolam and other benzodiazepines	IBW for continuous infusion
Atracurium/cisatracurium	TBW
Rocuronium/vecuronium	IBW
Suxamethonium	TBW (maximum dose 140 mg)
Fentanyl/alfentanil	TBW
Morphine	IBW
Remifentanil	LBM for continuous infusion
Paracetamol	IBW

IBW, ideal body weight; TBW, total body weight; LBM, lean body mass.
Reproduced from Bellamy M and Struys M, *Anaesthesia for the Overweight and Obese Patient*, Second Edition, by permission of Oxford University Press.

Anaesthesia was maintained using desflurane and remifentanil. Pressure-controlled positive pressure ventilation was used, with a PEEP of 10 cmH$_2$O. End-tidal carbon dioxide was maintained between 4.5 and 6.0 kPa. She was in a steep head-up position (reverse Trendelenburg) throughout. A warming blanket and fluid warmer were used intraoperatively.

❻ Expert comment
Ventilation techniques

Key to maintaining safe respiratory mechanics and adequate gas exchange is the 'open lung' technique. There has been much debate as to whether pressure-controlled or volume-controlled ventilation best fulfils these requirements. The evidence is scant, some studies suggesting better overall gas exchange or CO$_2$ clearance with pressure-controlled ventilation, whereas others suggest that there is no difference between techniques [28–30].

✪ Learning point Cardiovascular and respiratory effects of laparoscopy

- General anaesthesia in obese patients is associated with a 50% decrease in functional residual capacity, increased shunt fraction and increasing alveolar–arterial oxygen tension gradient. This is compounded by the pneumoperitoneum created in laparoscopic procedures. In extreme circumstances this can lead to hypoxia, hypercapnia, and eventually right heart failure and worsening of pulmonary hypertension [31].
- Blood gas sampling intraoperatively may be needed to accurately monitor the degree of hypercapnia.
- Ventilatory strategies include the use of PEEP and of vital capacity manoeuvres, which have been shown to be effective in preventing atelectasis and reducing postoperative complications in this group [32, 33]. However, these techniques may also result in a significant fall in cardiac output and necessitate the use of additional fluid or inotropes.

(continued)

• Pneumoperitoneum can cause compression of the inferior vena cava, increased systemic resistance and reduced cardiac output. These effects are added to by reverse Trendelenburg positioning and PEEP. Current practice does not routinely involve cardiac output monitoring although this may be considered in higher-risk patients undergoing more significant surgery.

✪ **Learning point** Analgesia

• Neuraxial techniques in obese patients may be very challenging to perform and tend to have a higher failure rate [34].
• Use of neuraxial analgesic techniques has declined with the increase in minimally invasive surgical techniques, which are associated with reduced postoperative pain and pulmonary complications.
• When neuraxial opioids are used it is usual to use a drug with limited duration in order to minimize any risk of delayed respiratory arrest; epidural infusions with local anaesthetic alone may have a role. Careful attention to the prevention of decubitus pressure sores in patients with reduced sensation secondary to neuraxial blockade is essential.
• Multimodal analgesia aims to reduce opioid requirements. The use of rectus abdominus sheath blocks and TAP blocks may help provide sub-umbilical analgesia. However, there is only limited evidence that the use of TAP blocks in abdominal surgery reduce opioid requirements [35].
• NSAID may increase the risk of postoperative renal dysfunction and should be used with caution where there are additional risk factors such as laparoscopy (raised intra-abdominal pressure) or pre-existing diabetic nephropathy [1].
• Patient-controlled analgesia with morphine, dosed according to IBW, is generally safe and effective, but requires careful monitoring especially in patients with OSA [36].
• Many clinicians consider using an increased dose of paracetamol on account of its increased clearance in obesity. Total perioperative doses as high as 4 g have been used in some centres [37]. A 2 g loading dose with a total of 5 g in 24 h was shown to be safe in 26 healthy subjects with blood concentrations below the toxic threshold and no adverse events [38]. It should be noted that this is an off-licence use.

❝ **Expert comment**

Use of neuraxial techniques in bariatric surgery has not gained widespread acceptance due to the short duration of hospital stay and rapid early mobilization, together with the technical challenges involved.

The use of opiates needs to be tailored to the individual and account taken of the environment in which the patient is to be nursed; for example, the patient with OSA is at increased risk; the patient who has undergone minimally invasive surgery may not require opioid medication.

These patients may be considered a high-risk extubation group and as such may benefit from the use of remifentanil to promote rapid waking at the end of surgery [16, 39].

Surgery was uneventful; a nasogastric tube was inserted prior to extubation, and following reversal of the NMBA she was woken and extubated in the sitting position, when wide awake. Postoperative analgesia was multimodal and included paracetamol, NSAID, morphine PCA and local anaesthetic to the wound. She was nursed on the HDU for 24 h. She was encouraged to mobilize by the nursing staff and physiotherapists. On the second postoperative day she underwent a gastrograffin swallow which did not demonstrate any anastomotic leak, and her nasogastric tube was removed. She was discharged home on the third postoperative day.

Discussion

Critical care requirement

Traditionally it has been considered mandatory for this group of patients to receive level 2 or 3 care. However, there is little evidence to support routine admission to HDU/intensive care unit, and standard current practice is to only admit patients with the following risk factors: intraoperative complications, unstable diabetes, symptomatic OSA, and super-morbid obesity.

The evidence for postoperative management has evolved as the case load and experience in this field has increased. A recent study suggested that limiting (elective) intensive care to those with severe OSA and/or BMI > 60 kg/m^2 did not increase either length of hospital stay or the overall incidence of postoperative pulmonary complications [40]. Another study found that OSA was not associated with an increase in pulmonary complications and that this group did not require routine admission to the intensive care unit [41].

⊕ **Clinical tip** Postoperative care

- Patients already established on home CPAP may benefit from being extubated straight on to a CPAP system. This may be needed for several postoperative nights, as OSA occurs during rapid eye movement sleep which is typically supressed for 4 or 5 days postoperatively and then shows rebound.
- CPAP does not increase the risk of anastomotic leak in these patients [42].
- Early mobilization should be encouraged to help with pulmonary function and to reduce the risk of venous thromboembolism.
- Good glycaemic control helps prevent wound infection and protects the myocardium during ischaemic episodes.

A Final Word from the Expert

Obese patients presenting for all types of surgery require meticulous preoperative assessment and perioperative care, and often present significant challenges to the anaesthetist not only because of their associated comorbidity but also the practical difficulties that anaesthesia presents. A sound understanding of the pathophysiology of obesity and its complications is essential to reduce risk. Although there are many sources of advice and guidance for safe anaesthesia in obese patients, including the AAGBI (2007 'glossy') [43] these guidelines cover organizational issues rather than giving 'hands-on' clinical advice. The Society for Obesity and Bariatric Anaesthetia (SOBA) has produced a single-page guidance document designed for use as a quick reference tool in the anaesthetic room [16]. Despite these, there is a paucity of good guidance, and a need for individual clinical experience as well as local policies and standard operating procedures.

With the rising prevalence of obesity and proven cost-effectiveness of bariatric surgery, demand for this type of procedure is likely to increase in the coming years. The development of multidisciplinary teams in weight reduction surgery, and of dedicated care pathways which include enhanced recovery programmes, are likely to increase safety and efficacy [44–46]. For a few selected patients it may be possible to streamline the process into a day-case procedure; perhaps for those with a BMI <40 kg/m^2, with no comorbidity and undergoing relatively simple surgery such as laparoscopic banding [15].

References

1. Lotia S, Bellamy MC. Anaesthesia and morbid obesity. *Cont Educn Anaesth Crit Care Pain* 2008;8:151–6.
2. NHS Information Centre [online]. *Statistics on obesity, physical activity and diet—England.* < http://www.ic.nhs.uk/pubs/opad12 >
3. Bellamy M, Struys M. *Anaesthesia for the overweight and obese patient.* Oxford: Oxford University Press; 2007.
4. Ogunnaike BO, Jones SB, Jones DB, Provost D, Whitten CW. Anesthetic considerations for bariatric surgery. *Anesth Analg* 2002;95:1793–1805.

5. Verselewel de Witt Hamer PC, Tuinebreijer WE. Preoperative weight gain in bariatric surgery. *Obes Surg* 1998;8:300–1.

6. Brodsky JB, Lemmens HJ, Brock-Utne JG, Vierra M, Saidman LJ. Morbid obesity and tracheal intubation. *Anesth Analg* 2002;94:732–6.

7. Neligan PJ, Porter S, Max B, Malhotra G, Greenblatt EP, Ochroch EA. Obstructive sleep apnea is not a risk factor for difficult intubation in morbidly obese patients. *Anesth Analg* 2009;109:1182–6.

8. Langeron O, Masso E, Huraux C, *et al*. Prediction of difficult mask ventilation. *Anesthesiology* 2000;92:1229–36.

9. Hardman JG, Wills JS, Aitkenhead AR. Investigating hypoxemia during apnea: validation of a set of physiological models. *Anesth Analg* 2000;90:614–18.

10. Royal College of Anaesthetists and Difficult Airway Society. Fourth National Audit Project. Cook TM, Woodall N, Frerk C editors. *Major complications of airway management in the United Kingdom. Report and findings.* London: Royal College of Anaesthetists; March 2011. < http://www.rcoa.ac.uk/nap4 >

11. Kripke DF, Ancoli-Israel S, Klauber MR, Wingard DL, Mason WJ, Mullaney DJ. Prevalence of sleep-disordered breathing in ages 40–64 years: a population-based survey. *Sleep* 1997;20:65–76.

12. Haines KL, Nelson LG, Gonzalez R, *et al*. Objective evidence that bariatric surgery improves obesity-related obstructive sleep apnea. *Surgery* 2007;141:354–8.

13. Liao P, Yegneswaran B, Vairavanathan S, Zilberman P, Chung F. Postoperative complications in patients with obstructive sleep apnea: a retrospective matched cohort study. *Can J Anaesth* 2009;56:819–28.

14. Gupta RM, Parvizi J, Hanssen AD, Gay PC. Postoperative complications in patients with obstructive sleep apnea syndrome undergoing hip or knee replacement: a case–control study. *Mayo Clin Proc* 2001;76:897–905.

15. Schumann R. Anaesthesia for bariatric surgery. *Best Pract Res Clin Anaesthesiol* 2011;25:83–93.

16. Society for Obesity and Bariatric Anaesthesia [website]. Single sheet summary—*The STOP-BANG assessment tool.* < http://www.sobauk.com/index.php?option = com_phocadownload&view = file&id = 3:single-sheet-guidelines&Itemid = 61 >

17. DeMaria EJ, Portenier D, Wolfe L. Obesity surgery mortality risk score: proposal for a clinically useful score to predict mortality risk in patients undergoing gastric bypass. *Surg Obes Relat Dis* 2007;3:134–40.

18. McCullough PA, Gallagher MJ, Dejong AT, *et al*. Cardiorespiratory fitness and short-term complications after bariatric surgery. *Chest* 2006;130:517–25.

19. Lerakis S, Kalogeropoulos AP, El-Chami MF, *et al*. Transthoracic dobutamine stress echocardiography in patients undergoing bariatric surgery. *Obes Surg* 2007;17:1475–81.

20. Wisen O, Hellstrom PM. Gastrointestinal motility in obesity. *J Intern Med* 1995;237:411–18.

21. Adams JP, Murphy PG. Obesity in anaesthesia and intensive care. *Br J Anaesth* 2000;85:91–108.

22. Jean J, Compere V, Fourdrinier V, *et al*. The risk of pulmonary aspiration in patients after weight loss due to bariatric surgery. *Anesth Analg* 2008;107:1257–9.

23. Clements RH, Yellumahanthi K, Ballem N, Wesley M, Bland KI. Pharmacologic prophylaxis against venous thromboembolic complications is not mandatory for all laparoscopic Roux-en-Y gastric bypass procedures. *J Am Coll Surg* 2009;208:917–21.

24. Jones JG, Sapsford DJ, Wheatley RG. Postoperative hypoxaemia: mechanisms and time course. *Anaesthesia* 1990;45:566–73.

25. Jense HG, Dubin SA, Silverstein PI, O'Leary-Escolas U. Effect of obesity on safe duration of apnea in anesthetized humans. *Anesth Analg* 1991;72:89–93.

26. Dixon BJ, Dixon JB, Carden JR, *et al*. Preoxygenation is more effective in the 25 degrees head-up position than in the supine position in severely obese patients: a randomized controlled study. *Anesthesiology* 2005;102:1110–15.

27. Coussa M, Proietti S, Schnyder P, *et al*. Prevention of atelectasis formation during the induction of general anesthesia in morbidly obese patients. *Anesth Analg* 2004;98:1491–5.

28. Cadi P, Guenoun T, Journois D, Chevallier JM, Diehl JL, Safran D. Pressure-controlled ventilation improves oxygenation during laparoscopic obesity surgery compared with volume-controlled ventilation. *Br J Anaesth* 2008;100:709–16.

29. De Baerdemaeker LE, Van der Herten C, Gillardin JM, Pattyn P, Mortier EP, Szegedi LL. Comparison of volume-controlled and pressure-controlled ventilation during laparoscopic gastric banding in morbidly obese patients. *Obes Surg* 2008;18:680–5.

30. Hans GA, Pregaldien AA, Kaba A, *et al*. Pressure-controlled ventilation does not improve gas exchange in morbidly obese patients undergoing abdominal surgery. *Obes Surg* 2008;18:71–6.

31. Nguyen NT, Wolfe BM. The physiologic effects of pneumoperitoneum in the morbidly obese. *Ann Surg* 2005;241:219–26.

32. Talab HF, Zabani IA, Abdelrahman HS, *et al*. Intraoperative ventilatory strategies for prevention of pulmonary atelectasis in obese patients undergoing laparoscopic bariatric surgery. *Anesth Analg* 2009;109:1511–16.

33. Whalen FX, Gajic O, Thompson GB, *et al*. The effects of the alveolar recruitment maneuver and positive end-expiratory pressure on arterial oxygenation during laparoscopic bariatric surgery. *Anesth Analg* 2006;102:298–305.

34. Dresner M, Brocklesby J, Bamber J. Audit of the influence of body mass index on the performance of epidural analgesia in labour and the subsequent mode of delivery. *Br J Obstet Gynaecol* 2006;113:1178–81.

35. Charlton S, Cyna AM, Middleton P, Griffiths JD. Perioperative transversus abdominis plane (TAP) blocks for analgesia after abdominal surgery. *Cochrane Database Syst Rev* 2010:CD007705.

36. Choi YK, Brolin RE, Wagner BK, Chou S, Etesham S, Pollak P. Efficacy and safety of patient-controlled analgesia for morbidly obese patients following gastric bypass surgery. *Obes Surg* 2000;10:154–9.

37. Enzor N, Johnston P, Bentley MR, Margarson MP. Pre-operative high-dose paracetamol is morphine-sparing in super-obese patients undergoing bariatric surgery. *Eur J Anaesthesiol* 2009;26:14AP2–4.

38. Gregoire N, Hovsepian L, Gualano V, Evene E, Dufour G, Gendron A. Safety and pharmacokinetics of paracetamol following intravenous administration of 5 g during the first 24 h with a 2-g starting dose. *Clin Pharmacol Ther* 2007;81:401–5.

39. Popat M, Mitchell V, Dravid R, Patel A, Swampillai C, Higgs A. Difficult Airway Society Guidelines for the management of tracheal extubation. *Anaesthesia* 2012;67:318–40.

40. El Shobary H, Backman S, Christou N, Schricker T. Use of critical care resources after laparoscopic gastric bypass: effect on respiratory complications. *Surg Obes Relat Dis* 2008;4:698–702.

41. Grover BT, Priem DM, Mathiason MA, Kallies KJ, Thompson GP, Kothari SN. Intensive care unit stay not required for patients with obstructive sleep apnea after laparoscopic Roux-en-Y gastric bypass. *Surg Obes Relat Dis* 2010;6:165–70.

42. Huerta S, DeShields S, Shpiner R, *et al*. Safety and efficacy of postoperative continuous positive airway pressure to prevent pulmonary complications after Roux-en-Y gastric bypass. *J Gastrointest Surg* 2002;6:354–8.

43. Association of Anaesthetists of Great Britan and Ireland [website]. *Peri-operative management of the morbidly obese patient.* < http://www.aagbi.org/sites/default/Obesity07.pdf >

44. Ronellenfitsch U, Schwarzbach M, Kring A, Kienle P, Post S, Hasenberg T. The effect of clinical pathways for bariatric surgery on perioperative quality of care. *Obes Surg* 2012;22:732–9.

45. Jacobsen HJ, Bergland A, Raeder J, Gislason HG. High-volume bariatric surgery in a single center: safety, quality, cost-efficacy and teaching aspects in 2,000 consecutive cases. *Obes Surg* 2012;22:158–66.

46 Lemanu DP, Srinivasa S, Singh PP, Johannsen S, MacCormick AD, Hill AG. Optimizing perioperative care in bariatric surgery patients. *Obes Surg* 2012;22:979–90.

CHAPTER 4

Neuroanaesthesia

Radiological coiling for cerebral aneurysm

Michele Kigozi

Expert Commentary Mary Newton
CPD Matrix Code: 2F01, 3F00, 3C00

Case history

A 50-year-old woman presented to the emergency department shortly after collapsing at home following the sudden onset of a severe headache associated with vomiting and a rapid reduction in conscious level.

On admission to hospital her conscious level was 13/15 on the Glasgow Coma Scale (GCS) (Eyes (E) = 3, Verbal (V) = 4, Motor (M) = 6) (see Chapter 8, Learning point, Glasgow Coma Score). Neurological examination demonstrated photophobia and neck stiffness, normal pupillary reflexes, and no focal or lateralizing neurological signs. The history and presentation were consistent with a diagnosis of subarachnoid haemorrhage (SAH). Blood pressure (BP) was elevated at 192/88 mmHg, but all other baseline observations were normal. The only abnormalities on admission blood tests were a raised white blood cell count (15 × 10^9/L) and hypomagnesaemia (0.49 mmol/L). The patient was a smoker of 30 cigarettes a day and was treated for hypertension with amlodipine and ramipril.

✪ Learning point Risk factors for subarachnoid haemorrhage (SAH)

Modifiable:
- Hypertension
- Smoking
- Cocaine abuse
- Oral contraceptive pill

Non-modifiable:
- Family history (5–20% of cases of SAH)
- Inherited connective tissue disorders, e.g. autosomal dominant polycystic kidney disease (2% of cases of SAH), Ehlers Danlos IV and neurofibromatosis type 1

An urgent non-contrast enhanced CT head scan was arranged. This confirmed the suspected diagnosis of SAH with no evidence of hydrocephalus (Figure 4.1). A subsequent CT angiogram showed an aneurysm of the left anterior communicating artery (Figures 4.2, 4.3). The patient was diagnosed with grade II SAH (using the World Federation of Neurological Surgeons (WFNS) clinical grading system) [1] (Learning point, Grading of SAH).

⊕ Clinical tip Transfer to a specialist neurosurgical centre

This patient was admitted directly to a tertiary referral neurosurgical centre. For those patients for whom this is not the case, prompt diagnosis, timely referral, and expedited transfer to a specialist neurosurgical centre should take place alongside patient stabilization and treatment. This will facilitate rapid treatment of the aneurysm which should take place within 48 h of the ictus [2].

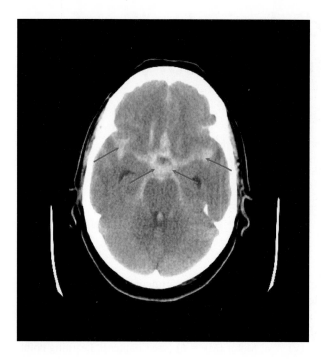

Figure 4.1 Unenhanced brain CT confirming subarachnoid haemorrhage. Arrows demonstrate subarachnoid blood—enhancing white appearance on CT.

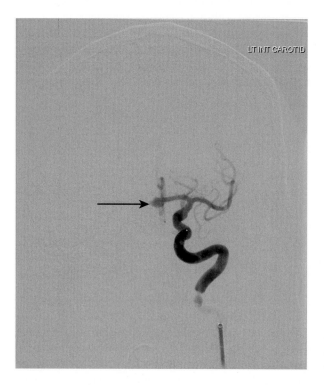

Figure 4.2 Digital subtraction angiogram (similar in appearance to CT angiogram) showing left anterior communicating artery aneurysm (arrow).

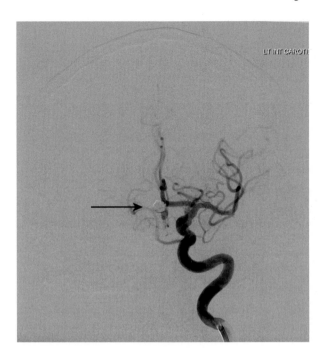

LT INT CAROTI

Figure 4.3 Digital subtraction angiogram showing left anterior communicating artery aneurysm occluded with coils (arrow).

★ **Learning point** Diagnosis of subarachnoid haemorrhage

Clinical presentation of SAH

SAH is usually accompanied by sudden onset of severe headache ('worst ever') lasting more than 1 h

± nausea and vomiting
± meningism
± transient or persistent loss of consciousness
± focal neurological deficit (including isolated cranial nerve palsies)
± epileptic seizures

Any reduction in conscious level should raise the clinical suspicion of hydrocephalus.

Investigations

Unenhanced CT of the head is the initial diagnostic tool of choice in all cases of SAH. Subarachnoid blood is quickly broken down and is almost completely reabsorbed within 10 days of SAH, therefore CT needs to be obtained and interpreted by an experienced radiologist without delay.

CT will miss ~2% of episodes of SAH within 12 h and 7% at 24 h.

Lumbar puncture (LP) is an important investigation used to exclude a diagnosis of SAH in patients with a convincing history but negative CT. The College of Emergency Medicine recommends a delay of at least 12 h between the onset of symptoms and performing the LP [3]. This delay is essential to allow for formation of bilirubin and oxyhaemoglobin (breakdown products of haemoglobin metabolism). These pigments give rise to a yellowish discolouration of cerebrospinal fluid (CSF) supernatant, known as xanthochromia, which can be detected in CSF for up to 2 weeks following SAH. The sample should be sent for spectrophotometry as this is more sensitive than visual inspection of the supernatant. All CSF samples sent for spectrophotometry should be centrifuged in the laboratory within 40 min of taking the sample; otherwise oxyhaemoglobin may form *in vitro* from a 'bloody tap'. Opening CSF pressure should be measured and documented.

> ✪ **Learning point**   Grading of subarachnoid haemorrhage
>
> The two most frequently used clinical grading scales for SAH are those of Hunt and Hess and the World Federation of Neurological Surgeons (WFNS) (Tables 4.1 and 4.2) [1, 4]. These correlate well with patient outcome and the risk of complications (elevated ICP, impaired cerebral autoregulation, cardiac dysfunction, hypovolaemia, and hyponatraemia). A clinical grading should be assigned as soon as possible after the diagnosis of SAH is made to optimize accurate communication between centres about patient status and to guide treatment.
>
> A third grading system, the Fisher scale (Table 4.3), uses a radiological (cranial CT) classification of SAH and is the best predictor of symptomatic cerebral vasospasm [5].
>
> **Table 4.1 Hunt and Hess grading scale for subarachnoid haemorrhage [4]**
>
> | Grade | Clinical description |
> |---|---|
> | I | Asymptomatic or minimal headache and slight nuchal rigidity |
> | II | Moderate-to-severe headache, nuchal rigidity, no neurological deficit other than cranial nerve palsy |
> | III | Drowsiness, confusion, or mild focal deficit |
> | IV | Stupor, moderate-to-severe hemiparesis and possibly early decerebrate rigidity and vegetative disturbances |
> | V | Deep coma, decerebrate rigidity and moribund appearance |
> | VI | Death |
>
> Reproduced from Hunt WE, Hess RM. Surgical risk as related to time of intervention in the repair of intracranial aneurysms. *Journal of Neurosurgery*, 28, 1, pp. 14–20, copyright 1968, with permission from the American Association of Neurological Surgeons.
>
> **Table 4.2 World Federation of Neurological Surgeons grading scale for aneurysmal subarachnoid haemorrhage [1]**
>
> | Grade | Glasgow Coma Scale | Motor deficit or dysphasia |
> |---|---|---|
> | I | 15 | Absent |
> | II | 13 or 14 | Absent |
> | III | 13 or 14 | Present |
> | IV | 7–12 | Present or absent |
> | V | 3–6 | Present or absent |
>
> Reproduced from 'Report of World Federation of Neurological Surgeons Committee on a Universal Subarachnoid Hemorrhage Grading Scale', *Journal of Neurosurgery*, 68, p. 985, copyright 1988, with permission from the American Association of Neurological Surgeons.
>
> **Table 4.3 Fisher grading scale of cranial CT [5]**
>
> | Grade | Findings on CT |
> |---|---|
> | 1 | No subarachnoid blood detected |
> | 2 | Diffuse or vertical layers <1 mm |
> | 3 | Localized clot and/or vertical layer >1 mm |
> | 4 | Intracerebral or intraventricular clot with diffuse or no SAH |
>
> Reproduced from Fisher C, et al., 'Relation of cerebral vasospasm to subarachnoid hemorrhage visualized by computerized tomographic scanning', *Neurosurgery*, 6, 1, pp. 1–9, Copyright 1980, with permission from the Congress of Neurological Surgeons.

❝ **Expert comment**
Prognostic factors in subarachnoid haemorrhage

The three main predictors of mortality and dependence following SAH are:

• Advanced age.
• Impaired level of consciousness on admission; a higher Hunt and Hess and WFNS grade (Tables 4.1 and 4.2).
• Large volume of blood on initial CT; higher Fisher grade (Table 4.3).

> ✪ **Learning point**   Causes of subarachnoid haemorrhage
>
> The most frequent cause of SAH is trauma. However, frequent causes of non-traumatic SAH are:
>
> • rupture of an intracranial ('berry') aneurysm (75–80%)
> • arteriovenous malformation (5%)
> • miscellaneous causes (15%), e.g. arterial dissections, vasculitides, haemorrhagic tumours, infective aneurysm, pituitary apoplexy, and cocaine abuse.

> ✪ **Learning point** Arterial blood supply of the brain
>
> The arterial supply to the brain is from both internal carotid arteries and the vertebrobasilar system. Anastomoses between the internal carotid arteries and the vertebrobasilar system form the circle of Willis. The majority of aneurysms are situated in one of the arteries of the circle of Willis. Aneurysms are more commonly found at arterial bifurcations as these are most prone to the intravascular shear stress induced by the haemodynamics of turbulent flow. 80–90% of intracranial aneurysms occur in the anterior (carotid) circulation (anterior and posterior communicating, or the middle cerebral artery). 10–20% of aneurysms are located in the posterior (vertebrobasilar) circulation.

Nimodipine was started (60 mg orally every 4 h). The patient was admitted to the neurosurgical ICU for BP control and a labetalol infusion was used to maintain a systolic BP of < 160 mmHg.

> ✪ **Learning point** Nimodipine
>
> Nimodipine is a voltage-gated calcium channel antagonist that inhibits calcium entry into smooth muscle cells and neurons. It is given routinely to all patients with SAH following the British aneurysm nimodipine trial in 1989 [6]. This double-blinded, placebo-controlled, randomized trial of nimodipine therapy (started within 96 h and continued for 21 days) versus placebo in 554 patients demonstrated a significant improvement in neurological outcome in patients on nimodipine. Nimodipine does not reduce the severity of cerebral vasospasm detected by angiography, but significantly reduces the incidence of cerebral infarction. The exact mechanism of action of nimodipine is unknown but in experimental models it has been shown to attenuate the increase in neuronal calcium that occurs after ischaemia.
>
> Nimodipine should be started as soon as SAH is diagnosed and continued for 21 days at a dose of 60 mg orally every 4 h. A dose of 30 mg 2 hourly can be used if hypotension occurs.

An arterial line was placed; the hypomagnesaemia was corrected and hydration was maintained with intravenous 0.9% sodium chloride. Intravenous paracetamol and low-dose oral morphine were administered for analgesia. The patient was maintained on strict bed rest and prescribed regular laxatives. Mechanical venous thromboembolic prophylaxis was started (compression and pneumatic devices). Neurological observations remained unchanged overnight.

> ✚ **Clinical tip** Acute management 'bundle' for subarachnoid haemorrhage
>
> **Monitoring**
> - Vital signs
> - GCS and pupillary size/response
> - Pain score
>
> **Investigations**
> - Unenhanced CT as soon as possible but within 24 h of onset of symptoms
> - Blood tests including: full blood count, urea and electrolytes, 'group and save'
> - ECG (repeat at 24 h intervals if abnormality detected)
> - Echocardiography (if clinical/radiographic signs of pulmonary oedema)
>
> **Therapy**
> - Nimodipine (oral 60 mg 4 hourly)
> - Strict bed rest with slight head-up position
> - Oxygen therapy to maintain SpO_2 ≥96% (or PaO_2 ≥11 kPa)
> - Normocarbia ($PaCO_2$ 4.5–5.5 kPa in ventilated patients)
> - Keep systolic BP >100 mmHg, <160 mmHg (tailor lower limit to pre-morbid BP; known hypertensive patients may need increased 'lower' limit due to shift of cerebral autoregulation curve). Treat sustained BP >160 mmHg cautiously to avoid hypotension
> - Analgesia: avoid NSAIDs until aneurysm occluded
>
> (continued)

⁕⁕ **Expert comment**

A major and frequently fatal early complication of aneurysmal SAH is re-bleeding. This is estimated to occur in up to 10% patients in the first 72 h following SAH [7] and is a reason for recommending early transfer to a specialist centre for treatment of SAH [2]. There is no evidence to prove that the rate of re-bleeding is increased with uncontrolled hypertension; however most centres aim to maintain systolic BP <160 mmHg in patients with unsecured ruptured aneurysms [8]. It is recommended that ruptured aneurysms are occluded early [8], within 48 h of the ictus [2].

- Antiemetics: avoid serotonin (5-HT₃) antagonists such as ondansetron if ECG evidence of prolonged QT interval (see Learning point, Cardiovascular and pulmonary complications following SAH)
- Intravenous fluids (0.9% sodium chloride) aiming for euvolaemia (maintenance fluid requirement 1.5 mL/kg/h)
- Strict record of fluid balance
- Blood glucose 6–10 mmol/L
- Laxatives
- Venous thromboembolism prophylaxis (mechanical methods only prior to aneurysm occlusion)

✪ **Learning point** Acute complications of subarachnoid haemorrhage

Neurological
- Hydrocephalus (15–20% of cases)
- Re-bleed (risk: day 1 = 5%, 1 month = 30%, after 6 months = 3% per year)
- Delayed cerebral ischaemia (DCI)/vasospasm (within 3–14 days, peak at 6–8 days. Incidence = 60–70% of patients with SAH)
- Cerebral oedema/infarction
- Seizures (5–8% of patients)

Medical
- Hyponatraemia: syndrome of inappropriate antidiuretic hormone (SIADH)/cerebral salt-wasting syndrome (CSWS)
- Hypernatraemia: diabetes insipidus (DI)
- Hypovolaemia (CSWS or DI)
- Hypomagnesaemia
- Neurogenic pulmonary oedema
- Cardiac dysfunction (ECG/echocardiography changes ± troponin rise)

The following morning (day 1) the neurovascular team (neuroradiologists and neurosurgeons) considered the aneurysm suitable for endovascular occlusion ('coiling'). The patient was unable to consent for the procedure so physician consent was undertaken in discussion with the family. The patient was transferred to the interventional radiology suite and prepared for general anaesthesia.

In addition to standard monitoring (oxygen saturation, end-tidal carbon dioxide, ECG, temperature) intra-arterial pressure monitoring was established. Induction and maintenance of anaesthesia was achieved by administration of propofol and remifentanil target-controlled infusions set sufficiently high to obtund the pressor response to tracheal intubation and placement of a nasogastric tube. Vecuronium was used to facilitate intubation. The patient's lungs were ventilated with an oxygen/air mix to maintain normoxia and normocarbia. A urinary catheter was placed to aid accurate fluid balance. Forced external air warming was used to maintain normothermia; temperature was monitored with a nasopharyngeal temperature probe.

✪ **Learning point** Endovascular ('coiling') versus surgical ('clipping') occlusion

The method of aneurysm exclusion chosen for a particular patient should be decided following discussion between neurosurgeons and neuroradiologists. The International Subarachnoid Aneurysm Trial (ISAT) published in 2002 randomized 2,143 patients with ruptured aneurysms to surgical clipping or endovascular coiling [9]. A total of 801 patients underwent a coiling procedure: of these, 190 were dependent or dead at 1 year (24%), compared with the 243 patients out of 793 (31%) who underwent a surgical clipping procedure: an absolute risk reduction for death or dependence at 1 year of 7%. The

(continued)

long-term ISAT results were published in 2005. These showed that significantly more (8.6%) patients in the coiled group needed treatment for a recurrence of the aneurysm (mean time 20.7 months following initial treatment). The re-bleed rate was low (0.6%) in coiled patients and not significantly different to that seen in the clipped group (0.3%). Limitations of the trial are that 88% of the randomized cases were WFNS grade 1 or 2, 52% of aneurysms were under 5 mm in size, and 97% were anterior circulation. The criticism is that these data are biased to small, anterior circulation aneurysms in good-grade patients, and thus not generalizable to the SAH population as a whole.

Advances in coil and stent technology (since the publication of ISAT) combined with increased expertise of radiologists have resulted in most aneurysms now being amenable to coiling, with the exception of some aneurysms of the middle cerebral bifurcation with complex anatomy. The less invasive nature of endovascular coiling, although unstudied, is likely to benefit patients with poor clinical grade and serious co-morbidity as well as those with aneurysms where surgical access is difficult (e.g. basilar tip) [10].

> ⭐ **Learning point** Coiling of an aneurysm
>
> Endovascular coiling is performed by an interventional neuroradiologist with the patient under general anaesthesia with guaranteed immobility. The procedure takes about 90 min, although this is largely determined by the accessibility of the aneurysm and experience of the operator. The femoral artery is cannulated and, under fluoroscopic guidance, a guiding catheter positioned in either the internal carotid or vertebral artery. A microcatheter is navigated into the aneurysm using bi-planar fluoroscopy and a pre-acquired fluoroscopic 'road map'. A very soft platinum coil is then introduced into the aneurysm. Once the coil has been optimally positioned within the aneurysm it is detached from its pusher wire at a specialized detachment zone (in most modern devices the coil is released from the pusher wire in the detachment zone by means of a thermo-mechanical cut). Once detached, the pusher wire is withdrawn under fluoroscopic guidance and the coil is left behind in the aneurysm (Figure 4.4). The coil leads to organization of thrombus in the aneurysm. Further coils are introduced into the aneurysm until the aneurysm is densely packed and no longer fills with blood. At this stage the aneurysm is excluded from the circulation and no longer at risk of rupture. Subsequently (after about 2 weeks) fibrosis of the aneurysm is completed and a functional endothelial membrane has formed across its neck.
>
> Some wide-necked aneurysms are treated with a combination of a stent and coils. A large variety of coils with different characteristics have been developed in recent years. This has resulted in most aneurysms now being amenable to endovascular coiling.
>
> Patients are followed up with angiography or magnetic resonance angiography at 6-monthly intervals following a coiling procedure to check for aneurysm recurrence. The recurrence rate is about 20% and about half of these will require further coiling [11, 12].

> 🗨 **Expert comment**
> Management of grade IV and V subarachnoid haemorrhage
>
> Before the introduction of endovascular occlusion ('coiling') of aneurysms, surgery ('clipping') was usually planned before day 4 or after day 10 following SAH to avoid the high-risk period for vasospasm. Most centres postponed surgery in poor-grade SAH (IV and V) patients until after day 10 and then only proceeded if there had been clinical improvement. During this time many patients died due to re-bleeding and/or vasospasm. Following early endovascular occlusion in association with supportive neurointensive care management, several centres have shown that just over 50% of patients with grade IV and V SAH survive with good functional outcome.

> 🗨 **Expert comment**
> There is no consensus about the use of anticoagulants or platelet anti-aggregation agents during coiling of ruptured aneurysms. Most centres use heparin to achieve an ACT of about two to three times normal around the time of first coil deployment and follow with the administration of aspirin shortly after this or at the end of the procedure [13].

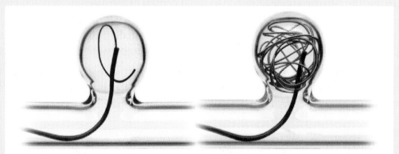

Figure 4.4 Schematic diagram of the placement of an endovascular platinum coil using a microcatheter. The catheter will then be withdrawn, leaving the coils within the aneurysm. The number of coils used will be dependent on the size of the aneurysm and radiological evidence of satisfactory occlusion of the aneurysm. Reproduced with kind permission from Stryker.

The patient received 5000 units of heparin after successful deployment of the first coil in the aneurysm to achieve an activated clotting time (ACT) between 250 and 300 s. ACT was monitored hourly to check that it remained within range.

> **✪ Learning point**   Principles of anaesthesia for endovascular occlusion ('coiling') of cerebral aneurysm
>
> General measures:
>
> - maintenance of adequate cerebral perfusion pressure (CPP = mean arterial pressure (MAP) – intracranial pressure (ICP))
> - avoidance of hypertension with stimulation (e.g. laryngoscopy, transfer of patient)
> - normocarbia and normoxia
> - normothermia
> - normoglycaemia
> - immobility
>
> Wherever possible, patients should be woken after the procedure to allow neurological assessment. The principles of anaesthesia would be the same for a surgical clipping procedure.

> **✚ Clinical tip**   Monitoring intracranial pressure (ICP) in sedated patients
>
> Patients with poor clinical grade SAH (WFNS grade IV and V) may require sedation and ventilation for airway protection and maintenance of oxygenation. Some will have an external ventricular drain (EVD) in place to manage hydrocephalus; the EVD can also be used to monitor ICP. In the absence of an EVD it is advisable to site an ICP measuring device as pressures >20 mmHg will necessitate further CT imaging to diagnose the cause. Without these measuring devices significant increases in ICP will only be determined by changes in pupillary size and response to light (late indicators of neurological deterioration) or by reducing/stopping sedation to assess neurological status. If ICP monitoring has been started before treatment for aneurysmal coil occlusion, this should be continued during the procedure. If, for any reason, sedation and ventilation need to be continued after the procedure, ICP monitoring should be continued until the patient's sedation can be reduced sufficiently to allow neurological assessment. When intra-procedural complications occur in patients without ICP monitoring or an EVD and a decision is made to keep the patient sedated and ventilated, an ICP monitoring device should ideally be sited (when the ACT has returned to normal) and continued until the patient can be assessed neurologically.

> **❝ Expert comment**
>
> Protamine should always be immediately available for the emergency reversal of heparin during endovascular coiling procedures. However, the decision to reverse heparin if intra-procedural aneurysm rupture occurs must be made in close consultation with the operating radiologist. Intra-procedural rupture occurs in ~2–3% of cases [14]. Practice varies; some radiologists will attempt to occlude the aneurysm as quickly as possible with coils without reversing the heparin whereas others will request that protamine is given in addition to rapid occlusion of the aneurysm.

Shortly after this, the procedure was complicated by rupture of the aneurysm and further SAH. This was associated with profound hypertension (systolic BP 220 mmHg) which was rapidly brought under control with repeated boluses of propofol (360 mg in total) and an increase in the rate of the remifentanil infusion. A decision was made not to reverse the heparin anticoagulation as rapid control of the bleeding was achieved by the neuroradiologist packing the aneurysm with coils.

At the end of the procedure both pupils were 5 mm in diameter and briskly reactive to light. Anaesthesia was continued while the patient underwent a post-procedure CT scan; this showed further subarachnoid blood around the aneurysm but no evidence of hydrocephalus. The patient was transferred back to the neurosurgical ICU where respiratory dysfunction required that sedation and ventilation continued.

> **✪ Learning point**   Complications of coiling
>
> Direct procedural complications
>
> Aneurysm rupture
>
> This is usually accompanied by an abrupt rise in arterial pressure ± bradycardia that requires immediate treatment. Propofol is often used in this scenario; very large doses may be required to maintain normotension. The radiologist may request reversal of heparin (1 mg protamine for every 100 units
>
> (continued)

heparin). Following rupture the radiologist will attempt urgent occlusion of the aneurysm with coils. As soon as possible (but without delaying the occlusion of the aneurysm) the patient's pupillary reflexes should be checked. Urgent CT should be performed as the findings may determine the need for neurosurgical intervention (placement of EVD or evacuation of haematoma).

Occlusive complications

In the event of vessel occlusion (by coil or thrombus) BP should be increased to maintain vessel patency and improve collateral flow. Malpositioned coils can usually be retrieved endovascularly. Intravenous antiplatelet agents (e.g. aspirin, glycoprotein IIb/IIIa inhibitors) can be used to facilitate dispersal of platelet aggregates by platelet inhibition.

Haemorrhage from a major non-cerebral vessel

Although rare, the team should be familiar with major haemorrhage protocols.

Indirect procedural complications

Contrast reactions

Iohexol is the most widely used non-ionic contrast media for angiography. Non-ionic media are associated with a lower incidence of mild to moderate anaphylactic reactions, although the incidence of fatal reactions is the same as that of ionic agents (1:10,000 exposures).

Contrast-induced nephropathy

Contrast-induced nephropathy (CIN) is a frequent cause of acute renal failure in hospital. Risk factors for development of CIN include pre-existing renal disease, diabetes mellitus, high dose of contrast, dehydration and co-administration of nephrotoxic drugs. The best prevention is optimal hydration and limitation of contrast dose. The administration of N-acetylcysteine or isotonic sodium bicarbonate may reduce the incidence of CIN but larger trials are needed to confirm any benefit.

> **❝ Expert comment**
>
> Low-grade pyrexia (in the absence of infection) frequently occurs following SAH. Several studies have shown that fever is independently associated with poor neurological outcome in this group [8, 15]. Infectious causes for temperature should be treated promptly. Antipyretic agents may help reduce fever (NSAIDs should be avoided until the aneurysm is secured). Surface cooling may be more effective, but shivering (and the consequent decrease in brain oxygen tension) must be avoided.

On admission to neurosurgical ICU, new-onset T-wave inversion was noted on a 12-lead ECG. This was associated with increasing difficulty in maintaining adequate oxygenation of the patient (65% inspired oxygen was required to obtain a PaO_2 of 8.8 kPa).

Significant increases in ventilator pressures and an increased respiratory rate were required to maintain normocarbia. Cardiac troponin I measured 12 h after aneurysm coiling was found to be three times the upper limit of normal. A chest X-ray demonstrated bilateral pulmonary infiltrates and increased vascular shadowing consistent with the diagnosis of pulmonary oedema. An echocardiogram performed the following day (day 2) showed regional wall motion abnormalities (RWMAs) involving the basal and middle portions of the anterior ventricular wall and an ejection fraction of 33%. The RWMAs did not correspond to a specific cardiac vascular territory. A diagnosis of neurogenic stunned myocardial syndrome was made. A noradrenaline infusion was commenced to maintain systolic BP. The cardiac index (using a LiDCO™ cardiac output monitor) was optimized by the addition of a dobutamine infusion.

Fluid balance was managed carefully to avoid hypovolaemia. Lung protective ventilation strategies were employed and the PaO_2 improved slightly over the next few hours; however, serial troponin I levels demonstrated a significant rise to a maximum level of 2.4 μg/L (upper limit of normal 0.04 μg/L in this laboratory assay).

> **✪ Learning point**   Cardiovascular and pulmonary complications following subarachnoid haemorrhage
>
> SAH induces massive stimulation of the central neuroendocrine axis, causing activation of the adrenal glands and increased sympathetic outflow [16, 17]. These effects occur frequently, particularly in patients with severe neurological insult in whom they are associated with increased morbidity and mortality [18].
>
> (continued)

Most complications are reversible and management is therefore supportive, with the focus being on treatment of the underlying brain injury.

ECG changes

ECG changes are seen in >90% of patients following SAH (including ST segment changes, T-wave changes, U waves, QT prolongation, sinus bradycardia and sinus tachycardia). Some may be difficult to distinguish from an acute ischaemic coronary event, and some cases of sudden death following SAH may be due to arrhythmias caused by QT prolongation. Most abnormalities improve as the neurological injury improves; persisting ECG abnormalities may raise concerns about poor overall outcome [16].

Arterial blood pressure changes and left ventricular dysfunction

Arterial BP changes and left ventricular dysfunction occur frequently following SAH [16–18]. Increased sympathetic tone at the time of haemorrhage may persist for up to 10 days and is often associated with hypertension (27%). In the acute phase of treatment before the aneurysm is secured, hypertension (>160 mmHg systolic) may need to be treated to reduce the risk of re-bleeding, but hypotension must be avoided. After the aneurysm has been secured, higher BPs may be accepted. If vasospasm is diagnosed, very high systolic pressures (180–200 mmHg) may be required in an attempt to reverse the signs of vasospasm.

A significant number of patients (18%) become hypotensive and may require fluids and vasopressor ± inotropic support to maintain arterial pressure. This is often due to left ventricular dysfunction which is seen in about 25% patients following SAH. It is primarily due to increased sympathetic outflow and an intense inflammatory response, both of which cause a pattern of reversible cardiac injury termed 'neurogenic stunned myocardium syndrome'. Typically the syndrome develops soon after SAH, in patients with no pre-existing history of ischaemic heart disease (although the two may coexist). The echocardiogram in neurogenic stunned myocardium syndrome shows RWMAs which do not correlate with coronary vascular territories. Although neurogenic stunned myocardium syndrome may cause a significant reduction in ejection fraction, there are only modest increases in cardiac troponin [16, 17]. Typically ventricular function improves within a few days with either no treatment or only supportive treatment.

Neurogenic pulmonary oedema

Neurogenic pulmonary oedema is a clinical syndrome characterized by the acute onset of pulmonary oedema following a significant insult to the central nervous system. SAH is the neurological insult most frequently associated with neurogenic pulmonary oedema; risk factors are increasing age, posterior circulation aneurysms and poor clinical and radiographic grade of SAH. Patients with neurogenic pulmonary oedema following SAH have a higher mortality rate [18].

The pathophysiology of neurogenic pulmonary oedema is not completely understood but four mechanisms have been demonstrated experimentally to cause it and a combination of these may be involved in most patients [16]:

- poor cardiac output: 'neurogenic stunned myocardium'
- hydrostatic forces: increased pulmonary capillary pressure from intense peripheral vasoconstriction
- localized increases in pulmonary capillary permeability: a direct effect in the pulmonary vascular bed (without systemic changes)
- pulmonary capillary endothelial damage: caused by the acute rise in BP resulting in an exudate

The diagnosis may be difficult. Typically neurogenic pulmonary oedema occurs within minutes or hours following SAH but may be delayed for up to 24 h. The classical symptoms and signs of pulmonary oedema are seen (e.g. hypoxia, bilateral hyperdense infiltrates, and increased vascular shadowing on chest X-ray). However, primary pulmonary complications are also frequently seen following SAH (in about 20% patients) and other causes of acute lung injury such as aspiration pneumonia should be excluded.

Management of neurogenic pulmonary oedema should focus on treating the underlying neurological problem, while maintaining cerebral oxygenation and minimizing pulmonary complications. Investigations should include echocardiography as patients with impaired ventricular function may benefit from inotropic and vasopressor support to maintain adequate BP. Careful fluid management is essential to maintain euvolaemia without worsening pulmonary oedema; hypovolaemia should be avoided as it is associated with a poor neurological outcome [18].

⑥ Expert comment

All cardiovascular complications following SAH are associated with an increased risk of death, poor neurological outcome, and DCI [18]. This probably reflects the severity of the underlying brain injury rather than the cardiovascular complication *per se*, although further studies are required to clarify this.

Table 4.4 Blood and urine test results

Parameter measured	Day 1, 08:00	Day 3, 16:00
Average urine output (mL/h)	40	250
Plasma sodium (mmol/L)	146	132
Urine sodium (mmol/day) (normal range 40–220 mmol/day)	Not measured	300
Urine osmolality (mOsm/kg) (normal random urine osmolality 50–1400 mOsm/kg)	Not measured	480

These results support a diagnosis of cerebral salt wasting syndrome. However, note that laboratory results for cerebral salt wasting are nearly identical to those of SIADH (syndrome of inappropriate anti-diuretic hormone), and accurate determination of volume status is key to distinguishing between these two conditions.

During this initial period of stabilization, the patient was ventilated and sedated with propofol and fentanyl. Sedation was weaned on day 4 to assess the patient's neurological state. The GCS remained low at 7: E = 2, V = T, M = 4. (The verbal score could not be assessed as the patient was intubated, hence the value 'T' which equates to a score of 1.) It was also noted that plasma sodium had fallen from 146 to 132 mmol/L in 8 h (Table 4.4). This was accompanied by a high total urine output (averaging 250 mL/h). Paired plasma and urine samples were taken for measurement of sodium and osmolality; results were consistent with a diagnosis of CSWS. Careful correction of fluid balance and sodium status was initiated with oral sodium supplements and intravenous 0.9% sodium chloride therapy.

> ✪ **Learning point** Sodium disturbances in subarachnoid haemorrhage
>
> Sodium disturbances are widespread following SAH [19]. Serum sodium and fluid balance should be monitored carefully. Severe disturbances in serum sodium require frequent measurement (at least twice daily) by the laboratory.
>
> Hyponatraemia (Na⁺ <135 mmol/L) is seen in 40% of patients and when severe may cause seizures and cerebral oedema. The two most frequent causes of hyponatraemia are CSWS and SIADH. CSWS causes loss of sodium (and subsequently water) via the kidneys and occurs in association with a variety of intracranial diseases including SAH. The aetiology of this condition is poorly understood, although excessive secretion of natriuretic peptides (atrial and brain) is thought to play a part. Both CSWS and SIADH cause hyponatraemia; SIADH is a 'volume-expanded' condition, whereas CSWS is a 'volume-contracted state' that involves renal loss of sodium.
>
> It is critical to distinguish between SIADH and CSWS (Table 4.5) as the treatment options are quite different. The treatment of SIADH normally requires fluid restriction but this should be avoided in patients following SAH, as hypovolaemia increases the incidence of DCI. CSWS requires sodium replacement combined with volume replacement [8]. In general, hyponatraemia must be corrected slowly (0.5 mmol/L/h; maximum total increase of 12 mmol/L in 24 h) to avoid causing central pontine myelinolysis. Some patients may have concurrent SIADH and CSWS; often SIADH predominates early on and CSWS becomes more significant a few days after SAH.
>
> Hypernatraemia (Na⁺ >145 mmol/L) is less prevalent following SAH than hyponatraemia and is usually due to osmotic diuretics or central DI. Serum sodium must be corrected slowly (0.5 mmol/L/h; maximum total decrease of 12 mmol/L in 24 h) even in the context of severe hypernatraemia (Na >160 mmol/L) as a rapid decrease in serum sodium may cause cerebral or pulmonary oedema. Severe disturbances in serum sodium require frequent monitoring and accurate fluid balance [19].

Over the next 24 h (day 5) the pupillary response to light became progressively more sluggish and repeat CT showed hydrocephalus. The patient was immediately transferred to the operating theatre for insertion of an EVD. Over the next 72 h, the GCS

Table 4.5 Changes seen in cerebral salt-wasting syndrome (CSWS) and syndrome of inappropriate antidiuretic hormone (SIADH)

	CSWS	SIADH
Urine output (0.5–1 mL/kg/h)[a]	High	Normal or low
Urine specific gravity (1010–1035)[a]	High	High
Urinary sodium (40–220 mmol/day)	High	High (concentrated)
Serum sodium (135–145 mmol/L)	Low	Low (dilutional)
Extracellular fluid volume	Low	High (retention)

[a] Specific gravity is the ratio of a liquid's density compared with a reference liquid (water) and therefore has no units.

improved to 10 and the patient was extubated. She remained on the neurosurgical ICU requiring careful fluid balance and monitoring of plasma sodium.

On day 12 after the SAH the patient developed right-sided weakness associated with right-sided hemi-neglect. This was thought to be due to DCI secondary to arterial vasospasm, a diagnosis that was supported by subsequent cerebral angiography. At the completion of angiography nimodipine was infused through the guiding catheter in the internal carotid artery at a rate of 0.1 mg/min. Additionally haemodynamic therapy ('triple-H' therapy; see Learning point, Management of DCI) was commenced; hypertension and haemodilution were established using 0.9% sodium chloride and noradrenaline infusions aiming for a systolic BP of 160 mmHg (from 120 mmHg). In line with current thinking and particularly in view of the previous cardiac dysfunction, euvolaemia rather than hypervolaemia was cautiously obtained and guided by cardiac output monitoring (LiDCO™) to optimize cardiac index and avoid fluid overload.

The neurological signs resolved completely with this treatment, supporting the diagnosis of DCI. The noradrenaline was weaned slowly over the following 2 days with no deterioration in the patient's neurological status. Haemoglobin was noted to have dropped from 10 to 8 g/dL over this 48 h period of aggressive fluid therapy; this was not corrected as the patient's neurological status remained stable. Drainage via the EVD slowed over this period. The patient's neurological state remained unchanged with the EVD clamped and the EVD was therefore removed on day 16. The patient was subsequently discharged to the ward on day 17 with a GCS of 12.

Subsequent recovery was uneventful. The patient's neurological status continued to improve and she was discharged home on day 32 with a GCS of 13 (E = 4, V = 4, M = 5). Functionally, she required supervision and assistance with all basic activities of daily living at this time.

> ✪ **Learning point** Delayed cerebral ischaemia
>
> Delayed cerebral ischaemia (DCI) often results in infarction and is a major cause of mortality and morbidity following SAH, accounting for 20% of cases of death/poor neurological outcome following SAH. DCI presents as a change in neurological status following the initial period of stabilization after other causes of neurological deterioration have been excluded including: hydrocephalus, cerebral oedema, electrolyte abnormalities, seizure activity, and pyrexia. Typical symptoms of DCI include agitation, altered consciousness, hemiparesis and aphasia. The peak onset of DCI is between days 3–14 following SAH [8] and it is more usually seen in patients presenting with large amounts of subarachnoid blood (Fisher grade 3 and 4). The cause of DCI is unknown. Angiographic vasospasm is seen in about 50% of patients following SAH [20]. About 40% patients with SAH have evidence of cerebral infarction on CT, but often areas of infarction occur in the absence of angiographic vasospasm or do not correspond with the territory of angiographic vasospasm. Microvascular dysfunction secondary to inflammation and thrombogenesis may be important in the pathogenesis of DCI. Histologically, changes are seen in the intima (thickening, loss of tight junctions), media (muscle hypertrophy and later necrosis) and adventitia (thickening), all of which contribute to luminal narrowing.

> **✪ Learning point** Prevention of delayed cerebral ischaemia
>
> Very little progress has been made in reducing the incidence of DCI. Although triple-H therapy may reverse the symptoms of DCI, the only treatment proven to reduce poor outcome following SAH is nimodipine (see Learning point, Nimodipine). Another potential treatment was magnesium, which is an N-methyl-D-aspartate receptor antagonist and a calcium channel blocker that is believed to have neuroprotective effects. In an initial phase II randomized clinical trial of magnesium in 283 patients with SAH, magnesium reduced the risk of DCI by 34%. This provided the rationale for the phase III clinical trial 'Magnesium in Aneurysmal Subarachnoid Hemorrhage II' (MASH II) [21]. This randomized SAH patients to receive either 64 mmol/day of intravenous magnesium or placebo, with the treatment starting within 4 days of SAH and continuing until day 20 post SAH. The primary outcome measure was poor outcome, defined as death or dependence (Rankin score >3 = moderately severe disability; unable to walk and attend to bodily needs without assistance, through to severe disability requiring constant nursing care) after 3 months. This multicentre trial enrolled 1204 patients in total and failed to show any difference between magnesium and placebo. The role of a statin in the prevention of DCI is under investigation. A large phase III study (STASH: SimvaSTatin in Aneurysmal Subarachnoid Haemorrhage) is nearing conclusion and should determine whether a 3-week course of simvastatin (40 mg given within 96 h of ictus and continued until day 21) will improve the long-term outcome in patients following SAH.

> **✪ Learning point** Management of delayed cerebral ischaemia
>
> Medical management of DCI involves initiation of triple-H therapy (hypertension, hypervolaemia and haemodilution) but there is only moderate quality evidence to support a benefit [22, 23]. Induced hypertension (160–200 mmHg systolic) has been shown to improve cerebral blood flow (CBF); patients who fail to respond to a vasopressor may respond to an inotrope. Hypervolaemia is associated with an increased complication rate (pulmonary and/or cerebral oedema) whereas hypovolaemia risks cerebral infarction and a worse outcome. For these reasons euvolaemia is now recommended. Several studies have shown improved cerebral oxygen delivery with haemoglobin of 10 g/dL when compared to 8 g/dL [24, 25]. Patients who fail to respond to medical therapy should be considered for endovascular management consisting of either intra-arterial vasodilator therapy or angioplasty or a combination of both. Again, there is no evidence to confirm a benefit from endovascular treatments.

> **✪ Learning point** Use of physiological monitoring and imaging in the diagnosis of delayed cerebral ischaemia
>
> These modalities are particularly important in sedated and poor-grade patients where accurate neurological assessment may not be possible.
>
> Transcranial Doppler (TCD) ultrasonography
> TCD is a non-invasive real-time monitor that provides indirect information about CBF. A low-frequency (2 MHz) ultrasound beam is directed through the thin-boned transtemporal window above the zygomatic arch. The mean red blood cell flow velocity (FV) in the study vessel is calculated from the shift in frequency of the Doppler signal. The middle cerebral artery is the easiest and most reliable artery to study (although the anterior and posterior cerebral arteries can also be studied).
>
> A baseline TCD examination should be performed as early as possible following SAH and then repeated daily in the high-risk period for vasospasm (day 3–12). An increase in FV to a velocity >120 cm/s predicts vasospasm. Using TCD helps to detect vasospasm before the onset of symptoms and allows early intervention.
>
> TCD has the advantage of being a non-invasive, inexpensive, bedside test with high specificity for proximal vessel spasm. However, TCD is less sensitive at detecting distal vessel spasm and varies with operator experience and the angle of insonation (angle between the ultrasound beam and vessel lumen).
>
> TCD is a valuable adjunct to neurological assessment especially in patients with a high risk of DCI (poor Fisher grade). High mean FV recordings may prompt the need for further imaging (CT angiogram or cerebral angiography). In patients with a demonstrable stenosis who have failed to respond to medical management (triple-H therapy) endovascular treatment (intra-arterial vasodilators and/or angioplasty) may be appropriate.
>
> (continued)

> **CT imaging in DCI**
>
> CT imaging should be instituted wherever there is delayed cerebral deterioration.
>
> Non-contrast head CT should be the initial evaluation in patients with a change in neurological status following SAH and/or TCD findings suggestive of DCI. In the absence of any other causes accounting for deterioration CT angiography (highly sensitive for severe vasospasm) and CT perfusion or cerebral angiography should be performed.

Discussion

The annual incidence of SAH in most populations is 10–16 cases per 100,000 population, with higher incidences seen in Finland and Japan. The incidence of SAH increases with age (mean age 55 years) and it has a female:male ratio of 3:2 [26].

The presentation of sudden onset, explosive ('worst ever') headache, lasting for more than an hour, remains a cardinal but non-specific feature in the diagnosis of SAH [27]. A period of unconsciousness occurs in almost half of patients with SAH, with one-third developing neurological deficits and 70% presenting with vomiting. There is no single sign or symptom pathognomonic of SAH. Headache is one of the most frequently reported symptoms in emergency departments; in one study 12% patients presenting with SAH were misdiagnosed [28]. Migraine was the most common incorrect diagnosis. Neurological complications occurred in 39% of these patients before they were correctly diagnosed (including re-bleeding in 21%). Misdiagnosis was more common in those who presented in good condition and was associated with increased morbidity and mortality. Seventy-three per cent of the misdiagnosed patients had not had CT. CT is therefore mandatory in all such presentations of headache, even with mild symptoms, to be followed by an LP delayed until at least 12 h post ictus if the CT is negative [29].

Outcome following SAH remains poor with a mortality rate of about 50% and an estimated 30% of survivors suffering moderate-to-severe neurological deficit. The major causes of mortality and morbidity associated with SAH are: death at time of bleed, re-bleeding (a significant number due to misdiagnosis), DCI and medical complications. An improvement in outcome from aneurysmal SAH will be brought about by: 1) identifying the cause of aneurysm formation, 2) lifestyle changes, 3) educating the public, 4) encouraging those with severe headache to attend hospital, 5) educating doctors to prevent misdiagnosis, the prevention of re-bleeding, and 6) reducing the incidence of DCI and medical complications.

Re-bleeding following SAH often occurs and, together with DCI, is the most frequently preventable cause of death in hospitalized patients. The risk is highest in the first 72 h (5–10% of patients) but particularly the first 24 h (5% of patients) following the ictus. Global brain oedema, hydrocephalus, hyponatraemia and seizures are more common after re-bleeding and contribute to the higher incidence of mortality and poor neurological outcome seen in this group of patients. Re-bleeding does not affect the incidence or timing of DCI [30].

The use of antifibrinolytics such as tranexamic acid has been shown to reduce the re-bleeding rate following SAH; however, their use is not generally recommended as studies on the use of antifibrinolytics demonstrated no outcome benefit, possibly due to an increased incidence of cerebral ischaemia [31, 32]. The only intervention shown to reduce the incidence of re-bleeding without adversely affecting outcome is early occlusion of the aneurysm, which remains the mainstay of treatment.

DCI (see Learning point, Delayed cerebral ischaemia) often results in infarction, and is a major cause of mortality and morbidity. The exact cause of DCI is unknown. Although arterial vasospasm is thought to play an important part, it has been recognized that only a proportion of patients with vasospasm will develop clinical symptoms of DCI, suggesting a more complex aetiology. Unfortunately, there has been little progress made in reducing the incidence of DCI. Although triple-H therapy may reverse the symptoms of DCI, the only treatment proven to reduce cerebral infarction and poor neurological outcome following SAH is nimodipine.

Medical complications of SAH occur frequently (pulmonary, cardiac, and electrolyte disturbances). Centres treating high volumes of patients with SAH have demonstrated reduced mortality and improved neurological outcome of patients with SAH. [2]. This may be due to increased access to neurointensivists in addition to neurovascular surgeons and interventional neuroradiologists.

✪ **Learning point**   Outcome following subarachnoid haemorrhage

The time-course of neurological and cognitive recovery after SAH is heterogeneous, with motor function recovering within the first 6 months and short-term memory being one of the last cognitive functions to recover.

Early indices of clinical outcome after SAH have been defined by the Glasgow Outcome Scale [33] and by modified Rankin Scores [34], both of which are specific to neurological disability and which are summarized in Tables 4.6 and 4.7, respectively.

Table 4.6 Glasgow Outcome Score [33]

Score	Definition
1	Dead
2	Vegetative state: unresponsive and unable to interact with environment
3	Severe disability: able to follow commands: unable to live independently
4	Moderate disability: able to live independently: unable to return to work/school
5	Good recovery: able to return to work or school

Reprinted from *The Lancet*, 305, 7905, Bryan Jennett and Michael Bond, 'Assessment of outcome after severe brain damage: a practical scale', pp. 480–484, Copyright 1975, with permission from Elsevier.

Table 4.7 Modified Rankin Score [34]

Score	Definition
0	No symptoms
1	No significant disability: able to carry out usual activities despite symptoms
2	Slight disability: able to look after own affairs, but unable to carry out all previous activities
3	Moderate disability: requires some help but able to walk unaided
4	Moderately severe disability: unable to attend to own bodily needs
5	Severe disability: requires 24 h nursing care
6	Dead

Reproduced from J C van Swieten, et al., 'Interobserver agreement for the assessment of handicap in stroke patients', Stroke, 19, 5, pp. 604–607, Copyright 1988, with permission from the American Heart Association.
Overall, 'poor' outcomes following SAH are: Glasgow Outcome Score 1–3, or Rankin Score 4–6.

A Final Word from the Expert

Aneurysmal SAH is a medical emergency that is frequently misdiagnosed. It continues to be a life-threatening condition. Approximately 10% patients with SAH die before reaching hospital from either catastrophic brain injury related to the haemorrhage or arrhythmia. The overall 30-day mortality rate is 45% with most of the in-hospital deaths attributable to re-bleeding or to DCI. An estimated one-third of survivors remain moderately-to-severely disabled. Early diagnosis of SAH and transfer to a specialist neurosurgical centre are essential. The priorities of management are to reduce the incidence of re-bleeding by early aneurysm occlusion (coiling or clipping) and to minimize the morbidity and mortality caused by delayed neurological deterioration (including hydrocephalus, electrolyte abnormalities, cerebral oedema and DCI) and other medical complications by their prompt recognition and treatment. Research continues in the area of aneurysmal SAH; more clinical trials are needed to provide evidence-based guidelines for the optimal management of this group of patients, most notably the prevention of re-bleeding, and the diagnosis and management of DCI (which account for the greatest mortality and morbidity following aneurysmal SAH).

The mortality from SAH has decreased in the last four decades, which many attribute to improved diagnosis (following the widespread introduction of CT and catheter angiography), early and improved aneurysm occlusion techniques, the introduction of nimodipine, and better management of medical complications.

References

1. Drake CG, Hunt WE, Sano K, Kassell N, Teasdale G, Pertuiset B. Report of a World Federation of Neurological Surgeons Committee on a universal subarachnoid haemorrhage grading scale. *J Neurosurg* 1988;68:985–6.
2. Consensus Conference on Neurovascular Services Executive Summary on Management of Subarachnoid Haemorrhage. London: British Society of Neuroradiology; October 2005. < http://www.bsnr.org.uk/guidelines/resources/Consensus_Conference_Summary.pdf >
3. Ferguson C. Guideline for the management of lone acute severe headache. London: College of Emergency Medicine; December 2009. < http://www.collemergencymed.ac.uk/Shop-Floor/Clinical%20Guidelines/ >
4. Hunt WE, Hess RM. Surgical risk as related to time of intervention in the repair of intracranial aneurysms. *J Neurosurg* 1968;28:14–20.
5. Fisher CM, Kistler JP, Davis JM. Relation of cerebral vasospasm to subarachnoid haemorrhage visualized by computerised tomographic scanning. *Neurosurgery* 1980;6:1–9.
6. Pickard JD, Murray GD, Illingworth R, *et al.* Effect of oral nimodipine on cerebral infarction and outcome after subarachnoid haemorrhage: British aneurysm nimodipine trial. *Br Med J* 1989;298:636–42.
7. Lord AS, Fernandez L, Schmidt JM, *et al.* Effect of rebleeding on the course and incidence of vasospasm after subarachnoid hemorrhage. *Neurology* 2012;78:31–7.
8. Diringer MN, Bleck TP, Hemphill JC, *et al.* Critical care management of patients following aneurysmal subarachnoid hemorrhage: recommendations from the Neurocritical Care Society's Multidisciplinary Consensus Conference. *Neurocrit Care* 2011;15:211–40.
9. Molyneux AJ, Kerr RS, Yu LM, *et al.* International subarachnoid aneurysm trial (ISAT) of neurosurgical clipping versus endovascular coiling in 2143 patients with ruptured intracranial aneurysms: a randomised comparison of effects on survival, dependency, seizures, rebleeding, subgroups, and aneurysm occlusion. *Lancet* 2005;366:809–17.

10. Valee JN, Aymard D, Vicaut E, Reis M, Merland JJ. Endovascular treatment of basilar tip aneurysms with guglielmi detachable coils: predictors of immediate and long-term results with multivariate analysis—6-year experience. *Radiology* 2003;226:867–79.

11. Priebe HJ. Aneurysmal subarachnoid haemorrhage and the anaesthetist. *Br J Anaesth* 2007;99:102–18.

12. Varma MK, Price K, Jayakrishnan V, Manickam B, Kessell G. Anaesthetic considerations for interventional neuroradiology. *Br J Anaesth* 2007;99:75–85.

13. Ro B, Reul J. World Federation of Interventional and Therapeutic Neuroradiology. *Guidelines for peri- and intra-procedural anticoagulation and antiaggregation.* < http://www.wfitn.org/Anticoagulation-Protocols/guidelines-for-peri-and-intra-procedural-a nticoagulation-and-antiaggregation.html >

14. Luo CB, Teng M-H, Chang FC, Lin CJ, Guo WY, Chang CY. Intraprocedure aneurysm rupture in embolization: clinical outcome with imaging correlation. *J Chinese Med Assoc* 2012;75:281–5.

15. Wartenberg KE, Schmidt JM, Claassen J, *et al.* Impact of medical complications on outcome after subarachnoid hemorrhage. *Crit Care Med* 2006;34:617–23.

16. Gregory T, Smith M. Cardiovascular complications of brain injury. *Cont Educn Anaesth Crit Care Pain* 2012;12:67–71.

17. Davison DL, Terek M, Chawla LS. Neurogenic pulmonary edema. *Crit Care* 2012;16:212–19.

18. van der Bilt IA, Hasan D, Vandertop WP, *et al.* Impact of cardiac complications on outcome after aneurysmal subarachnoid hemorrhage: a meta-analysis. *Neurology* 2009;72:635–42.

19. Peets A, Zygun D. Electrolyte disorders. In: Gupta A, Gelb A editors. *Essentials of neuroanaesthesia and neurointensive care.* London: Saunders; 2008. p. 241–6.

20. Rabinstein AA, Friedman JA, Weigand SD, *et al.* Predictors of cerebral infarction in aneurysmal subarachnoid hemorrhage. *Stroke* 2004;35:1862–6.

21. Dorhout Mees SM, on behalf of the MASH-II study group. Magnesium in aneurysmal subarachnoid hemorrhage (MASH II) phase III clinical trial. *Int J Stroke* 2008;3:63–5.

22. Origitano TC, Wascher TM, Reichman OH, Anderson DE. Sustained increased cerebral blood flow with prophylactic hypertensive hypervolemic hemodilution ("triple-H" therapy) after subarachnoid hemorrhage. *Neurosurgery* 1990;27:729–39.

23. Sen J, Belli A, Albon H, *et al.* Triple-H therapy in the management of aneurysmal subarachnoid haemorrhage. *Lancet* 2003;2:614–21.

24. Dhar R, Allyson Z, Videen TO, *et al.* Red blood cell transfusion increases cerebral oxygen delivery in anemic patients with subarachnoid hemorrhage. *Stroke* 2009;40:3039–44.

25. Naidech AM, Drescher J, Ault ML, Shaibani A, Batjer HH, Alberts MJ. Higher hemoglobin is associated with less cerebral infarction, poor outcome, and death after subarachnoid haemorrhage. *Neurosurgery* 2006;59:775–9.

26. Linn FH, Rinkel GJ, Algra A, van Gijn J. Incidence of subarachnoid haemorrhage: role of region, year, and rate of computed tomography: a meta analysis. *Stroke* 1996;27:625–9.

27. Linn FH, Rinkel GJ, Algra A, van Gijn J. Headache characteristics in subarachnoid haemorrhage and benign thunderclap headache. *J Neurol Neurosurg Psychiatry* 1998;65:791–3.

28. Kowalski RG, Claassen J, Kreiter KT, et al. Initial misdiagnosis and outcome after subarachnoid haemorrhage. *J Am Med Assoc* 2004;291:866–9.

29. Van der Wee N, Rinkel GJ, Hasan D, van Gijn J. Detection of subarachnoid haemorrhage on early CT: is lumbar puncture still needed after a negative scan? *J Neurol Neurosurg Psychiatry* 1995;58:357–9.

30. Harrod C, Bendok BR, Batjer HH. Prediction of cerebral vasospasm in patients presenting with aneurysmal subarachnoid haemorrhage: a review. *Neurosurgery* 2005;56:633–54.

31. Van Rossum J, Wintzen AR, Endtz LJ, Schoen JH, de Jonge H. Effect of tranexamic acid on rebleeding after subarachnoid hemorrhage: a double-blind controlled clinical trial. *Annals of Neurology* 1977;2:238–42.

32. Gaberel T, Magheru C, Emery E, Derlon JM. Antifibrinolytic therapy in the management of aneurysmal subarachnoid hemorrhage revisited. A meta-analysis. *Acta Neurochirurgica* 2012;154:1–9.

33. Jennett B, Snoek J, Bond MR, Brooks N. Disability after severe head injury: observations on the use of the Glasgow Outcome Scale. *J Neurol Neurosurg Psychiatry* 1981;44:285–93.

34. Van Swieten JC, Koudstaal PJ, Visser MC, Schouten HJA, van Gijn J. Interobserver agreement for the assessment of handicap in stroke patients. *Stroke* 1988;19:604–7.

4.2 Anaesthesia in the head-injured patient

Paul James

❝ Expert Commentary Iain Moppett
CPD Matrix Code: *2A02, 2F01, 2F03, 3A10, 3F00, 3C00*

Case history

An ambulance pre-alert call triggered the assembly of the trauma team to the emergency department resuscitation room of a tertiary neurosurgical referral centre with the imminent arrival of a 25-year-old Caucasian male. Injuries were sustained following a high-speed collision on his mountain bike with a tree. On scene the paramedics reported that he was initially combative and agitated, but rapidly deteriorated while in transit.

On arrival in the emergency department the patient was assessed by the trauma team in accordance with a framework set out in the *Advanced trauma life support* manual, following an ABC approach. The trauma team worked in parallel—the anaesthetist took responsibility for airway and breathing management; an orthopaedic trainee was responsible for gaining intravenous access and taking bloods; one emergency department nurse attached monitoring while another acted as scribe to ensure that all details were recorded. The trauma team leader directed and co-ordinated the team members as necessary.

On assessment of the patient there were signs of intermittent upper airway obstruction. The cervical spine was immobilized with a hard, close-fitting cervical collar, blocks and tape. Breathing was laboured with a respiratory rate of 8, but chest movement was symmetrical. Auscultation of his chest revealed transmitted upper airway noise; no clinical evidence of chest trauma was found. Peripheral oxygen saturation was 95 % with 15 L/min oxygen inspired via a non-rebreathing facemask. Non-invasive BP was 102/47 mmHg with a MAP of 65 mmHg, and pulse rate 108 beats/min. GCS was calculated as 7/15 (eyes 1, voice 2, and motor response 4). The patient's pupils were examined and the left was found to be dilated and sluggishly responsive to light, the right more responsive and less dilated. There were obvious signs of external head trauma with a large left frontal laceration, periorbital swelling and ecchymosis. Blood glucose was 8.4 mmol/L on finger-prick testing.

❝ Expert comment

The history is very important in trauma. Always try to ensure that as much information as possible is obtained from the ambulance crew.

❝ Expert comment

A significant number of patients with traumatic brain injury (TBI) 'talk and die' which offers hope that it may be possible to lessen the consequences of the primary injury.

❝ Expert comment

TBI is often associated with significant extracranial injuries; around 1 in 20 patients with severe TBI have cervical spine injury, usually at higher levels (occiput to C3). While severity of brain injury is the major factor determining death in around one-third of patients with major trauma, safe and expectant management of the cervical spine is mandatory to avoid causing avoidable spinal cord injury.

❝ Expert comment

Hypotension, hypoxia and hyperglycaemia are all associated with a worsened outcome following TBI. On arrival this patient is not significantly hypotensive or hypoxic, but the presence of localizing pupillary signs and a low GCS are strongly suggestive of intracerebral mass effect.

✪ Learning point Prehospital airway management

Early recognition of impending airway compromise is essential to preventing secondary brain injury. Prehospital airway management may be required. NCEPOD [1] reported that one in eight trauma patients arrived to hospital with partially or completely obstructed airways. The report also highlighted unsatisfactory airway management in 7% of cases. Intubation remains the gold standard, but there may be a role for supraglottic airways in the prehospital environment [2] or in the difficult airway scenario. In the emergency department the rate of difficult intubation may be as high as 8.5% [3].

Large-bore venous access was obtained in the right antecubital fossa and bloods were taken for full blood count, urea and electrolytes, clotting screen, 'group and screen' and a venous blood gas. There were no other obvious signs of external injury. The patient was estimated to weigh 85 kg. In light of the impending complete airway compromise, depressed GCS, and the clinical signs of raised ICP the decision was made to secure his airway, institute rescue measures to reduce presumed intracranial hypertension, and arrange urgent brain imaging.

✪ Learning point Indications for CT head scan following traumatic head injury

UK guidelines recommend an urgent CT head scan be performed for any patient with traumatic head injury and a presenting GCS of ≤12. For patients with GCS ≥13, a CT head scan may still be indicated if other clinical features are present (Table 4.8).

Table 4.8 Indications for CT head scan following traumatic head injury: SIGN and NICE guidance [4]

GCS	SIGN guidelines	NICE guidelines
15	• Age >65 years and loss of consciousness or amnesia • Retrograde amnesia >30 min • Clinical evidence of a skull fracture • Any seizure • Dangerous mechanism of injury or significant assault • Anticoagulation	• Age >65 years • Coagulopathy • Dangerous mechanism of injury (motor vehicle vs pedestrian, fall from height >1 m or >5 steps)
13–14	• No improvement within 1 h of clinical observation or 2 h of injury	• At 2 h after head injury in the emergency department
13–15	• Base of skull or depressed skull fracture • Suspected penetrating injuries • Deteriorating consciousness • New focal neurological signs • A history of coagulopathy with loss of consciousness, amnesia or any neurological feature • Severe and persistent headache • Two distinct episodes of vomiting	• Suspected open skull fracture or depressed fracture • Post-traumatic seizure • Any signs of basal skull fracture • Focal neurological deficit • More than one episode of vomiting • 30 min amnesia

NICE, National Institute for Health and Care Excellence; SIGN, Scottish Intercollegiate Guidelines Network. Reproduced with permission from 'Guideline 110 Early Management of Patients with Acute Head Injury', 2009, SIGN, and National Institute for Health and Clinical Excellence (2007) Adapted from 'CG56 Head injury: Triage, assessment, investigation and early management of head injury in infants, children and adults', London: NICE. Available from http://guidance.nice.org.uk/CG56.

✪ Learning point Intracranial pressure (ICP)

ICP is the pressure exerted on the cerebral tissues, and is related to the volume of the constituents within the skull (brain, blood, and CSF). Once identified, raised ICP must be aggressively treated; sustained ICP >20 mmHg is associated with worsened neurological outcome [5]. Those patients showing a response to treatment for raised ICP have a significant reduction in the risk of death compared with those who do not [6].

Following 3 min of preoxygenation, anaesthesia was induced with alfentanil 30 microgram/kg, thiopentone 3 mg/kg, and suxamethonium 1.5 mg/kg.

The neck collar was removed prior to induction of anaesthesia and airway management with manual in-line stabilization substituted until intubation was complete. Cricoid pressure was applied, and tracheal intubation followed the cessation of fasciculation. His airway was secured with a size 8 cuffed tracheal tube. Once tracheal tube position was confirmed clinically and with end-tidal carbon dioxide monitoring, intermediate-acting neuromuscular blockade (atracurium 50 mg) was given to prevent coughing and facilitate ventilation. Sedation was started with a propofol infusion. The tracheal tube was secured with tape to avoid venous obstruction and the patient's trolley placed in reverse Trendelenburg at 30°. Given the clinical signs of raised ICP, urgent neurosurgical advice was sought. The on-call neurosurgical registrar suggested immediate measures to reduce ICP and urgent imaging. Mannitol 0.5 g/kg was given intravenously and the patient prepared for transfer for urgent CT. Ventilation with the transfer ventilator was set to achieve an end-tidal carbon dioxide of between 4.0 and 5.0 kPa. The right radial artery was cannulated to establish intra-arterial BP monitoring, initial BP 108/51 mmHg (MAP 66). Appropriate bolus doses of vasopressor (metaraminol) were used to maintain an estimated CPP of between 50 and 70 mmHg (i.e. MAP 70–90 mmHg assuming an ICP of 20 mmHg). Arterial blood gas analysis was performed to confirm concordance with arterial carbon dioxide tension. Inspired oxygen was titrated to maintain peripheral oxygen saturations of > 95 %.

⊕ **Clinical tip**   Spinal injury

All patients requiring urgent tracheal intubation following a head injury should be considered to have a full stomach. Securing the airway invariably requires a rapid sequence induction. They must also be presumed to have an underlying cervical spine injury until definitive imaging is obtained. The incidence of cervical injury is greater in those involved in motor vehicle-related trauma, or those with an initial GCS ≤8 [8]. Patients presenting with significant head injury may also have multiple other injuries.

✪ **Learning point**   Induction agents

No consensus exists as to the ideal induction agent for the head-injured patient and there has been no demonstrable effect of specific anaesthetic agents on outcome following head injury. It is important to appreciate the different pharmacodynamic and pharmacokinetic properties. In deciding which agent to use it remains pertinent to consider:

- avoidance of increases in ICP during airway manipulation
- preservation of adequate CPP
- preservation of normal cerebral autoregulation

Thiopentone, propofol and etomidate all decrease ICP, $CMRO_2$ and CBF [9]. 'Propofol may also have free radical scavenging and anti-inflammatory properties' [10].

Ketamine is emerging as an attractive option, partly because it causes limited compromise to the cardiovascular system. It has long been avoided due to an association with increased CBF and increased ICP. However, a recent review [11] points to safe use under conditions of controlled ventilation with co-administration of a γ-aminobutyric acid receptor agonist (e.g. benzodiazepines). In laboratory findings [12] ketamine has neuroprotective properties, and 'S(+)-ketamine additional neuroregenerative effects, even when administered after onset of a cerebral insult' [11].

In practice, the safest agent to use is probably the one with which the anaesthetist is most familiar. The emergency department is not a good place to start trying out new techniques.

✪ **Learning point**   Avoiding hypotension

At all times measures should be taken to avoid hypotension. CPP = MAP – ICP. There is overwhelming evidence that, at any time, systolic BP <90 mmHg in the head-injured patient is significantly detrimental:

- In 717 cases reviewed from the Traumatic Coma Data Bank [13], hypotension was associated with a 150% increase in mortality.
- The occurrence of intraoperative hypotension has been shown to confer a threefold increase in mortality [14]. The duration of hypotension is directly correlated with worsened outcomes.
- Hypotension occurring late, such as on ICU, also carries a significant increase in mortality and morbidity [15].
- CPP should be maintained between 50 and 70 mmHg [16].

The patient was transferred to CT fully monitored. CT was performed revealing a large left-sided acute subdural haematoma (SDH) with significant midline shift (Figure 4.5). A minimally displaced linear right temporal bone fracture was also commented on. The cervical spine and thoracolumbar spine were imaged with helical CT at the same time. The whole spine was cleared later that day after a radiologist skilled in neuroradiology reported the images. On-site neurosurgical opinion was sought; after review of the images, the decision was made to emergently evacuate the haematoma.

❝ **Expert comment**

The debate continues over clearing the cervical spine in obtunded patients. Caution is well-founded given that an incorrectly treated cervical spine injury may lead to significant morbidity. Equally, inflicting prolonged immobilization until a patient is 'awake' carries significant risks (pressure sores, raised ICP [17, 18], airway access problems, difficult central venous access, and increased staff demands for log rolling). Guidelines [19] and reviews of the available evidence [20, 21] exist with the general consensus that in these patients it is acceptable to clear the cervical spine with a helical CT scan reported by a radiologist skilled in musculoskeletal or neuroradiology. The role of routine MRI scanning of the cervical spine in obtunded trauma patients is unclear. The use of plain X-rays for clearing the thoracolumbar spine in obtunded trauma patients is now not advised in favour of CT [21].

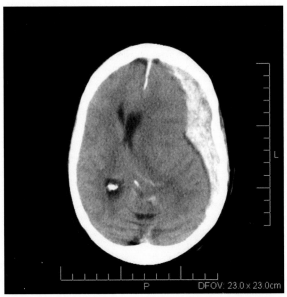

Figure 4.5 CT head showing a large left-sided acute, traumatic subdural haematoma and significant midline shift.

> ⭐ **Learning point** Indications for surgery in acute traumatic subdural haematoma
>
> Intracranial haemorrhage complicates severe TBI in 25–45% of cases. It is seen in 3–12% of moderate TBI and 1 in 500 patients with mild TBI [22].
>
> Indications for surgery in acute SDH [23] are as follows:
>
> - Acute SDH >10 mm thick and/or midline shift >5 mm regardless of GCS
> - GCS <9 with SDH of <10 mm or <5 mm midline shift if GCS has dropped by 2 points from injury or pupil signs
> - Evacuation should occur as soon as possible when surgical indications are met

> ➕ **Clinical tip** Pupil size
>
> Regular assessment and documentation of pupil size and reactivity is important in diagnosing clinical deterioration.

Full monitoring was retained and the patient transferred directly from the CT scanner to the neurosurgical theatre. On arrival in theatre the patient was transferred to the operating table, and placed on the theatre ventilator. Ventilator settings were adjusted to maintain an end-tidal carbon dioxide of around 4.5 kPa; an arterial blood gas sample was taken at the time to confirm concordance with arterial carbon dioxide tension.

> ⭐ **Learning point** Ventilation in traumatic brain injury
>
> - Avoidance of hypoxia is crucial, and inspired oxygen concentration should be titrated to maintain an arterial oxygen saturation >90% (PaO_2 >60 mmHg/8.0 kPa) at all times [24].
> - Hypercapnia induces cerebral vasodilatation. In the injured brain this can lead to a significant increase in ICP and subsequent reduction in cerebral perfusion.
> - Current UK guidance suggests maintaining $PaCO_2$ between 4.5 and 5.0 kPa [25]. Once a mainstay of cerebral resuscitation, hyperventilation and subsequent hypocapnia have been proven to lead to cerebral vasoconstriction and worsening perfusion. Hyperventilation should therefore be avoided routinely [26].
> - Hyperventilation use should be reserved for short-term control of ICP or briefly to aid surgical exposure. In the event of prolonged hyperventilation, cerebral oxygenation monitoring should be employed.

Propofol sedation was stopped, sevoflurane started aiming for an end-tidal concentration equating to 0.8 minimum alveolar concentration (MAC) and a remifentanil target-controlled infusion (50 µg/mL) started at target effect-site concentration of 4 ng/mL.

★ Learning point Maintenance of anaesthesia (Table 4.9)

It is widely acknowledged that volatile agents reduce $CMRO_2$. As a consequence of cerebral vasodilatation CBF and ICP are elevated. These effects can be attenuated with concentration <1 MAC.

Total intravenous anaesthetic (TIVA) techniques, usually propofol with a short-acting opioid, reduce CBF, ICP, and $CMRO_2$. Techniques for neuroanaesthesia with either TIVA, inhalational agents or a mixture of the two have been described. Despite the differences, there is no evidence that anaesthetic technique is an independent factor in intraoperative brain swelling in neurosurgery [27].

The use of nitrous oxide is controversial. It has been linked to elevated ICP, increased CBF, increased $CMRO_2$ and impairment of cerebral autoregulation [28], but none of these effects has been shown to be important in clinical practice, where the concomitant use of other agents influences the effects of nitrous oxide [29, 30].

Remifentanil has emerged as a useful agent in neuroanaesthesia. Its nature as a potent, rapidly acting opioid renders it adept at reducing the pressor response to highly stimulating insults (such as surgery or tracheal suctioning). Its effects on cerebral autoregulation and carbon dioxide reactivity are neutral [31]. Provided arterial carbon dioxide is controlled it has little effect on CBF [32].

Table 4.9 Effects of anaesthetic agents on cerebral physiology

Agent	Intracranial pressure	Cerebral blood flow	Cerebral metabolic requirement for oxygen	Other effects
Propofol	↓	↓	↓	Maintains or improves cerebral autoregulation
Etomidate	↓	↓	↓	Adrenal suppression Maintains systemic haemodynamic stability
Thiopentone	↓	↓	↓	
Ketamine	↑	↑	↔	Maintains systemic haemodynamic stability More recent evidence has prompted a reappraisal of the potential usefulness of ketamine
Remifentanil	↔	↔ (provided $PaCO_2$ is controlled)	↔	
Isoflurane	↑	↑	↓	Changes are dose dependent, especially above 1.5 MAC
Sevoflurane	↑	↑	↓	
Desflurane	↑	↑	↓	

Further neuromuscular blockade was given and a nerve stimulator was placed to monitor neuromuscular function. A second 14G cannula was sited and an infusion of Hartmann's solution was started slowly. The patient's scalp was infiltrated with lidocaine and adrenaline and he was then prepped and draped ready for surgery. Just prior to commencement of surgery, remifentanil target-controlled infusion was increased to 6 ng/mL until the dura was exposed. It was subsequently titrated to maintain systolic BP and MAP within desired limits. The patient underwent a left frontoparietal craniotomy (Figure 4.6).

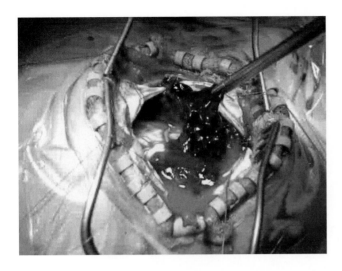

Figure 4.6 Craniotomy and removal of subdural haematoma.

Following evacuation of the haematoma a subdural pressure device was inserted and connected to a monitor for ongoing measurement of ICP to guide management on the neurointensive care unit. Pupils were examined and found to be equal and reactive to light. The patient was transferred from the operating theatre to the ICU.

Upon arrival to ICU he was sedated with propofol and alfentanil following the unit protocols. Ventilation was continued to maintain desired arterial carbon dioxide tension monitored by regular blood gas analysis. A right-sided subclavian central line was inserted. The patient was subsequently maintained in 30° head-up position.

Seventy minutes after arrival, ICP suddenly rose to 29 mmHg accompanied by a dilated unreactive right pupil. An arterial blood gas was checked, and arterial carbon dioxide tension was found to be 4.8 kPa with a satisfactory oxygen tension. BP started to fall and a vasopressor (noradrenaline) was commenced. ICP remained high, prompting further treatment. Boluses of propofol were given to little effect, followed by a bolus dose of atracurium. An atracurium infusion was then started with peripheral nerve stimulation monitoring, aiming for deep neuromuscular block with a depth of less than two twitches on train of four. A further dose of mannitol (0.5 mg/ kg) was also administered.

With the raised ICP not responding to rescue therapies, emergent CT scanning was organized after discussion with the neurosurgical team. He was transferred with rescue measures ongoing. CT scan revealed a large right temporal extradural haematoma with significant midline shift along with evidence of the prior surgery. He was rapidly transferred directly back to theatre for further evacuation of the haematoma.

⊗ **Learning point**   Management of intracranial hypertension

Intracranial hypertension is common following TBI, with diffuse tissue swelling often precipitating further secondary insults. The potential for re-bleeding must always be considered and access to emergent CT scanning is vital.

Current treatment of uncontrolled intracranial hypertension is undergoing intensive scrutiny. Standard medical therapy aims to reduce ICP through adherence to the basic principles of all

(continued)

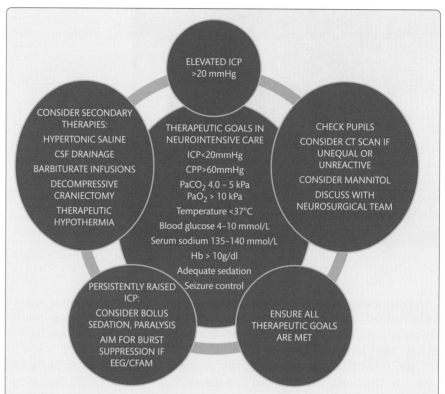

Figure 4.7 Therapeutic goals and schematic for the treatment of elevated intracranial pressure (ICP) in neurointensive care. CSF, cerebrospinal fluid; CPP, cerebral perfusion pressure; CT, computed tomography; EEG, electroencephalogram; CFAM, cerebral function analysis monitor. Data from Guidelines for the Management of Severe Traumatic Brain Injury, Third Edition, Brain Trauma Foundation. https://www.braintrauma.org/pdf/protected/Guidelines_Management_2007w_bookmarks.pdf.

neuroanaesthesia: avoidance of secondary insults and optimizing cerebral perfusion (Figure 4.7). Using sedation reduces the cerebral metabolic demand and facilitates ventilation for control of arterial carbon dioxide tension. The aim of paralysis is to avoid coughing or straining which may raise the ICP. Deep sedation with barbiturates finds its roots nearly 50 years ago. In various studies it has been shown to reduce cerebral metabolism. Despite this, the Cochrane review [33] reveals there is no conclusive evidence that barbiturate therapy improves outcomes. Hypotension, offsetting or even worsening the positive effects of barbiturates on CPP, can occur in up to 25% of patients [33].

Close liaison with surgical colleagues is paramount. Prompt recognition of mass lesions and expedient evacuation are the most effective measures for ICP control. Surgical management is also an option for intractable intracranial hypertension, especially if the first-tier therapy has failed. Decompressive craniectomies have been used in TBI patients, with a wide range of outcomes. High-quality (level I) positive evidence, however, remains elusive. The most recent evidence comes from the Decompressive Craniectomy in Diffuse Traumatic Brain Injury (DECRA) trial [34]. They reported on 155 patients randomized either to standard therapy or to bitemporal decompressive craniectomy. Encouraging results on ICP control and length of ventilation-days and ICU stay are tempered by worsened long-term outcomes in the surgical group. The Randomised Evaluation of Surgery with Craniectomy for Uncontrollable Elevation of Intra-Cranial Pressure (RESCUE-ICP) trial is seeking to clarify the position of surgery in these patients, investigating decompressive surgery versus optimal medical therapy. Recruitment is ongoing and the results are awaited.

⑥ Expert comment

Although monitoring of ICP has not of itself been shown to be of benefit, the outcomes in units which use it as part of their brain injury protocol are better than those that do not. The choice of monitoring device is dependent on the surgeon and the patient. EVDs have the advantage that CSF can be removed therapeutically, but are more invasive than ICP sensors ('bolts') which can be inserted at the bedside in critical care.

> **⊗ Learning point**   Pathophysiology of traumatic brain injury
>
> Classically this has been divided into two distinct periods:
>
> - The *primary injury* represents the direct mechanical damage, subjecting the brain tissue to shearing and compressive forces. The resulting cascade of neurodestructive events is prompted by physical destruction of cell membranes, and loss of ionic homeostasis, causing inflammation, neuronal swelling and hypoperfusion [35, 36]. Little can be done therapeutically to influence this.
> - The *secondary injury* is the consequence of further physiological insults, such as hypoperfusion and hypoxia, to already 'at-risk' brain tissue. Techniques that prevent secondary brain injury form the tenets of anaesthesia care for the head-injured patient.

> **⊗ Learning point**   Hyperosmolar therapies
>
> There remains controversy as to the most effective hyperosmolar therapy. Hypertonic saline and mannitol have both been shown to aid reduction in ICP. Randomized trials have suggested that hypertonic saline solutions may be superior to mannitol. This view is supported by Cochrane review [37] and meta-analysis [38] but as yet no definitive answer from a large, multicentre, randomized controlled trial exists.

> **⊗ Learning point**   Glycaemic control
>
> Hyperglycaemia following head injury is associated with an increase in morbidity and mortality: 'Any episode of hyperglycaemia ($\geq$11.1 mmol/L or 200 mg/dL) is associated with 3.6-fold increased risk of hospital mortality in patients with severe TBI' [39]. Elevated plasma glucose leads to an increase in glycolysis, resulting in 'metabolic acidosis within brain parenchyma, overproduction of reactive oxygen species and ultimately neuronal cell death' [40]. Avoidance of hypoglycaemia is of course equally important. There is currently little evidence addressing the specific issue of perioperative glycaemic control in the head-injured patient; extrapolating data from other areas of practice (e.g. intensive care), it would seem prudent to maintain serum glucose <10 mmol/L [41].

Discussion

Head injury is the leading worldwide cause of mortality in patients aged < 45 years. The most frequent causes of head injury are falls and motor vehicle collisions. In the UK it is estimated that roughly one million people attend emergency departments with head injury per year [42]. Up to 10% of these are classified as moderate or severe (GCS < 12 and < 9, respectively). In data extracted from the UK trauma audit research network, between 2005 and 2006, severe isolated TBIs carried a mortality of 23% [43]. Morbidity from head injury carries a large socio-economic burden. In one study [44] survival with moderate or severe disability was 47% following mild injury and similar to that after moderate (45%) or severe injury (48%). These statistics equate to an incidence of 100–150 per 100,000 (0.1–0.15%) population per year newly disabled young people and adults [44].

As understanding of brain injury expands, work is being directed to specific pathological processes. However, as yet there remains no therapeutic panacea. Current focus of research is the effect of therapeutic hypothermia on outcomes following head injury. It has been found to 'reduce cerebral metabolism, reduce excitatory neurotransmitter release, and attenuate changes in blood–brain permeability' [45]. Definitive evidence of benefit remains hard to pin down, but ongoing large multicentre trials (e.g. Eurotherm 32–35) aim to finally answer the question.

This case illustrates the management of a patient with an isolated traumatic head injury, from admission to hospital to definitive surgical management. It highlights the fact that anaesthesia for the head-injured patient should focus on optimizing physiological variables, and minimizing secondary insult in the 'at-risk' brain [46]. Clinical diligence must be paid to the avoidance of hypoxia, hypotension, hypercapnia (and hypocapnia) and hyperglycaemia. The management of unexpected postoperative intracranial hypertension is discussed, and the need for early CT re-scanning is highlighted.

Applying these principles and the introduction of clinical guidelines (Table 4.10) has had a significant effect on outcomes following head injury.

Table 4.10 Summary of recommendations from the Brain Trauma Foundation [47]

Physiological parameter	Level of evidence	Recommendation
Blood pressure and oxygenation	I	–
	II	Avoid hypotension (SBP <90 mmHg)
	III	Oxygenation should be monitored. Avoid hypoxia (PaO_2 <60 mmHg or oxygen saturations <90%)
		Jugular venous saturations <50% or brain tissue oxygen tension <15 mmHg require treatment
Hyperosmolar therapy	I	–
	II	Mannitol is effective for control of raised ICP (0.25 g/kg to 1.0 g/kg)
	III	Use should be restricted to patients with progressive deterioration not attributable to extracranial cause
Prophylactic hypothermia	I	–
	II	
	III	Not significantly associated with reduced mortality compared with normothermic controls. May be associated with a reduction in mortality if cooling is for >48 h
Intracranial pressure monitoring	I	–
	II	ICP monitoring in all patients with GCS 3–8 and an abnormal CT scan
		ICP >20 mmHg should trigger treatment
	III	Indicated in TBI patients with a normal CT scan if two or more of the following exist: • age >40 years • unilateral or bilateral motor posturing, or • hypotension (SBP <90 mmHg)
Cerebral perfusion pressure	I	–
	II	Avoid aggressive measures to maintain CPP >70 mmHg (with fluids or vasopressor) to lessen the risk of adult respiratory distress syndrome (ARDS)
	III	Avoid CPP <50 mmHg
Hyperventilation	I	–
	II	Hyperventilation ($PaCO_2$ <25 mmHg) is not recommended
	III	Hyperventilation should be avoided in the first 24 h following TBI. If hyperventilation is used, jugular venous oxygen saturations or brain tissue oxygen tension measurements are recommended
Steroids	I	The use of steroids is not recommended for improving outcome or reducing raised ICP. High-dose methylprednisolone is associated with increased mortality.

Data from Brain Trauma Foundation, 'Guidelines for the management of severe traumatic brain injury', New York: BTF; 2007 https://www.braintrauma.org/pdf/protected/Guidelines_Management_2007w_bookmarks.pdf

A Final Word from the Expert

TBI is unfortunately still a widely occurring and devastating injury, particularly in young men. There is no magic bullet which 'cures' TBI. However, careful attention to detail throughout the patient's care will probably improve outcomes overall.

Important points to remember in managing these patients are:

1. TBI is often associated with other major injuries and these should be actively excluded/ managed during initial management.

2. Hypoxia and hypotension should be assiduously avoided as they are associated with worsened outcome.

3. Simple things are often overlooked which can make a difference such as head-up tilt, avoidance of venous compression and checking the blood glucose.

TBI is a team affair which necessitates good communication between ambulance personnel, emergency department, radiology, anaesthesia, theatres, neurosurgery and critical care. In the midst of this, it is easy to forget the relatives who will need someone to look after them too.

The outcome following TBI is slowly improving with reductions in the number of deaths and people left with significant injury, but it is still poor. Most of these improvements are believed to have come from better supportive care in ICU and adherence to carefully considered clinical protocols for management.

References

1. National Confidential Enquiry into Patient Outcome and Death (2007). *Trauma: who cares?* London: NCEPOD; 2007. < http://www.ncepod.org.uk/2007report2/Downloads/SIP_summary.pdf >

2. Hammell CL, Henning JD. Prehospital management of severe traumatic brain injury. *Br Med J* 2009;338:1262–6.

3. Fourth National Audit Project of the Royal College of Anaesthetists and Difficult Airway Society. Cook TM, Woodall N, Frerk C editors. *Major complications of airway management in the United Kingdom. Report and findings*. London: Royal College of Anaesthetists; March 2011. < http://www.rcoa.ac.uk/node/4211 >

4. National Institute for Health and Care Excellence. *Head injury: Triage, assessment, investigation and early management of head injury in infants, children and adults*. London: NICE; 2007. < http://publications.nice.org.uk/head-injury-cg56/guidance#assessment-and-investigation-in-the-emergency-department >

5. Ji-Yao Jiang, Guo-Yi Gao, Wei-Ping Li, Ming-Kun Yu, Cheng Zhu. Early indicators of prognosis in 846 cases of severe traumatic brain injury. *J Neurotrauma* 2002;19:869–74.

6 Farahvar A, Gerber LM, Chiu Y-L, *et al*. Response to intracranial hypertension treatment as a predictor of death in patients with traumatic brain injury. *J Neurosurgery* 2011;114:1471–8.

7. Association of Anaesthetists of Great Britain and Ireland. *Recommendations for the safe transfer of patients with brain injury*. London: AAGBI; 2006. < http://www.aagbi.org/sites/default/files/braininjury.pdf >

8. Holly LT, Kelly DF, Counelis GJ, Blinman T, McArthur DL, Cryer HG. Cervical spine trauma associated with moderate and severe head injury: incidence, risk factors, and injury characteristics. *J Neurosurg* 2002;96:285–91.

9. Turner BK, Wakim JH, Secrest J, Zachary R. Neuroprotective effects of thiopental, propofol, and etomidate. *AANA J* 2005;73:297–302.

10. Fukuda S, Warner DS. Cerebral protection. *Br. J. Anaesth.* 2007;99:10–17.

11. Himmelseher S, Durieux ME. Revising a dogma: ketamine for patients with neurological injury? *Anesth Analg* 2005;101:524–34.

12. Shapira Y, Lam AM, Engl CC, *et al.* Therapeutic time window and dose response of the beneficial effects of ketamine in experimental head injury. *Stroke* 1994;25:1637–43.

13. Chesnut RM, Marshall L, Klauber MR, *et al.* The role of secondary brain injury in determining outcome from severe head injury. *J Trauma* 1993;34:216–22.

14. Pietropaoli JA, Rogers FB, Shackford SR, Wald SL, Schmoker JD, Zhuang J. The deleterious effects of intraoperative hypotension on outcome in patients with severe head injuries. *J Trauma* 1992;33:403–7.

15. Chesnut RM, Marshall SB, Piek J, Blunt BA, Klauber MR, Marshall LF. Early and late systemic hypotension as a frequent and fundamental source of cerebral ischemia following severe brain injury in the Traumatic Coma Data Bank. *Acta Neurochir Suppl (Wien)* 1993;59:121–5.

16. Bratton SL, Chestnut RM, Ghajar J, *et al.* Brain Trauma Foundation; American Association of Neurological Surgeons; Congress of Neurological Surgeons; Joint Section on Neurotrauma and Critical Care, AANS/CNS. Guidelines for the management of severe traumatic brain injury blood pressure and oxygenation. *J Neurotrauma* 2007;24:S7–13.

17. Raphael JH, Chotai R. Effects of the cervical collar on cerebrospinal fluid pressure. *Anaesthesia* 1994;49:437–19.

18. Hunt K, Hallsworth S, Smith M. The effect of rigid collar placement on intracranial and cerebral perfusion pressure. *Anaesthesia* 2001;56:511–13.

19. Morris C, Guha A, Farquhar I. *Evaluation for spinal injuries among unconscious victims of blunt polytrauma: a management guideline for intensive care.* February 2005. < http://www.ics.ac.uk/EasysiteWeb/getresource.axd?AssetID = 479&type = full&servicetype = Attachment >

20. Morris CGT, McCoy E. Clearing the cervical spine in unconscious polytrauma victims, balancing risks and effective screening. *Anaesthesia* 2004;59:464–82.

21. Plumb JOM, Morris CG. Clinical review. Spinal imaging for the adult obtunded blunt trauma patient: update from 2004. *Intensive Care Med* 2012;38:752–71.

22. Bullock MR, Chesnut R, Ghajar J, *et al.* (Surgical Management of Traumatic Brain Injury Author Group). Surgical management of acute subdural hematomas. *Neurosurgery* 2006;58(3 Ch 1):S2-1–S2-3.

23. Bullock MR, Chesnut R, Ghajar J, *et al.* (Surgical Management of Traumatic Brain Injury Author Group). Surgical management of acute subdural hematomas. *Neurosurgery* 2006;58(3 Ch 3):S2-7–S2-15.

24. Bratton SL, Chesnut RM, Ghajar J, *et al.* Brain Trauma Foundation. Guidelines for the management of severe traumatic brain injury. I. Blood pressure and oxygenation. *J Neurotrauma* 2007;24:S14–20.

25. Association of Anaesthetists of Great Britain and Ireland. *Recommendations for the safe transfer of patients with brain injury.* London: AAGBI; May 2006.

26. Coles JP, Fryer TD, Coleman MR, *et al.* Hyperventilation following head injury; effects on ischemic burden and cerebral oxidative metabolism. *Crit Care Med* 2007;35:568–78.

27. Rasmussen M, Bundgaard H, Cold GE. Craniotomy for supratentorial brain tumors; risk factors for brain swelling after opening the dura mater. *J Neurosurg* 2004;101:621–6.

28. Hancock SM, Nathanson MH. Nitrous oxide or remifentanil for the "at risk" brain. *Anaesthesia* 2004;59:313–15.

29. Strebel S, Kaufman M, Baggi M, Zenklusen U. Cerebrovascular carbon dioxide reactivity during exposure to equipotent isoflurane and isoflurane in nitrous oxide anaesthesia. *Br J Anaesth* 1993;71:272–6.

30. Inaba S, Sato J, Aono M, Numata T, Nishino T. Combined effects of nitrous oxide and propofol on the dynamic cerebrovascular response to step changes in end tidal PCO_2 in humans. *Anesthesiology* 2003;98:633–8.

31. Ostapkovich ND, Baker KZ, Fogarty-Mack P, Sisti MB, Young WL. Cerebral blood flow and CO_2 reactivity is similar during remifentanil/N_2O and fentanyl/N_2O anesthesia. *Anesthesiology* 1998;89:358–63.

32. Engelhard K, Reeker W, Kochs E, Werner C. Effect of remifentanil on intracranial pressure and cerebral blood flow velocity in patients with head trauma. *Acta Anaesthesiol Scand* 2004;48:396–99.

33. Roberts I. Barbiturates for acute traumatic brain injury. *Cochrane Database Syst Rev* 2000;(2):CD000033.

34. Cooper J, Rosenfeld JV, Murray L, *et al.* Decompressive craniectomy in diffuse traumatic brain injury. *N Engl J Med* 2011;364:1493–1502.

35. Bouma GJ, Mulzelaar JP, Choi SC, Newlon PG, Young HF. Cerebral circulation and metabolism after severe traumatic brain injury;the elusive role of ischemia. *J Neurosurg* 1991;75:685–93.

36. Werner C, Engelhard K. Pathophysiology of traumatic brain injury. *Br J Anaesth* 2007;99:4–9.

37. Wakai A, Roberts IG, Schierhout G. Mannitol for acute traumatic brain injury. *Cochrane Database Syst Rev* 2007;(1):CD001049.

38. Kamel H, Navi BB, Nakagawa K, Hemphill JC 3rd, Ko NU. Hypertonic saline versus mannitol for the treatment of elevated intracranial pressure: a meta-analysis of randomized clinical trials. *Crit Care Med* 2011;39:554–9.

39. Griesdale DE, Tremblay MH, McEwen J, Chittock DR. Glucose control and mortality in patients with severe traumatic brain injury. *Neurocrit Care* 2009;11:311–16.

40. Zygun DA, Steiner LA, Johnston AJ, *et al.* Hyperglycemia and brain tissue pH after traumatic brain injury. *Neurosurgery* 2004;55:877–81; discussion 882.

41. Griesdale DE, Tremblay MH, McEwen J, Chittock DR. Glucose control and mortality in patients with severe traumatic brain injury. *Neurocrit Care* 2009;11:311–16.

42. van Dijk G. Head injury, the bare essentials. *Pract Neurol* 2011;11:50–5.

43. Gabbe BJ, Lyons RA, Lecky FE, *et al.* Comparison of mortality following hospitalisation for isolated head injury in England and Wales, and Victoria, Australia. *PLoS One* 6(5):e20545.

44. Thornhill S, Teasdale G, Murray G, *et al.* Disability in young people and adults one year after head injury: prospective cohort study. *Br Med J* 2000;320(7250):1631–5.

45. Curry P, Viernes D, Sharma D. Perioperative management of traumatic brain injury. *Int J Crit Illness Injury Sci* 2011;1:27–35.

46. Moppett IK. Traumatic brain injury: assessment, resuscitation and early management. *Br J Anaesth* 2007;99:18–31.

47. Brain Trauma Foundation. *Guidelines for the management of severe traumatic brain injury*. New York: BTF; 2007. < https://www.braintrauma.org/pdf/protected/Guidelines_Management_2007w_bookmarks.pdf >

CHAPTER 5

Obstetric anaesthesia

CASE

5.1 Obstetric haemorrhage: planning a safe delivery

Phoebe Syme

Expert Commentary David Bogod

CPD Matrix Code: *2B02, 2B03, 2B05, 3B00*

Case history

A 32-year-old, gravida 1, woman was referred to the obstetric anaesthetic department for preoperative assessment for caesarean section.

Her first delivery had been by emergency caesarean section due to fetal distress, and was conducted under epidural anaesthesia, with no reported surgical or anaesthetic complications. While under ultrasound surveillance for a low-lying placenta during her current pregnancy, she presented to obstetric services with painless vaginal blood loss at 33 weeks of gestation. There was no other medical or obstetric history. She was admitted for observation and monitoring, and prescribed intravenous steroids. During this time her haemoglobin and haemodynamic condition remained stable. The vaginal blood loss initially settled, but at 37 weeks two small-volume bleeds occurred over a period of 12 h. Her haemoglobin was stable at 11 g/dL. Her blood pressure was 122/70 and her heart rate 86 beats/min. No blood products were administered. A colour Doppler ultrasound done at 32 weeks of gestation had shown major placenta praevia with part in an anterior position but did not demonstrate abnormal placental adhesion (Figure 5.1). In view of this no further imaging was undertaken. Caesarean section was planned for the following morning. Consent was obtained for a caesarean section by the obstetric team and included full explanation of the bleeding risk, potential requirement for blood transfusion, invasive monitoring, intensive care admission and progression to hysterectomy as a life-saving procedure. After a full discussion of the anaesthetic options with the anaesthetic consultant, the patient chose to proceed with regional anaesthesia (RA) but understood that conversion to general anaesthesia (GA) was a possibility.

Learning point Causes of antepartum haemorrhage

Antepartum haemorrhage is defined as bleeding from the genital tract after the 24th week of pregnancy. Causes include:

- Placenta praevia: maternal haemorrhage (usually painless) from separation of a placenta implanted abnormally low in the uterus
- Placental abruption: maternal haemorrhage (often associated with abdominal pain) from abnormal separation of a normally placed placenta
- Vasa praevia (rare): fetal haemorrhage from abnormally located fetal vessels coursing through the membranes close to the cervical os
- Uterine rupture in women with previous caesarean section
- Local causes: vulval or cervical infection, trauma or tumour
- Heavy show

Clinical tip Anaemia

A physiological anaemia occurs in pregnancy as plasma volume increases to a greater extent than red cell mass. Other common causes of anaemia in pregnancy, including iron and folate deficiency, should be actively sought and treated.

❝ **Expert comment**

A fundamental aspect of this case is the need to plan for potential haemorrhage. Early involvement of the anaesthetic team allows for preoperative planning which starts with taking a detailed medical and obstetric history. When haemorrhage occurs it can be massive, both in volume and in rate, and requires a multidisciplinary approach to bleeding control and replacement of blood loss. All hospitals should have major haemorrhage protocols in place, specifying lines of communication and transfusion guidelines. The case requires attendance of anaesthetic and obstetric consultants, supported by other suitably senior trainees, alongside experienced midwifery staff. Cross-matched blood (4–6 units) should be present before starting the procedure, blood bank alerted, and senior haematology staff standing by. Transfusion services need to be warned if massive haemorrhage is suspected or occurs, and portering staff will be required promptly. An on-site high-dependency facility is a necessary prerequisite, and interventional radiology, if available, should be alerted.

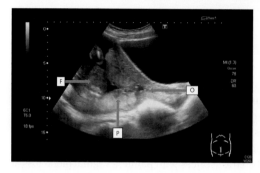

Figure 5.1 Ultrasound image of placenta praevia at 20 weeks of gestation showing a major placenta praevia (complete coverage of the os).
F, fetus; O, cervical os; P, placenta.

⭐ **Learning point** Definitions

Placenta praevia

A placenta inserted wholly or in part in the lower segment of the uterus. Major placenta praevia exists when the placenta covers the cervical os; otherwise the condition is described as a partial or minor placenta praevia [1].

Placenta accreta, increta, percreta

These terms describe a morbidly adherent placenta. A normal placenta will separate promptly following delivery along a natural cleavage plane along the decidua basalis of the uterus. The chorionic villi of the placenta may occasionally invade into the myometrium (placenta accreta). If invasion crosses the myometrium this is termed placenta increta. Percreta is the most severe form as the placenta invades through the endometrium, myometrium and beyond the uterine serosa. Involvement of the bladder or rectum is a risk with this variant. The term placenta accreta can be used to refer to all variants [1].

⭐ **Learning point** Imaging the placenta

All women who have had a previous caesarean section must have their placental site determined. This is a key recommendation from the 2003–2005 CEMACH report, Saving Mothers' Lives.

The chance of a placenta praevia being morbidly adherent rises rapidly with the number of previous caesarean sections. Normally 3%, the chance rises to 11% with one previous section, 40% with two, and 61% with three [2].

Further imaging using colour Doppler ultrasound or magnetic resonance imaging (MRI) is required to determine the presence of an abnormally inserted placenta.

In most situations requests for additional placental imaging using MRI are reserved for those with equivocal results on ultrasound scan. This decision is usually made by the obstetric team; however, the implications of failing to identify a morbidly adherent placenta are significant for the anaesthetic team as well.

> ### ✪ Learning point   Care bundles for high-risk caesarean section [1]
>
> The National Patient Safety Agency (NPSA) and Royal College of Obstetricians have described a 'care bundle' to be implemented during caesarean section for all cases of suspected placenta accreta. The care bundle is also recommended for cases of placenta praevia with a history of previous caesarean section (as in this case), or for cases of anterior placenta underlying a caesarean scar. The components of the bundle include:
>
> - consultant obstetrician planned and directly supervising delivery
> - consultant anaesthetist planned and directly supervising anaesthetic care at delivery
> - blood and blood products available
> - multidisciplinary involvement in preoperative planning
> - preoperative patient discussion and consent includes possible interventions (such as hysterectomy, leaving the placenta in place, cell salvage and interventional radiology)
> - local availability of a critical care bed

At nine o'clock the following morning the patient arrived for her elective caesarean section. In preparation for surgery the rapid transfusion and cell salvage equipment was primed.

In attendance were: a consultant obstetrician and consultant anaesthetist, a trainee from each specialty, a senior midwife and student, and the theatre team including an extra member of staff trained in cell salvage. The haematology laboratory and portering staff had been informed of the potential need for blood products. Four units of blood were cross-matched and transferred to the refrigerator in the delivery suite. A team brief using the World Health Organization checklist took place prior to the patient arriving, with further checks on arrival (anaesthetic sign in) and prior to the start of surgery (surgical time out).

> ### ✪ Learning point   Intraoperative cell salvage [3]
>
> Intraoperative cell salvage (ICS) allows re-transfusion of autologous blood, which previously would have been lost during the course of the operative procedure. Potential benefits include reducing anaemia, eliminating the inherent risks of allogeneic blood transfusion and reducing costs. The circuit contains a dual-lumen suction device, anticoagulant, filters, collection chamber, centrifuge, and saline washers (Figure 5.2). Concerns regarding the safety of cell salvage in obstetric practice focus on the inadvertent transfusion of amniotic fluid and fetal blood cells. Amniotic fluid contains proteolytic enzymes that can activate clotting when within the maternal circulation. Concerns over iatrogenic amniotic fluid embolism have not been borne out in practice, and the use of ICS during obstetric haemorrhage is recommended by the American Society of Anesthesiologists, the Centre for Maternal and Child Enquiries (CMACE), the National Institute for Health and Care Excellence, the Obstetric Anaesthetists Association, and the Association of Anaesthetists of Great Britain and Ireland. The reporting of maternal mortality via the CMACE and near miss data via the United Kingdom Obstetric Surveillance System (UKOSS) will continue to generate information regarding the safe use of ICS (see Learning point, UK Obstetric Surveillance System).
>
> The amniotic fluid load in the salvaged blood is reduced by using separate suction for the amniotic fluid and a LeukoGuard® RS filter (Pall Medical, Portsmouth, UK) in the blood-giving set. It should be noted that use of the leukocyte depletion filter limits the flow of salvaged blood (82 mL/min) compared to the 200 μm filter in a standard blood-giving set.
>
> Cell salvage equipment is unable to distinguish fetal from maternal red blood cells. In the situation of a Rhesus-negative mother with a Rhesus-positive fetus, the induction of maternal Rhesus antibodies by transfusion of fetal red blood cells has the potential to cause haemolytic disease of the newborn in future pregnancies. The risk is reduced by administration of Anti-D, which should be given after obstetric haemorrhage whether or not cell salvage is employed.
>
> (continued)

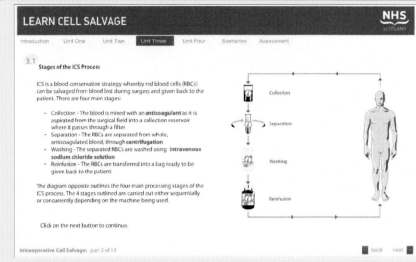

Figure 5.2 Stages of intraoperative cell salvage. E-learning module, Learn Cell Salvage, available (requires registration) via e-Learning for Healthcare: http://www.e-lfh.org.uk (Blood transfusion: Blood 07 – Learn Cell Salvage). Reproduced with permission from Better Blood Transfusion, SNBTS.

Salvaged blood contains red cells suspended in 0.9% saline (haematocrit: 50–70%). It is important to be aware that since only the red cell component is re-transfused correction of coagulopathy may still be required.

The transfusion of autologous blood should follow the same safety protocols as for allogeneic (donor) blood. The salvaged blood should be labelled with the patient identification data and an expiry time. The blood should be prescribed, and positive patient identification should be confirmed prior to transfusion. Salvaged blood should not be stored in the refrigerator but should be kept with the patient at all times.

The rising costs of allogeneic blood (about £125 per unit red cells) compared with the relatively low cost of the disposable element of the cell salvage machine (about £80) may result in considerable cost savings, but a trial including suitable economic evaluation is currently lacking.

Two large-bore (14G) cannulae were placed followed by a spinal anaesthetic using 0.5% levobupivacaine 2.5 mL and diamorphine 300 μg. A fluid co-load (1000 mL Hartmann's solution) and a phenylephrine infusion were commenced to offset the anticipated hypotension associated with spinal anaesthesia. After an appropriate block developed surgery began. A 2.4 kg baby was delivered uneventfully 12 min after knife to skin. An initial 5 units of oxytocin, given over 1 min, was followed with an oxytocin infusion running at 10 units/h.

> ✪ **Learning point** Choice of anaesthetic technique
>
> The choice of RA versus GA for caesarean section when there is high risk of significant haemorrhage is not fully resolved (Table 5.1). Many anaesthetists prefer GA when the risk of massive haemorrhage is increased, citing potential problems with hypotension from the sympathetic block induced by RA. Current evidence, however, indicates that RA is safe, but not superior to GA in placenta praevia. A retrospective survey of 350 cases of caesarean section for placenta praevia conducted over a 14-year period identified a 60% rate of RA, with just over 2% requiring conversion to GA [4]. The case-mix included both elective and emergency surgery, and seven cases of placenta accreta were diagnosed at
>
> (continued)

Table 5.1 Comparison of general and regional anaesthesia

General anaesthesia (GA)		Regional anaesthesia (RA)	
Pro	Con	Pro	Con
Avoids emergency conversion if surgery is prolonged or difficult or massive haemorrhage mandates a GA	Serious risks of GA (aspiration, allergy, failed intubation etc.)	Mother awake for the birth of her child enabling early feeding/bonding. Presence of partner	Risk of hypotension due to sympathetic block. This can be disastrous in an already hypovolaemic patient.
GA as the primary technique avoids excessive hypotension associated with the combination of sympathetic block from RA combined with GA	Increased requirement for postoperative opioid analgesia	Improved early postoperative analgesia	Single-shot spinal technique may not provide adequate block time if surgery is prolonged or complicated
	Increased postoperative nausea and vomiting	Avoids serious risks of GA, although conversion to GA is always a risk	Serious risks of RA (high block, nerve damage, etc.)

delivery. Of these seven, two had RA despite the requirement for peripartum hysterectomy. Although there is some evidence of an increased need for transfusion in patients who receive GA, this may reflect the more severe end of the spectrum as RA is converted to GA [4]. A combined spinal–epidural technique can be used to overcome concerns regarding the length of surgery.

It should be remembered that in an emergency situation, producing a sympathetic block in an already hypovolaemic patient by use of RA can be disastrous.

The anaesthesia for caesarean section when a placenta accreta has been diagnosed preoperatively has also been debated. Most in this situation would advocate a general anaesthetic technique since there is significant risk of massive haemorrhage with the possibility of progression to hysterectomy [5]. Authors of a Canadian case series, however, suggested that neuroaxial anaesthesia was an acceptable alternative. The series identified 23 cases of whom 17 primarily had RA; the rate of conversion to GA was high at nearly 30% [6].

Other factors influencing the decision between GA and RA include the urgency of surgery, likelihood of massive haemorrhage, presence of coagulopathy, haemodynamic instability, expected duration of surgery and the patient's wishes.

Whenever RA is chosen, conversion to GA may still be required if blood loss is excessive, if the patient is not coping, or if extensive intra-abdominal manipulation is required. Preparation should be made to undertake GA in a timely fashion, and for those patients where GA may prove complicated, early GA needs to be considered with adequate back-up plans in place.

The patient developed a tachycardia (110–125 bpm) following the oxytocin bolus; this was assumed to be a drug side-effect. Blood loss at this stage was estimated at 600 mL based on the blood in suction devices. A further 1000 mL of Hartmann's solution was infused over 10 min. Despite this the patient required increasing amounts of phenylephrine to maintain a systolic blood pressure above 90 mmHg. She became anxious and began to complain of nausea. This was communicated to the surgical team who requested pharmacological management for uterine atony. A further 5 unit dose of oxytocin was followed after 5 min by an intramuscular dose of ergometrine (500 μg). The surgical team informed the anaesthetic team that the uterus was atonic, and that the placenta was not delivered with standard cord traction. Blood loss was ongoing but after a further 2 min the surgeon was successful in finding a plane of cleavage and the placenta was delivered. At that stage the decidual bed appeared not to be bleeding. The diagnosis of placenta accreta was dismissed. Her haemoglobin was recorded at 7.9 g/dL on a point-of-care device. No near patient-testing for coagulation was available so blood samples were sent to the laboratory for a coagulation screen (activated partial thromboplastin time (APTT), prothrombin time (PT), and fibrinogen) and a full blood count.

Initial blood results (Table 5.2) became available 45 min after they were sampled. Management of coagulation prior to this was empirical. Over the course of the next 60 min, 4 units of blood and 2 units of fresh frozen plasma (FFP) were transfused along with the return of 300 mL of cell salvaged blood, aiming for a haemoglobin of 10 g/dL (due to risk of further bleeding) and maintenance of normal coagulation.

Table 5.2 Intraoperative blood test results

Full blood count	Clotting studies	Renal function and electrolytes
Hb 7.7 g/dL	PT 11.8 s	Na 144 mmol/L
Platelet count 111 × 10^9 /L	APTT 38.2 s	K 5.3 mmol/L
WCC 7.2 × 10^9 /L	Fibrinogen 2.6 g/L	Urea 5.8 mmol/L
		Creatinine 81 µmol/L
		Calcium 2.2 mmol/L

❝ Expert comment

Estimation of blood loss can be inaccurate, and underestimation occurs commonly. Studies from military trauma victims demonstrating a mortality benefit from increasing the plasma component of transfusion have led to a 1:1 transfusion ratio (packed red cells:plasma) being recommended by some [8]. Studies in civilian trauma centres have not reproduced these results [9]. Further evaluation of the optimal transfusion ratio is required in both trauma and obstetric populations. Many hospital haematology departments now provide 'trauma boxes' containing blood and FFP in a ratio of 1:1 or 2:1 for multiple trauma cases, and these are suitable for major haemorrhage in the maternity unit.

✪ Learning point　Management of massive blood loss

Therapeutic goals of management of massive blood loss are:

- Maintenance of tissue perfusion and oxygenation by restoration of blood volume and haemoglobin.
- Arrest of bleeding by treating any obstetric, traumatic or surgical cause.
- Judicious use of blood component therapy to correct coagulopathy.
- Avoiding acidaemia, hypothermia and hypocalcaemia are vital to prevent coagulopathy.

A guideline for management of postpartum haemorrhage (PPH) produced by the Royal College of Obstetricians and Gynaecologists (RCOG) suggests the following principles for blood product transfusion [7]:

- 4 units of FFP for every 6 units of red cells or 12–15 mg/kg of FFP if PT/APTT >1.5 × normal
- Platelets if platelet count <50 × 10^9/L
- Cryoprecipitate if fibrinogen <1 g/dL

✪ Learning point　Point-of-care testing

Point-of-care testing of haemoglobin using either a blood gas analyser or haemoglobinometer such as a HemoCue® (HemoCue Ltd, Dronfield, UK) device has become increasingly common. The accuracy of such devices has been compared with laboratory tests and found to correlate well. New to the market are non-invasive continuous haemoglobin monitors using a finger probe similar to a pulse oximeter (multi-wavelength spectrophotometric method). Currently these track trends better than absolute values and are not in common use.

Point-of-care testing of coagulation using thromboelastography (TEG® Hemonetics Corporation, Braintree, MA, USA) or thromboelastometry (ROTEM®, TEM International, Munich, Germany) can reveal the extent and type of coagulopathy within 20 min. These real-time monitors of whole blood coagulation require training prior to their use, and although they have been widely used in cardiac and liver surgery they are rarely available on obstetric units and no protocols for their use is such settings have been established.

At this point the placenta had been delivered, the uterus had contracted, bleeding was seemingly controlled (haemoglobin was 10.1 g/dL measured on a point-of-care device), and the patient was maintaining a systolic blood pressure of 110 mmHg without vasopressor support. The wound was closed and the patient cleaned and transferred to a ward bed.

On transfer to the bed the patient vomited. Non-invasive blood pressure estimation was slow and the radial pulse was weak. She was immediately transferred back to the operating table and the surgical team was recalled. Their assessment revealed a high, boggy uterus and vaginal bleeding of ~ 400 mL consistent with uterine atony. During the 10 min period of assessment and resuscitation the patient required a fluid bolus and ephedrine to maintain an adequate blood pressure. The obstetric team then elected to re-open. The block height was no longer adequate for the procedure and a general anaesthetic was administered (rapid sequence induction followed by volatile maintenance). Treatment for uterine atony and continued bleeding was both pharmacological and surgical.

⊗ **Learning point**   Causes of postpartum haemorrhage

The four Ts:

- Tone: uterine atony
- Tissue: retained products
- Trauma: tear or injury to the genital tract
- Thrombin: abnormalities of coagulation

⊗ **Learning point**   Treatments for uterine atony

Pharmacological

- Oxytocin is a naturally occurring polypeptide hormone produced by the hypothalamus, then stored in the posterior pituitary. It acts on specific receptors in the myometrium to cause uterine contraction. Side-effects include tachycardia, hypotension, and tachyarrhythmias
- Ergometrine is an ergot alkaloid. It directly stimulates the uterine smooth muscle causing contraction. Side-effects include hypertension (vasoconstriction by stimulation of alpha-adrenergic and serotoninergic receptors and inhibition of endothelial-derived relaxation factors), nausea, and vomiting.
- Misoprostol is a synthetic prostaglandin E_1 analogue (PGE_1). It acts on receptors on the myometrium leading to uterine contraction. Side-effects include diarrhoea, pyrexia, and shivering.
- Carboprost is a synthetic prostaglandin $F_{2\alpha}$ analogue ($PGF_{2\alpha}$) causing uterine contraction, probably by a direct effect on the myometrium. Side-effects include stimulation of the smooth muscle of the gastrointestinal tract, arterioles, and bronchioles. Whereas some obstetricians prefer direct myometrial injection, this can lead to cardiovascular instability and bronchospasm. Intramuscular injection is safer, but its short half-life may require repeat administration every 10 min. As it can precipitate severe bronchospasm in patients with asthma, it should only be used with caution and when the benefits outweigh the risk.

Surgical and radiological treatment for postpartum haemorrhage: see Table 5.3

Bleeding continued despite further pharmacological treatment for uterine atony (sublingual misoprostol, then intramuscular carboprost) and replacement of blood and blood products (10 units packed red cells and cell-salvaged blood, 4 units FFP, 1 adult unit platelets, and 6 units cryoprecipitate on the advice of a haematologist). Calcium chloride 10 mmol was used to treat hypocalcaemia diagnosed on a blood gas. The bleeding was thought to originate from the placental site. Surgical attempts to halt the bleeding included the insertion of a Rusch balloon (hydrostatic balloon catheter)

⊕ **Clinical tip**   Estimating blood loss

Blood loss in obstetric scenarios is often underestimated. In a 2006 study 12 simulated obstetric clinical scenarios were reproduced with spillage of known quantities of blood (examples: blood on the floor, saturated surgical swabs, clotted blood in a kidney dish). More than 100 health professionals were then asked to estimate blood loss in each scenario, and these were compared with the actual blood loss. In five of the 12 scenarios blood loss was significantly underestimated and in none of the scenarios was blood loss overestimated. Pictorial guidelines were produced to facilitate visual estimation of blood loss [10].

⊕ **Clinical tip**   Early diagnosis of postpartum haemorrhage

The importance of early diagnosis and treatment of PPH is emphasized in the 2006–2008 maternal mortality review [11]. Delay of >2 h between delivery and placement of uterine compression sutures is independently associated with an increased risk of hysterectomy [12]. Early warning scores modified for obstetric practice (Maternity Early Warning Scores: MEWS) are used in many centres. To correct bleeding early monitoring must be both performed and acted upon.

Table 5.3 Second-line therapies for postpartum haemorrhage [13]

Procedure	Description
Intrauterine balloon tamponade	Inflated in the uterus, exerting pressure on the interior of the uterus
	Can be used following vaginal delivery
	Relatively non-invasive
	Examples include Rusch or Bakri balloon
Uterine compression suture	Sutures placed externally on the uterus
	Several techniques described, including B Lynch suture
	No data to support the use of one technique over another
Interventional radiology	Radiological procedures vary but usually accessed via the femoral artery
	Can be unilateral or bilateral
	Internal iliac artery or uterine artery
	Balloon catheter inserted and/or embolization procedure undertaken
Pelvic vessel ligation	Surgical procedure
	Internal iliac artery, uterine artery, hypogastric artery, or ovarian artery ligated
	Can impair future radiological procedures
rFVIIa	Recombinant activated Factor VII
	'Off-label' use
	Risk of thromboembolic complications

and failure of that to halt the bleeding required the surgeon to re-open the abdomen to allow definitive management. Examination of the uterus on re-opening revealed continued uterine atony. A B Lynch suture was placed but the patient continued to require vasopressor support, her haemoglobin dropped further and the decision was made to perform a hysterectomy. Following subtotal hysterectomy the patient stabilized. Although she was transferred to the intensive care unit intubated she was soon extubated, and was discharged to the ward on the second postoperative day. Venous thromboembolism prevention took the form of TED stockings preoperatively and for the first postoperative day. Low-molecular-weight heparin at prophylactic dose was started on the second postoperative day and continued for seven days. She did not require a return to theatre or suffer any further complications during her inpatient stay.

> **✪ Learning point** Fibrinogen
>
> Correction of coagulopathy is critical to arrest of haemorrhage. Levels of fibrinogen are a useful marker of haemostatic compromise [14]. Hypofibrinogenaemia (<2 g/dL) is traditionally treated by large volume administration of FFP (up to 30 mL/kg is required to increase fibrinogen level by 1 g/dL), or cryoprecipitate (13 units = 260 mL to increase fibrinogen level by 1 g/dL). More recently fibrinogen concentrate, derived from plasma from pooled non-UK donors, has been used to correct congenital and acquired hypofibrinogenaemia [15]. Fibrinogen concentrate is not frozen for storage, so its main advantage is rapid availability in a small volume (100 mL contains 2 g fibrinogen). It should be noted that the normal values for fibrinogen in late pregnancy (4–7 g/L) are higher than in the non-pregnant population (2–4 g/L).

Discussion

In the UK, major obstetric haemorrhage occurs in around 3.7 per 1000 births (95% CI: 3.4–4.0). In the CMACE 2006–2008 report there were nine direct deaths and two late direct deaths related to obstetric haemorrhage [11]: a mortality rate of 0.39 per 100,000 maternities (95% CI: 0.20–0.75); ~0.1% of all cases of major obstetric haemorrhage. Of these 11 women, three had morbidly adherent placentas. The wide gap between the incidence of major haemorrhage and its resultant mortality is a testament to the teams involved in the care of the bleeding patient. However, substandard care was identified in two-thirds of cases resulting in death and in four of these it was considered that different treatment may have altered the outcome.

Peripartum hysterectomy leading to the loss of fertility should be discussed antenatally with patients who are at high risk of haemorrhage. In some cases it may be appropriate to proceed immediately to hysterectomy if the placenta is found to be morbidly adherent; even then surgery may be technically difficult.

A national population-based descriptive study from UKOSS identified 315 women who underwent peripartum hysterectomy for uncontrolled haemorrhage [16]: 53% because of uterine atony and 38% due to a morbidly adherent placenta. The mortality associated with peripartum hysterectomy was < 1%. In 29 of the 315 women, the sole treatment was hysterectomy. The cause of haemorrhage in these women was placenta accreta (66%), uterine rupture (14%), fibroids (14%), and infection (14%). Early decision to proceed to hysterectomy resulted in a significant reduction in transfusion requirements. In these cases the women were not significantly older or more highly parous. Information on maternal views gathered preoperatively can help guide surgical decision-making, although, in cases where uterine conservation is important, early hysterectomy may not be an option. Pharmacological management of uterine atony is advised in the RCOG guideline for the treatment of PPH secondary to placenta accreta due to the relatively atonic lower uterine segment; however, in this UKOSS study, no reduction in transfusion of packed red cells, platelets, or cryoprecipitate was noted in bleeding placenta accreta patients when managed with uterotonics compared with the 25% of similar patients who did not receive these agents (though more FFP was used in this group).

✪ Learning point   UK Obstetric Surveillance System [17]

UKOSS was launched in 2005, a joint initiative between the National Perinatal Epidemiology Unit and the RCOG. It is a surveillance system designed to improve the cost-effectiveness, efficiency, and ease of data collection on rare conditions of pregnancy and the peripartum. Nominated clinicians, including anaesthetists, midwives, obstetricians and risk managers in every consultant-led maternity unit in the UK (a total of 226 in 2007) use a tick-box report card to indicate the number of cases of the conditions under surveillance on a monthly basis (even if that number is zero). Up to five reminders are sent, and return rates of reporting cards often exceed 90%. For those units reporting a case, a more detailed data collection form is sent, requesting further details such as confirmation of case definition, prognostic factors, management and outcomes. The data collected by UKOSS has provided information on the natural history, prognosis, risk factors, and adherence to evidence-based practice around several rare conditions. Data can be used for case–control and cohort studies (controls are identified and data collected in a similar manner).

Interventional radiology

The uterine artery usually arises from the anterior division of the internal iliac artery but there can be considerable anatomical variation. There is often a large collateral supply with anastomoses between the right and left uterine arteries and the ovarian arteries. Potential interventional radiological procedures include insertion of balloon catheters into the internal iliac arteries or uterine arteries, or more permanent embolization procedures. Embolization can be achieved using gelatin sponges which will allow recanalization of the vessel in a number of weeks. The timing of the procedure also varies, with either insertion of balloons prophylactically prior to caesarean section or following development of PPH. Balloon catheters can be left in position for up to 24 h postoperatively allowing re-inflation to control postoperative haemorrhage while further intervention is arranged. In the case described here interventional radiology was not used. Consideration of its use was recommended in Good Practice guidance from the RCOG in 2007 [18] but availability around the country is variable. A postal survey reported that only 31% of responding units had experience with interventional radiology. Fewer than one-third of these units reported 24 h availability, most frequently due to lack of personnel [19]. In the case described there was no interventional radiology available. Evidence for its efficacy is limited to case series, predominantly from large tertiary centres. In view of the potential for collateral supply, surgical ligation is not always successful for haemorrhage cessation; reported success rates for surgical uterine artery ligation have been as low as 36% [13]. Success rates for radiological procedures, however, have been reported to be as high as 100% [20]. Ischaemic phenomena such as uterine necrosis, lumbar plexus ischaemia, and gluteal pain can occur following interventional radiological procedures. Fetal compromise from uterine artery spasm is also a recognized complication, and continuous fetal monitoring is advised when balloon catheters are placed prophylactically. In one case-series of 11 women, two deliveries were expedited because of fetal bradycardia [21].

Recombinant Factor VIIa and tranexamic acid

The use of recombinant activated Factor VII in massive obstetric haemorrhage is controversial. Guidelines have been published from a multidisciplinary group in Australasia convened by the manufacturers [22]. The level of evidence supporting its use is currently low, being limited to case reports and case series with one non-randomized study. The consensus group recommended considering rFVIIa prior to hysterectomy if PPH continues despite replacement of blood components and surgical interventions. The suggested dose is 90 μg/kg repeated at 20 min if necessary. This is an off-label use and adverse effects include increased risk of thromboembolism.

Tranexamic acid is an antifibrinolytic agent commonly used for menorrhagia; it exerts its effect by blocking lysine binding sites on plasminogen molecules. Fibrinolysis is inhibited and excessive or recurrent bleeding is reduced. The large CRASH study (Clinical Randomisation of an Antifibrinolytic in Significant Haemorrhage) in trauma victims demonstrated a significant improvement in mortality following early administration (within 3 h) of injury without an increase in thromboembolism [23]. Evidence for effectiveness in major obstetric haemorrhage is lacking. The WOMAN trial (World Maternal Antifibrinolytic Trial) is an international double-blinded, placebo-controlled trial currently underway, comparing the effect of tranexamic acid to placebo; primary outcome measures are death and hysterectomy [24].

A Final Word from the Expert

It is easy to be lulled into a false sense of security in the obstetric unit, where routine caesarean sections in healthy women follow each other without incident day after day. But it should be remembered that a substantial proportion of the increased cardiac output of the term pregnant woman goes to the uterus (10–20% of cardiac output), with the result that haemorrhage can be torrential and difficult to control. Blood loss is frequently underestimated at and after caesarean section, since dilution with amniotic fluid makes it difficult to assess volume, and a healthy woman can tolerate losses of 2 L or more before she decompensates. A concealed blood loss can be particularly hard to detect, and it should be remembered that there are more organs than the uterus which can bleed; splenic artery aneurysm rupture is largely a specific complication of pregnancy and features in several issues of the Confidential Enquiry into Maternal Deaths. Management follows simple principles: volume replacement; restoration of coagulation; adequate correction of anaemia; surgical intervention to stop the source.

References

1. Royal College of Obstetricians and Gynaecologists. *Green-top Guideline No. 27: Placenta praevia accreta and vasa praevia: diagnosis and management*. London: RCOG; 2011.
2. Silver RM, Landon MB, Rouse DJ, *et al*. National Institute of Child Health and Human Development Maternal–Fetal Medicine Units Network. Maternal morbidity associated with multiple repeat caesarean deliveries. *Obstet Gynecol* 2006;107:1226–32.
3. Learn Cell Salvage eLearning module. *E-Learning for healthcare*. < http://www.e-lfh.org.uk >
4. Parekh N, Husaini SWU, Russell IF. Caesarean section for placenta praevia: a retrospective study of anaesthetic management. *Br J Anaesth* 2000;84:725–30.
5. Wise A, Clark V. Challenges of major obstetric haemorrhage. *Best Pract Res Clin Obstet Gynaecology* 2010;24:353–65.
6. Lilker SJ, Meyer RA, Downey KN, Macarthur AJ. Anesthetic considerations for placenta accreta. *Int J Obstet Anesth* 2011;20:288–92.
7. Royal College of Obstetricians and Gynaecologists. *Green-top Guideline No. 52: Prevention and management of postpartum haemorrhage*. London: RCOG; 2009.
8. Borgman MA, Spinella PC, Perkins JG, *et al*. The ratio of blood products transfused affects mortality in patients receiving massive transfusions at a combat support hospital. *J Trauma* 2007;63:805–13.
9. Scalea TM, Bochicchio KM, Lumpkins K, *et al*. Early aggressive use of fresh frozen plasma does not improve outcome in critically injured trauma patients. *Ann Surg* 2008;248:578–84.
10. Bose P, Regan F, Paterson-Brown S. Improving the accuracy of estimated blood loss at obstetric haemorrhage using clinical reconstructions. *Br J Obstet Gynecol* 2006;113:919–24.
11. Centre for Maternal and Child Enquiries (CMACE). Saving Mothers' Lives: reviewing maternal deaths to make motherhood safer: 2006–08. The Eighth Report on Confidential Enquiries into Maternal Deaths in the United Kingdom. *Br J Obstet Gynecol* 2011;118 (Suppl 1):1–203.
12. Kayem G, Kurinczuk JJ, Alfirevic Z, Spark P, Brocklehurst P, Knight M. Uterine compression sutures for the management of severe postpartum haemorrhage. *Obstet Gynecol* 2011;117:14–20.
13. Kayem G, Kurinczuk JJ, Alfirevic Z, Spark P, Brocklehurst P, Knight M. Specific second-line therapies for postpartum haemorrhage: a national cohort study. *Br J Obstet Gynecol* 2011;118:856–64.
14. De Lloyd L, Bovington R, Kaye A, *et al*. Standard haemostatic tests following major obstetric haemorrhage. *Int J Obstet Anesth* 2011;20:135–41.
15. Bell SF, Rayment PW, Collins PW, Collis RE. The use of fibrinogen concentrate to correct hypofibrinogenaemia rapidly during obstetric haemorrhage. *Int J Obstet Anesth* 2010;19:218–34.
16. Knight M, on behalf of UKOSS. Peripartum hysterectomy in the UK: management and outcomes of the associated haemorrhage. *Br J Obstet Gynecol* 2007;114:1380–7.
17. UK Obstetric Surveillance System. < http://www.npeu.ox.ac.uk/ukoss >
18. Royal College of Obstetricians and Gynaecologists. Royal College of Radiologists. British Society of Interventional Radiology. *Good Practice. No. 6. The role of emergency and elective interventional radiology in postpartum haemorrhage*. London: RCOG; 2007. < www.rcog.org.uk/womens-health/clinical-guidance/ role-emergency-and-elective-interventional-radiology-postpartum-haem >
19. Webster VJ, Stewart R, Stewart P. A survey of interventional radiology for the management of obstetric haemorrhage in the United Kingdom. *Int J Obstet Anesth* 2010;19:278–81.
20. Gonsalves M, Belli A. The role of interventional radiology in obstetric hemorrhage. *Cardiovasc Intervent Radiol* 2010;33:887–95.
21. Sadashivaiah J, Wilson R, Thein A, McLure H, Hammond CJ, Lyons G. Role of prophylactic uterine artery balloon catheters in the management of women with suspected placenta accreta. *Int J Obstet Anesth* 2011;20:282–7.

22. Welsh A, McLintock, C, Gatt S, Somerset D, Popham P, Ogle R. Guidelines for the use of recombinant activated factor VII in massive obstetric haemorrhage. *Aust NZ J Obstet Gynaecol* 2008;48:12–16.

23. CRASH-2 trial collaborators, Shakur H, Roberts I, Bautista R, *et al.* The importance of early treatment with tranexamic acid in bleeding trauma patients: an exploratory analysis of the CRASH-2 randomised controlled trial. *Lancet* 2011;377:1096–1101.

24. Shakur H, Elbourne D, Gülmezoglu M, *et al.* The WOMAN Trial (World Maternal Antifibrinolytic Trial): tranexamic acid for the treatment of postpartum haemorrhage: an international randomised, double blind placebo controlled trial. *Trials* 2010;11:40.

5.2 Category 1 caesarean section: treating mother and child

Dom Hurford

Expert Commentary Paul Howell
CPD Matrix Code: *1B02, 2B02, 2B05, 3B00*

Case history

At 18:00 a 28 year-old primiparous woman at 39 weeks of gestation was admitted to the Delivery Suite having gone into spontaneous labour 6 h earlier. On initial assessment she was contracting regularly and her cervix was 8 cm dilated. Four hours later cervical dilatation was unchanged, and after discussion with the obstetricians the patient agreed to a syntocinon infusion to augment labour, but at that stage declined an epidural. Continuous cardiotocograph (CTG) monitoring was started at this point.

Two hours later the CTG showed some decelerations of the fetal heart rate which coincided with contractions (see an example of a CTG trace in Figure 5.3). As these recovered with contraction cessation the management plan remained the same. However, over the subsequent hour these decelerations lengthened and deepened, and at 01:10 there was a persistent fetal bradycardia to 60 beats/min which did not recover. The obstetrician was called urgently and a decision was made to perform a category 1 caesarean section (CS).

> **Expert comment**
>
> Patients receiving syntocinon for induction or augmentation of labour may expect to experience increasingly painful contractions, and be at increased risk of requiring assisted delivery or emergency CS. For this reason it is worthwhile discussing and encouraging early placement of an epidural. This is a good opportunity to give the patient relevant patient information leaflets (e.g. free download from the Obstetric Anaesthetists' Association (OAA) website [1])

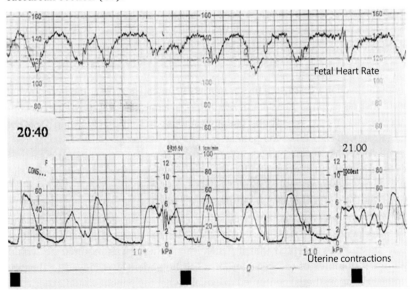

Figure 5.3 An example of a CTG trace showing late decelerations. Reproduced with permission from: PROMPT Course Manual (Second Edition), ISBN 978-1-906985-63-9, August 2012, RCOG Press.

⊙ **Learning point** Classification of urgency of caesarean section

For many years, 30 min has been used as the standard goal for the 'decision to delivery interval' at emergency CS. A four-tier classification for the urgency of delivery of the fetus, based on clinical need rather than time intervals, was described in 2000, and this system has now entered clinical practice in the UK [2]. Each category reflects a balance between the safe care of the mother and the degree of urgency to deliver the baby although interpretation of the groupings is still open to debate (Table 5.4).

Table 5.4 Classification of urgency of caesarean section

Category of urgency	Implication
1	Immediate threat to life of woman or fetus
2	Maternal or fetal compromise which is not immediately life-threatening
3	Needing early delivery but no maternal or fetal compromise
4	At a time to suit the woman and maternity services

Reproduced from Lucas DN, Yentis SM, Kinsella SM et al., 'Urgency of caesarean section: a new classification', *Journal of the Royal Society of Medicine*, 93, pp. 346–350, copyright 2000, with permission from SAGE Publications.

The National Institute for Health and Care Excellence (NICE) has recently updated its 2004 CS guidelines and seems rather ambivalent about the use of the 30 min target. It is clear that even 30 min may be too long in certain situations (e.g. catastrophic maternal haemorrhage or persistent fetal bradycardia), and they refer to a category 1 CS being performed as 'quickly as possible after making the decision'. However, they do note the usefulness of decision-to-delivery time of 30 min as an auditable measure of an obstetric unit's overall performance [3].

Categories are useful for audit purposes, but in reality there is a spectrum of urgency based upon the presence and extent of maternal or fetal compromise. In 2010 the RCOG together with the Royal College of Anaesthetists produced a joint document in support of this concept: 'Classification of Urgency of Caesarean Section – a continuum of risk (Good Practice No. 11)' [4]. The document encourages the move away from time-based classifications towards a spectrum of urgency adding in a colour coded guide: red for emergency "crash" CS, through yellow to green for planned elective cases. The overall aim is for teams to consider the individual risk in each case and thereby use the appropriate techniques and urgency for each case, for instance avoiding general anaesthesia when time allows for a regional technique. Within the new classification there are calls for the retention of the colloquial term 'crash section' for the extremely urgent case that needs immediate delivery to distinguish from other less urgent category 1 cases [5]. The effectiveness of this new classification (or any other) is dependent on prompt, clear and effective communication amongst the team caring for the patient, most particularly between obstetrician and anaesthetist.

The midwife in charge instigated the local protocol for category 1 CS and fast-bleeped the anaesthetist on-call and the theatre team. At the same time the obstetrician consented the mother for the operation. The anaesthetist arrived quickly onto Delivery Suite and introduced himself to the patient.

The anaesthetist established which intrauterine fetal resuscitation (IUFR) measures had been commenced, including whether the syntocinon infusion was turned off, and began a rapid assessment of the patient. As expected the patient and her partner were both very anxious and it was difficult to fully assess and discuss the potential events in detail. The obstetrician was anxious to expedite transfer of the patient to theatre and this was started whilst the anaesthetist was talking to the patient. The partner wished to come to theatre but accepted that if general anaesthesia was required he would leave. Within 10 minutes of the decision for a CS the patient was moved to theatre. During transit the anaesthetist continued to explain what the patient would experience and gained verbal consent.

✪ Learning point Initial management of category 1 caesarean section [2, 6, 7]

If at any stage difficulty is anticipated, call for help early.

Assessment

- Past medical history: pre-pregnancy and current medical issues
- Drug history
- Allergies
- Previous anaesthetics/complications for patient or family

Examination

- Formal examination of the airway including: Mallampati class, neck mobility, thyromental distance and dentition

Administration

- Drugs: Ranitidine 50mg IV and metoclopramide 10mg IV

Discussion

- Consent for both regional and general anaesthesia—see later but emphasis on regional anaesthesia where possible
- Options for analgesia after CS

As an ideal, both should be discussed, however informed consent for anaesthesia is the priority, whereas discussing issues such as analgesia and antiemetics is dependent on the time available, i.e. degree of urgency.

Initial management should include:

- Reduce risk of hypotension using:
  o intravenous ephedrine or phenylephrine infusion
  o volume preloading (or co-loading) with crystalloid
  o 15° left lateral tilt
- Pre-oxygenation with rapid sequence induction (RSI) for all general anaesthetics

❝ Expert comment

The combination of pain and administered opioids (systemic or epidural) may delay gastric emptying in labour, increasing the risk of pulmonary aspiration if general anaesthesia is necessary. If not previously given in labour, ranitidine should be given before emergency CS to reduce the risk of acid aspiration, and metoclopramide is recommended as a prokinetic.

The number of documented cases of pulmonary aspiration are few, and as a result there is increasing pressure in some units to relax the fasting rules for 'low risk' women in labour. However, the Confidential Enquiries have repeatedly shown that pulmonary aspiration has not gone away altogether and is still an important cause of maternal death [8].

❝ Expert comment

Aortocaval compression is a significant issue for both mother (hypotension, low cardiac output) and particularly the distressed baby (utero-placental perfusion) and tilt is very important in reducing this.

✪ Learning point Intrauterine fetal resuscitation [9–11]

During labour, physiological changes lead to a reduction in oxygen delivery to the fetus. In severe cases this can lead to fetal compromise with fetal distress and bradycardia. The aim of IUFR is to improve fetal oxygen delivery during fetal distress or placental disruption, such as a placental abruption. There are six key interventions, which can be remembered using the acronym SPOILT [11]:

- **S**top syntocinon infusion
- **P**osition: left lateral or other aortocaval displacement method
- **O**xygen: 15 L/min via Hudson mask with reservoir bag
- **I**ntravenous fluid bolus: 1 L crystalloid (Hartmann's solution)
- **L**ow blood pressure: control with vasopressor as required
- **T**ocolysis: Terbutaline 0.25 mg subcutaneously (0.5 mL of 1 mL ampoule) or GTN sublingual spray (initial two puffs, repeated after 1 min until contractions stop, to a maximum three doses)

Reprinted from *Anaesthesia and Intensive Care Medicine*, 11, 7, NK. Weale, SM. Kinsella, 'Intrauterine fetal resuscitation', pp. 262–265, Copyright 2010, with permission from The Medicine Publishing Company Ltd and Elsevier.

✚ Clinical tip Tilt

When tilting the table or using a wedge look at the mother's abdomen from the head-end of the table and ensure that 'the bump' looks tilted over. Also use a lateral board to prevent the obese mother from rolling off the operating table (it has happened).

(continued)

There is some debate as to the impact of administrating maternal oxygen to improve fetal oxygen delivery. The pragmatic approach taken by many is that it is unlikely to cause harm, contributes to preoxygenating the mother, is relatively simple to do and is potentially beneficial. The authors would encourage this practice and emphasise that maternal hypoxia should certainly be avoided and treated whenever it occurs.

❖ Learning point   Consent

Time constraints often limit a full and detailed discussion, particularly before emergency general anaesthesia. Whatever the time constraints it is important to explain as much as is possible. A brief description of spinal or general anaesthesia, including risks and side effects, is important. Depending upon available time it is worth considering including the following areas regarding general anaesthesia: the need for RSI, the common risks of sore throat, poorer pain control afterwards (TAP block and PCA), postoperative nausea and vomiting, and the very rare risks of awareness and aspiration pneumonia.

For a regional technique, including a rapid sequence spinal, areas to highlight include the need to remain still during needle placement, remaining awake during the operation, partner can be present, unusual sensations of pushing and pulling but ideally no pain, and the potential side-effects and risks including: failure and the need for conversion to general anaesthesia, hypotension, shivering, post-dural puncture headache, and nerve injury (very rare).

Consent for a category 1 section is difficult to achieve and as such, despite all efforts, there is often an element of treating the patient in their best interest. The balance between informing the mother of the risks involved and keeping an already extremely anxious mother calm can be hard to achieve.

❝ Expert comment

If time allows patient information leaflets (e.g. from the OAA website [1]) may be given to the patient.

❝ Expert comment

It is disappointing how often patients with fetal distress are transferred to the operating theatre flat on their backs on the bed—this should never happen—they should always be transferred in the lateral position—and the anaesthetist accompanying the patient from delivery suite to the theatre should ensure this is so.

❝ Expert comment

Reassessing the CTG on arrival in theatre is VERY important. It is not uncommon for the fetal bradycardia or other cause for concern to have recovered when the patient is assessed in theatre, and this is likely to significantly reduce the pressure from the obstetricians to administer a 'crash' general anaesthetic. ALWAYS get the obstetricians to quickly check the fetal heart before a 'crash' category 1 CS.

On arrival in theatre the patient was transferred from her bed to the theatre table in the left lateral position.

Oxygen at 15 L/min flow rate was continued via a Hudson mask with a reservoir bag. At this stage the anaesthetist asked for the CTG trace to be reassessed [9].

The CTG showed an improvement in fetal heart rate to 120 bpm. The 16G IV cannula in situ was flushed to confirm patency. After discussion between the senior obstetrician and the anaesthetist it was decided there was enough time to attempt spinal anaesthesia.

Whilst preparations were made for spinal anaesthesia the team completed an abridged emergency WHO checklist.

❖ Learning point   WHO checklists

Since the national adoption of the WHO checklist, an obstetric-specific version has been promoted by the NPSA [12], and many hospitals have also developed their own individual variations. The extent of checks deemed essential prior to an emergency operation varies. Many argue that it is during emergency cases that mistakes are more likely to occur, and that therefore greater time should be spent on this aspect of theatre governance. The minimal requirements potentially include: confirmation of the patient's name against a name band, any known allergies, confirmation of the planned operation, and that a consent form has been signed.

A phenylephrine infusion (100 microgram/mL) was attached to the patient's IV cannula, to be started at a rate of 20 mL/h immediately after the spinal anaesthetic was administered, according to local protocol. Intravenous Hartmann's solution (1 L) was started at a rapid rate.

> **Expert comment**
>
> Phenylephrine has been shown to correct maternal hypotension during regional anaesthesia more effectively than ephedrine, with less fetal acidosis and better correction of the maternal nausea and vomiting associated with hypotension.
>
> Administration of phenylephrine by infusion has also been shown to be more effective than using boluses and is preferred by some anaesthetists. Care should be taken to avoid excessive vasoconstriction leading to rebound hypertension, bradycardia, and a fall in maternal cardiac output.
>
> A pragmatic solution for many anaesthetists which minimises the risks of haemodynamic instability is to draw up both phenylephrine and ephedrine syringes and treat hypotension according to maternal heart rate: HR >100 beats/min give phenylephrine, HR <100 beats/min give ephedrine boluses.

With the patient in the left lateral position the anaesthetist prepared for the spinal using standard hand washing, gloves, gown, mask, and hat.

> **Expert comment**
>
> Most anaesthetists currently appear to prefer the sitting position for siting spinal and epidural blocks and consider it is easier to define the midline, particularly in obese patients.
>
> Advocates of the lateral position argue it is an easier position for many women to assume, and easier and quicker when transferring a patient from a bed onto the operating table.
>
> There are some situations which are less well suited to the sitting position (e.g. umbilical cord prolapse), and also some evidence that uteroplacental perfusion is better in the lateral position compared to sitting [13].
>
> The relative benefits and disadvantages of lateral vs. sitting positions remain controversial [14, 15]. Ultimately, in these urgent situations the prime consideration is to consider in which position the anaesthetist is most likely to be successful in getting the spinal in: that will be determined by personal preference and experience.

> **Expert comment**
>
> Chlorhexidine in alcohol is now considered more effective than iodine for skin preparation, and there is some evidence to suggest that 2% chlorhexidine is more effective than the 0.5% solution. However, there are concerns that 2% chlorhexidine is more neurotoxic than 0.5%. Currently no data exist regarding whether this is a significant clinical risk for spinal and epidurals but most manufacturers of chlorhexidine 2% recommend that it is not used for 'lumbar puncture' and this therefore makes it unsuitable for both spinal and epidural anaesthesia [16].

The patient's back was cleaned with 0.5% chlorhexidine solution in alcohol and left to dry.

Lidocaine 1% was prepared for local infiltration. The anaesthetic assistant helped position the patient appropriately with legs flexed and chin tucked onto the chest as much as was possible. A sterile sheet, with a central hole, was placed over the patient's lumbar region with the hole at the level of L3/4 after careful palpation and determination of Tuffier's line. Despite the time needed for preparation of the spinal the time elapsed since calling for the CS was about 20 min. The anaesthetist was unable to site the spinal needle on the first attempt and confirmed with the obstetrician that there was enough time before undertaking a second attempt.

During this attempt (with the patient more tightly positioned) the CTG trace developed a persistent fetal bradycardia. The anaesthetist therefore abandoned the attempted spinal and proceeded to general anaesthesia.

> **Expert comment**
>
> It is very important to keep good communication between the obstetrician and anaesthetist whilst attempting a 'rapid sequence spinal'. If there is a high chance of having to convert to general anaesthesia it may be prudent to preoxygenate the patient during the attempt at spinal anaesthesia.

> **Learning point** Pros and cons of spinal anaesthesia for category 1 caesarean section
>
> There are a number of reasons why regional anaesthesia is preferable to general anaesthesia for category 1 CS, these include [17, 18]:
>
> 1. Aspiration risk reduced.
> 2. Failed intubation and failed ventilation risk avoided.
> 3. 'Awareness' avoided (though inadequate blockade may also lead to distress).
> 4. Mother awake and involved.
>
> (continued)

5. Partner able to remain present.
6. Less sleepy baby.
7. Early maternal-baby bonding.
8. Postoperative analgesia improved by neuraxial opioid.
9. Postoperative nausea and vomiting reduced.
10. Venous thromboembolism risk reduced and early mobilization possible.

Disadvantages to regional anaesthesia include:

1. Risk of failed or inadequate block.
2. Sympathetic block with associated hypotension, nausea and vomiting. Sequelae to mother and baby reduced by co-loading with crystalloid and early vasopressor administration.
3. Duration of spinal block and operation both variable, although the majority of CS are performed within the predicted 2 h window of the neuraxial (spinal) block.
4. High blocks with associated respiratory compromise.
5. Post dural puncture headache.
6. Rare serious complications of neuraxial blocks (e.g. nerve damage): discussed in the NAP3 report [19].

There are also situations where regional anaesthesia is contraindicated and general anaesthesia is the preferred option.

1. Maternal choice or refusal.
2. Infection at the injection site.
3. Significant coagulopathy (e.g. pre-eclampsia, abruption).
4. Cardiovascular instability due to haemorrhage.
5. Local anaesthetic allergy.
6. Raised ICP.

Relative contraindications to neuraxial block include:

1. Language barrier.
2. Neurological disease.
3. Significant spinal deformity/previous surgery (increased risk of failure and perhaps complications).
4. Maternal pyrexia (if possible wait until antibiotics are administered).
5. Systemic sepsis.

In all these circumstances each case must be judged individually.

✪ Learning point   Rapid sequence spinals (RSS) [20, 21]

An increasingly popular variation to the technique of spinal anaesthesia used in an emergency is the 'rapid sequence spinal'.

- Non-touch technique is adopted.
- Sterile gloves are used but no gown.
- Patient's skin is swabbed once with chlorhexidine in alcohol.
- One attempt to site a spinal needle at L3/4 (unless alteration in position would allow a successful second attempt).
- Local anaesthetic is injected as usual, with opioid if time allows.
- Fentanyl has been advocated as it is easier to add to the injectate and more rapid in onset and therefore useful for preventing visceral pain when the block is below T4.

RSS was first described in 2003 and since then there have been supporters and challengers of its role. RSS describes an approach to administering spinal anaesthesia in an emergency situation in order to mitigate the risks of general anaesthesia while also enabling prompt delivery of the baby. Critics cite a potential for increased risk of infection due to use of a non-touch technique (using sterile gloves and chlorhexidine as a single application, but not the other components regarded as standard for aseptic procedures). Proponents suggest that in balancing risks the avoidance of general anaesthesia outweighs the theoretical risks attributed to RSS. RSS requires involvement of the whole theatre team and communication is an essential component. RSS is not for the inexperienced practitioner and should only be introduced after appropriate team training.

> **✪ Learning point** Indications for general anaesthesia [19, 20]
>
> 1. Maternal choice after full consent.
> 2. Immediacy of anaesthesia with no time to perform regional anaesthesia.
> 3. Failed regional anaesthesia.
> 4. Coagulopathy (significant).
> 5. Raised ICP.
> 6. Cardiovascular instability.
> 7. Systemic sepsis.
> 8. Relative contraindication for regional after assessment (see above list).
>
> There are no definitive contraindications to general anaesthesia, only a weighing up of the risks for the individual patient and adaptation of pharmacological agents used depending upon allergy and complications (e.g. malignant hyperthermia). Sometimes general anaesthesia is rightly the chosen technique simply because regional anaesthesia cannot be guaranteed to be deployed and successful with the same speed. Deaths included in recent Centre for Maternal and Child Enquiries (CMACE) reports show predominant direct anaesthetic causes are: unrecognised oesophageal intubation, pulmonary aspiration of gastric contents and failure of ventilation. This further highlights the importance of early antacid therapy and the essential requirement for end-tidal carbon dioxide monitoring during intubation.

The necessity to change to general anaesthesia was briefly explained to the patient, and her partner was escorted from theatres by a member of staff. The patient was re-positioned supine with a 15° left tilt to displace the uterus and minimise aortocaval compression. She was given 30 mL of 0.3 M sodium citrate to drink.

Preoxygenation was performed with a tightly fitting anaesthetic facemask (FiO_2 = 1.0 at 15 L/min). The operating table was positioned head up to aid intubation and reduce the risk of aspiration. Two pillows were used to optimise the position of the patient's airway; one under the shoulders and the other behind the neck to create an exaggerated flexed neck and extended head position. Patient monitoring consistent with AAGBI guidelines (ECG, oxygen saturation, non-invasive blood pressure monitoring and capnography) was established during preoxygenation. The team prepared for RSI and the anaesthetic assistant identified the cricoid cartilage. After 3 min preoxygenation (and with an end-tidal oxygen fraction of >90%) the patient was reassured once more prior to induction of anaesthesia.

An RSI was performed with cricoid pressure applied (10 N before loss of consciousness, increasing to 30 N as consciousness was lost [22]).

Thiopentone (450 mg) was administered, rapidly followed by 100 mg suxamethonium.

> **❝ Expert comment**
>
> In obese patients requiring an RSI the standard dose of 100 mg suxamethonium may not be enough.

After 30 s a Macintosh 3 blade was used for laryngoscopy. The anaesthetist could only obtain a grade 4 view despite adjusting the assistant's cricoid pressure themselves. The anaesthetist attempted to intubate blindly with a gum elastic bougie (GEB) but on railroading a tracheal tube this was found to be in the oesophagus and was removed. At this stage the anaesthetist asked a theatre team member to call the anaesthetic consultant for help.

A second intubation attempt was made with a McCoy blade but the view was not improved. Neither further adjustment of the patient's head position nor temporary release of cricoid pressure improved the laryngeal view.

> **❝ Expert comment**
>
> In the case of a really urgent RSS it may be sensible to keep it simple and just give a slightly higher dose of spinal bupivacaine (e.g. 3.0 mL heavy bupivacaine 0.5 %) with no opioid.

> **❝ Expert comment**
>
> It is worth noting that a significant number of studies have shown that spinals are associated with more acidotic babies compared to general anaesthesia, and that purely for the baby (particularly the stressed baby) general anaesthesia may be best. However, this issue is not yet fully resolved, and where possible regional techniques are generally still considered best all-round, as they are much better and safer for the mother in the emergency situation (and hence for the baby and family overall).

> **❝ Expert comment**
>
> On the premise that citrate is worth giving, and since a woman who collapses during the operation or needs rapid conversion to general anaesthesia for any reason may not be in a position to drink it (or the anaesthetist may forget to give it in the panic that ensues), it is recommended that *all* women at CS (even elective) be given citrate before the spinal goes in!

> **❝ Expert comment**
>
> Poorly applied cricoid pressure is widely recognized as a significant factor in difficult and failed intubation, and it is worthwhile having regular training of operating department practitioners and anaesthetic assistants in the use of this technique, both in terms of positioning, and the force to apply – use simple weighing scales (10 N ≡ 1 kg, 30 N ≡ 3 kg).

> **❝ Expert comment**
>
> It is very important to call for help at an early stage! Call for any colleague close by, as well as the consultant, and alert the obstetric team to the fact that the anaesthetist is having airway difficulties.

> ⊗ **Learning point** Grade of laryngoscopy
>
> Cormack and Lehane originally described their four-point grading of view at laryngoscopy as indicative of the degree of difficulty with intubation, especially in the obstetric population (see Case 1.2, Figure 1.5).
>
> - Grade 1. Most of the glottis is visible. Should be no difficulty.
> - Grade 2. Posterior extremity of glottis only is visible. Potential for slight difficulty.
> - Grade 3. Epiglottis only can be seen and no part of the glottis visible. Potentially severe difficulty in intubation.
> - Grade 4. No view of any glottic structures. Severe difficulty in securing the airway likely.
>
> While this grading system is widely used there is little robust evidence that the changes in grade correlate with changes in intubation difficulty. The grading system is also poorly recalled by many anaesthetists. Several other grading classifications have been advocated [23].
>
> Reproduced from RS Cormack and J Lehane, 'Difficult tracheal intubation in obstetrics', *Anaesthesia*, 39, 11, pp. 1105–1111, Copyright © 1984, John Wiley and Sons and The Association of Anaesthetists of Great Britain and Ireland, with permission.

Expert comment

At this point it is vital to turn attention to oxygenation of the patient: the Confidential Enquiries into maternal mortality have repeatedly taught us that patients die from failure to oxygenate not failure to intubate. Obstetric patients desaturate exceedingly quickly, so prompt action is required.

The patient remained apnoeic and her oxygen saturations fell rapidly below 90%. The anaesthetist stopped trying to intubate and attempted to ventilate the patient's lungs manually with a facemask and anaesthetic circuit. This was difficult despite inserting an oropharyngeal airway and the oxygen saturations continued to fall.

The anaesthetist then elected to try an SAD; cricoid pressure was released to allow this to be done [24]. Due to the emergency nature of the surgery and the risk of pulmonary aspiration, a ProSeal™ Laryngeal Mask Airway (PLMA, Intavent Direct, Maidenhead, UK) was chosen and this was inserted easily and enabled ventilation of the lungs. A regular end-tidal carbon dioxide trace was observed, oxygen saturations improved, and bilateral air entry was heard on chest auscultation.

Expert comment

A number of second-generation SAD are now available which are probably better suited to the obstetric patient (with potential aspiration risk) than the LMA classic™ (cLMA), particularly where there is a drain tube which may be used to pass a gastric tube to aspirate gastric contents. The majority of published work is on the PLMA [25] which has a larger mask than the cLMA and a posterior cuff, both of which contribute to the increased airway seal. Other devices such as the i-gel™ (Intersurgical, Wokingham, UK) and the LMA Supreme® (Intavent) may be useful, although none will work in all patients.

With the airway maintained with an SAD the decision now was whether to proceed with the operation or to abandon and wake the mother up.

Expert comment

The question of whether to proceed or wake the mother up is difficult, (particularly for the solo trainee working out-of-hours), and may be associated with considerable pressure from the obstetricians. The decision will be based on a combination of personal experience of the anaesthetist, the clinical indication for CS, and the apparent effectiveness/stability of the airway control.

In view of the potential risks of loss of the airway and aspiration, there is a strong argument to support waking the mother up unless the operation is itself potentially lifesaving for the mother (i.e. haemorrhage, collapse). Waking the mother up is widely considered the safest option for the mother, and trainees should be assured by their departmental supervisors that they will always get support for waking a mother up in the situation of a failed intubation if they consider this the safest thing to do.

In addition, if there is any doubt about the correct placement and effectiveness of airway devices, there is no justification for continuing with the operation, and the patient should be woken up.

The question of whether to attempt intubation (blind or with a fibreoptic scope) through an effective SAD is also controversial, and there is a strong conservative argument to say 'keep things simple' and 'if the SAD is working well, don't fiddle with it'. A maternal death was reported in the 2006–2008 Confidential Enquiry when unrecognised oesophageal intubation occurred via an effective SAD [8].

In view of the clinical situation, the good seal achieved by the SAD and ease of ventilation, the anaesthetist opted to continue, and gave atracurium for muscle paralysis and commenced controlled ventilation with isoflurane 2% to achieve a MAC 1.0.

Ⓒ Expert comment

The decision whether to ventilate or allow spontaneous breathing is also controversial, and traditional teaching is to maintain deep anaesthesia with spontaneous ventilation to minimise the risk of inflating the stomach and increasing the risk of aspiration. However, with the increasingly obese population who may not self-ventilate effectively, and more effective second generation SADs, controlled ventilation with muscle paralysis is probably to be preferred in most situations.

If spontaneous ventilation is chosen, the patient must be kept sufficiently deeply anaesthetised to minimise the risk of coughing/breath-holding/regurgitation etc.

The surgeon was informed that the airway was secured and surgery commenced. The baby was successfully delivered within 3 min of the first surgical incision and immediately assessed by the attending paediatrician. The 1 min Apgar score was 9 and no further intervention was required. When the umbilical cord was clamped, following delivery, 5 mg of intravenous diamorphine was administered and the patient's volatile concentration (1.0 MAC) was confirmed. At the end of the operation the anaesthetist performed bilateral TAP blocks for postoperative analgesia, each with 20 mL of 0.25% levobupivacaine injected under ultrasound guidance.

✪ Learning point Transversus abdominis plane (TAP) block

TAP blocks may be used as part of the multimodal approach to analgesia after CS, and are particularly useful after general anaesthesia when there has been no opportunity to administer neuraxial opioids. Local anaesthetic blockade of the anterior abdominal wall sensory nerves has been shown to reduce the need for postoperative opiates and can last up to 36 h, although 12 h is more usual [26, 27]. TAP blocks are performed at the end of a CS using an aseptic technique. The target site is between the internal oblique and transversus abdominis planes (Figure 5.4). An appropriately long (~ 80 mm) nerve block needle is required and ultrasound guidance improves procedure efficacy and safety.

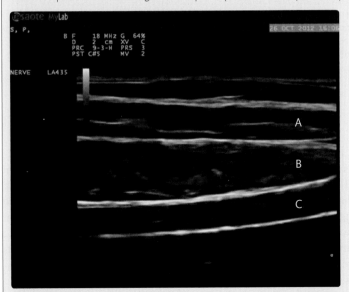

Figure 5.4 Ultrasound scan of abdominal wall prior to placement of a TAP block. (A) External oblique. (B) Internal oblique. (C) Transversus abdominis.

(continued)

If the urgency of surgery precluded obtaining consent for TAP blocks then proceeding in the patient's best interests is generally considered acceptable as adequate analgesia in these patients can be difficult to achieve. Contraindications include: patient refusal, allergy to local anaesthetic, and infection at the injection site [28]. Before administering any local anaesthetic it is advisable to check whether local anaesthetic has been administered by the surgeons and ensure the total dose of local anaesthetic lies within the total safe cumulative limit.

At the end of surgery, residual neuromuscular blockade was assessed using a train-of-four stimulus from a nerve stimulator, three twitches were seen, and neostigmine/glycopyrronium was administered. The mother was extubated when fully conscious in the left lateral position. Bed tilt, head down position, and suction were all available for this stage of anaesthesia.

⓬ Expert comment

The 2006–2008 Confidential Enquiry provides a reminder that aspiration is still a significant issue and may occur at extubation as well as at intubation [8].

Before leaving theatre the team completed the WHO checklist 'sign out' confirming the operation performed, that surgical counts were correct, and highlighted concerns for recovery. The lead obstetrician, anaesthetist, scrub nurse, ODP, midwife, and theatre runners all participated in this sign out. Issues included: postoperative fluids, analgesia, and prescribing low-molecular-weight heparin (LMWH).

An hour later the patient was comfortable in recovery. She was pain-free and with regular paracetamol and diclofenac prescribed and it was judged there was no need for a morphine PCA device. Oral morphine (10–20 mg) was prescribed as required up to a maximum frequency of 2-hourly. She and her baby were discharged from the recovery room to the ward an hour later.

✪ Learning point   Recovery

In all post-theatre recovery areas, one-to-one nursing is required until the mother has achieved full airway control, can communicate effectively and is cardiovascularly stable. According to NICE guidelines observations (respiratory rate, blood pressure, heart rate, pain and sedation scores) should be performed every 30 min for the first 2 h then hourly if stable [3]. There is no mention of oxygen saturation measurement in the NICE guidelines but in line with postoperative guidelines from the AAGBI this seems an appropriate observation to include. Appropriate pain relief needs to be discussed and prescribed [29].

Discussion

Failed obstetric intubation

In 2007–2008, of 649,837 obstetric deliveries, 2,454 (0.37%) patients had a general anaesthetic [30, 31]. Failed intubations have consistently been reported as being higher in the obstetric than the general population, 1:249 to 1:238 in the UK [32, 33]. The reasons for this higher rate are not fully established but physiological and anatomical changes in the mother together with the anxiety uniquely associated with obstetric emergency intubation are likely key elements [33]. The majority of general anaesthetics in obstetrics occur in category 1 CS, and one centre reported 78% of their intubations were for this specific group [34].

There is no established guideline for failed intubation management of obstetric patients, although the OAA and the DAS are currently working to create one. On their website, the OAA has collated a number of different hospital guidelines and described features they liked, disliked or were unsure about, but as yet a cohesive algorithm has not been developed [35]. Because of this it is hard to be didactic for this particular case study, though certain themes are worth exploring.

There will always remain a role for general anaesthesia in CS, most notably when a patient refuses a regional technique, but other reasons also prevail: low platelets in HELLP syndrome, abnormal clotting, spinal fusion surgery (where the anaesthetist fails to site a neuraxial block) or inadequate regional blockade. It is noteworthy that, as the use of spinal anaesthesia and adoption of 'rapid sequence spinals' in emergency settings increases, the use of general anaesthesia for CS and the exposure of trainees to emergency obstetric intubation will decrease.

There is increasing availability of a wide array of adjuncts designed to improve the rate of successful intubation. Videolaryngoscopes are the most widely available of these adjuncts and several studies have shown a clear improvement in Cormack and Lehane laryngeal view with use of specific scopes [36]. However, whilst they have been shown to improve the view in many circumstances, they have not yet been shown to consistently increase the success rate at intubation. Factors such as learning curve for the use of each videolaryngoscope and the fact that tube manipulation is not performed under direct vision mean that an improved laryngeal view may not translate into improved intubation success. In view of the learning curve for these devices, there is an argument that anaesthetists should become skilled in the use of a videolaryngoscope in low-risk cases and then progress to using this for potentially complicated obstetric intubations, both elective or emergency, in order to achieve a minimal standard of competency with them in this setting [5]. Unfortunately the current evidence does not enable a clear recommendation to be made as to which videolaryngoscope should be chosen for this purpose.

Other relevant adjuncts include the range of head and neck supports to aid ideal positioning of the patient, particularly if obese, prior to intubation, the Oxford HELP pillow (Head Elevating Laryngoscopy Pillow, Alma Medical, UK) being one such device (Figure 5.5).

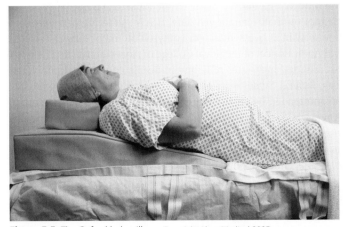

Figure 5.5 The Oxford help pillow. Copyright Alma Medical 2005.

The Difficult Airway Society Rapid Sequence Induction Guidelines (DAS RSI) describe a staged management for failed intubation during RSI in the non-obstetric population [37]. Because of the lack of obstetric-specific guidelines these DAS non-pregnant guides are often referred to despite the fact that there are differences in the potential management of these two populations. The initial intubation plan (plan A) prescribes a maximum of three attempts at intubation, the use of adjuvants (such as the bougie) and optimizing the patient's position. This is also the accepted practice with obstetric patients.

In the DAS 'routine intubation' guideline, failed primary intubation (plan A) is followed by a secondary intubation attempt (plan B). This is absent in the RSI guideline and after failing to intubate the next step is oxygenation (plan C). Oxygenation can be achieved by facemask ventilation and waking the patient or by insertion of an SAD. If an SAD is chosen and a stable airway is achieved the decision as to whether to continue with surgery or wake the patient logically follows.

There are many opinions as to the optimal SAD to use to rescue the obstetric airway. The Proseal® (PLMA) has been the most widely described in the literature, in particular for its improved airway seal and potential increase in protection against aspiration [25, 38–40]. A recent survey showed that a significant majority of trainees would use a PLMA when they were unable to intubate in a category 1 CS [41]. Other second-generation SADs are also very popular. Other second generation SADs include both the Supreme LMA and i-gel. There is limited evidence available at present on which to judge which device to use in the emergency setting. Specifically in the obstetric population there is almost none.

A number of techniques have been described to assist in the placement of each different SAD. One particular technique for the PLMA is railroading it over a gum elastic bougie placed in the oesophagus, which is associated with an increased first attempt success rate [42]. Further details are beyond the remit of this chapter. The technique should only be used by those who are trained appropriately.

The important message with airway management is to keep it simple, have the right equipment and to be skilled in the use of this equipment before an event like this occurs.

Plan C describes maintaining oxygenation and ventilation (whether with facemask, cLMA or PLMA) and waking the patient up [31]. This can be a difficult decision in the face of a profound fetal bradycardia but the mother's life must take precedence.

If at any stage a 'cannot intubate–cannot ventilate' (CICV) situation develops then prompt implementation of Plan D is essential – cricothyroidotomy or surgical airway. The recent 4th National Audit Project of the Royal College of Anaesthetists and Difficult airway Society (NAP4) reported high rates of failure in needle cricothyroidotomy performed by anaesthetists. Several causes were identified, including poor technique and training. NAP4 has recommended better training for anaesthetists in management of the CICV situation. Any anaesthetist covering an obstetric unit is exposed to the risk of having to manage an unexpectedly difficult airway, and should therefore receive training in needle cricothyroidotomy and surgical airway techniques [43]. The take home message is always the same: death occurs from failure to oxygenate not failure to intubate.

It should also be remembered that in a perimortem/maternal cardiac arrest situation, delivery of the baby forms part of the resuscitation of the mother, and may improve the chances of survival of mother and baby.

A Final Word from the Expert

Management of category 1 CS can be very demanding, and requires continual reassessment as well as good communication both with the patient as well as the whole theatre team. It is essential to try and maintain a calm methodical approach during these cases. Calling early for help is mandatory and is to be expected not only from trainees but also from consultants who need a second pair of hands. The care of the mother and baby is paramount but the conflict between their respective needs may sometimes make the necessary decisions harder to take.

References

1. Obstetric Anaesthetists' Association. *Information for mothers*. < http://www.oaa-anaes. ac.uk/content.asp?ContentID = 83 >
2. Lucas DN, Yentis SM, Kinsella SM, *et al*. Urgency of caesarean section: a new classification. *J R Soc Med* 2000;93:346–350.
3. National Institute for Health and Care Excellence. *CG132 Caesarean section*; 2011. < http:// publications.nice.org.uk/caesarean-section-cg132 >
4. Royal College of Obstetricians and Gynaecologists. *Classification of urgency of caesarean section—a continuum of risk* (Good Practice No. 11); 2010. < http://www.rcog.org.uk/ classification-of-urgency-of-caesarean-section-good-practice-11 >
5. Howell P. *Obstetric anaesthesia: change, what change?* Royal College of Anaesthetists. Bulletin 63, September 2010. < http://www.rcoa.ac.uk/document-store/ bulletin-63-september-2010 >
6. University Hospitals Bristol NHS Foundation Trust. *Department of Obstetric Anaesthesia Guidelines 2009*.
7. Obstetric Anaesthetists' Association. *Antacid prophylaxis*. < http://www.oaa-anaes.ac.uk/ content.asp?ContentID = 334 >
8. Cantwell R, Clutton-Brock T, Cooper G, *et al*. Saving Mothers' lives: reviewing maternal deaths to make motherhood safer: 2006–2008. The Eighth Report of the Confidential Enquiries into Maternal Deaths in the United Kingdom. *Br J Obstet Gynaecol* 2011;118:1–203.
9. Thurlow J, Kinsella SM. Intrauterine resuscitation: active management of fetal distress. *Int J Obstet Anesth* 2002;11:105–16.
10. Obstetric Anaesthetists' Association. Intrauterine resuscitation. < http://www.oaa-anaes. ac.uk/content.asp?ContentID = 427 >
11. Weale NK, Kinsella SM. Intrauterine fetal resuscitation. *Anaesth Intens Care Med* 2010;11:262–5.
12. UK National Health Service. WHO surgical safety checklist: for maternity cases only. < http://www.nrls.npsa.nhs.uk/resources/type/guidance/?entryid45 = 83972 >
13. Suonio S, Simpanen AL, Olkkonen H, Haring P. Effect of the left lateral recumbent position compared with the supine and upright positions on placental blood flow in normal late pregnancy. *Ann Clin Res* 1976;8:22–6.
14. Tsen LC. Neuraxial techniques for labor analgesia should be placed in the lateral position. *Int J Obstet Anesth* 2008;17:146–9.
15. Polley LS. Neuraxial techniques for labor analgesia should be placed in the lateral position. *Int J Obstet Anesth* 2008;17:149–52.
16. Cook TM, Fischer B, Bogod D, *et al*. Antiseptic solutions for central neuraxial blockade: which concentration of chlorhexidine in alcohol should we use? *Br J Anaesth* 2009;103:456–7.
17. Harries S, Garry M, Ratnalikar V. Anaesthesia for caesarean section: regional anaesthesia. In: Clyburn P, Collis R, Harries S, Davies S editors. *Obstetric anaesthesia*. Oxford: Oxford University Press; 2008.

18. Collis R, Evans M, Farley C, Chethan D. Anaesthesia for caesarean section: general anaesthesia. In: Clyburn P, Collis R, Harries S, Davies S editors. *Obstetric anaesthesia*. Oxford: Oxford University Press; 2008.

19. Cook TM, Counsell D, Wildsmith JA. Major complications of central neuraxial block: report on the Third National Audit Project of the Royal College of Anaesthetists. *Br J Anaesth* 2009;102:179–90.

20. Scrutton M, Kinsella SM. The immediate caesarean section: rapid-sequence spinal and risk of infection. *Int J Obstet Anesth* 2003;12:143–4.

21. Kinsella SM, Girgirah K, Scrutton MJL. Rapid sequence spinal anaesthesia for category-1 urgency caesarean section: a case series. *Anaesthesia* 2010;65:664–9.

22. Vanner RG, Asai T. Safe use of cricoid pressure. *Anaesthesia* 1999;54:1–3.

23. Cook TM. A new practical classification of laryngeal view. *Anaesthesia* 2000;55:274–9.

24. Li CW, Xue FS, Xu YC, *et al*. Cricoid pressure impedes insertion of, and ventilation through, the ProSeal laryngeal mask airway in anesthetized, paralyzed patients. *Anesth Analg* 2007;104:1195–8.

25. Halaseh BK, Sukkar ZF, Hassan LH, Sia AT, Bushnaq WA, Adarbeh H. The use of ProSeal laryngeal mask airway in caesarean section—experience in 3000 cases. *Anaesth Intens Care* 2010;38:1023–8.

26. Farragher RA, Laffey JG. Postoperative pain management following cesarean section. In: Sorten G, Carr DB, Harmon D, Puig MM, Browne J editors. *Postoperative pain management: an evidence-based guide to practice*. Philadelphia: Elsevier/Saunders; 2006.

27. McDonnell JG, Curley G, Carney J, *et al*. The analgesic efficacy of transversus abdominis plane block after cesarean delivery: a randomized controlled trial. *Anesth Analg* 2008;106:186–91.

28. Obstetric Anaesthetists' Association. *TAP blocks*. < http://www.oaa-anaes.ac.uk/content. asp?ContentID = 389 >

29. Obstetric Anaesthetists' Association. *Analgesia post LSCS*. < http://www.oaa-anaes.ac.uk/ content.asp?ContentID = 388 >

30. UK National Health Service, Information Centre for Health and Social Care. *Anaesthetics used before or during delivery by method of onset of labour and method of delivery, 2008–09* (Table 6). < http://www.hesonline.nhs.uk >

31. UK National Health Service, Information Centre for Health and Social Care. *NHS Maternity Statistics, England: 2007–08*. < http://www.ic.nhs.uk/ >

32. Barnardo PD, Jenkins JG. Failed tracheal intubation in obstetrics: a 6-year review in a UK region. *Anaesthesia* 2000;55:690–4.

33. Rahman K, Jenkins JG. Failed tracheal intubation in obstetrics: no more frequent but still managed badly. *Anaesthesia* 2005;60:168–71.

34. Searle R, Lyons G. Vanishing experience in training for obstetric general anaesthesia: an observational study. *Int J Obstet Anesth* 2008;17:233–7.

35. Obstetric Anaesthetists' Association. *Failed intubation*. < http://www.oaa-anaes.ac.uk/ content.asp?ContentID = 357 >

36. C-MAC™ Karl Storz Video Laryngoscopes. D Blade Product Information. Karl Storz (Germany); 2010.

37. Difficult Airway Society. *Rapid sequence induction—guidelines*. < http://www.das.uk.com/ guidelines/rsi.html >

38. Cook TM, Lee G, Nolan JP. The ProSeal™ laryngeal mask airway: a review of the literature. *Can J Anesth* 2005;52:739–60.

39. Keller C, Brimacombe J, Lirk P, Puhringer F. Failed obstetric tracheal intubation and postoperative respiratory support with the proseal laryngeal mask airway. *Anesth Analg* 2004;98:1467–70.

40. Awan R, Nolan JP, Cook TM. Use of a ProSeal laryngeal mask airway for airway maintenance during emergency Caesarean section after failed tracheal intubation. *Br J Anaesth* 2004;92:144–6.

41. Hurford D, Streets C, Laxton C. Use of LMA following failed intubation and CMACE. *Anaesthesia* 2011;66:752–3.
42. Brimacombe J, Keller C, Judd DV. Gum elastic bougie-guided insertion of the ProSeal laryngeal mask airway is superior to the digital and introducer tool techniques. *Anesthesiology* 2004;100:25–9.
43. Cook TM, Woodall N, Frerk C. Major complications of airway management in the UK: results of the 4th National Audit Project of the Royal College of Anaesthetists and the Difficult Airway Society. Part 1. Anaesthesia. *Br J Anaesth* 2011;106:617–31.

CHAPTER 6

Paediatric anaesthesia

6.1 Magnetic resonance imaging and the neonate

Erica Dibb-Fuller

Ⓘ Expert Commentary Hugo Wellesley
CPD Matrix Code: *2A08, 2D02, 3D00*

Case history

An ex-premature infant was scheduled for magnetic resonance imaging (MRI) of his brain under general anaesthesia. At birth he was 30 weeks plus 3 days of gestation and weighed 1.2 kg, but on presentation for his scan his postmenstrual age was 42 weeks and he weighed 2.8 kg. He was born by spontaneous vaginal delivery after premature rupture of membranes due to maternal infection. He required resuscitation at birth and was intubated, given surfactant therapy and ventilated for 3 weeks. During this time he suffered an episode of necrotizing enterocolitis (NEC), which responded to medical treatment, and he underwent surgery for ligation of a patent ductus arteriosus (PDA) which was uncomplicated. After one failed extubation, he was extubated successfully on to nasal continuous positive airway pressure (CPAP). He required this for the following 2 weeks, after which it was weaned off. Since then, he had been self-ventilating on nasal prong oxygen of 0.25 L/min (giving an estimated FiO_2 of 0.29) [1] and had a diagnosis of bronchopulmonary dysplasia (BPD). He was receiving oral and nasogastric feeds, and was being treated with domperidone and ranitidine for management of gastro-oesophageal reflux. He had had a grade II intraventricular haemorrhage (IVH) diagnosed by cranial ultrasound performed at 1 week of age, as part of routine screening, but there had been no other neurological concerns.

☻ Learning point Complications of prematurity

Preterm birth (before 37 weeks gestation) accounts for 75% of perinatal mortality. Risk factors for premature delivery include maternal hypertension, pre-eclampsia, multiple pregnancy, intrauterine growth restriction, maternal diabetes, malnutrition, and infection (e.g. chorioamnionitis and especially malaria or human immunodeficiency virus infection in developing countries). In developed countries morbidity and mortality rates reduce significantly with increasing gestational age beyond 23 weeks, and after 32 weeks of gestation outcomes are similar to those of term infants. Complications of prematurity depend on the gestational age and birth weight. Neonatal mortality rates for the UK vary from 903 per 1000 live births at <24 weeks of gestation to 0.9 per 1000 (a 1000-fold fall) for gestation >36 weeks [2].

Respiratory system

Alveoli start to form at around 17 weeks and even at term there are only 10% of the final adult number of alveoli. Surfactant is produced by type II alveolar cells and is insufficient before 32–34 weeks of gestation, predisposing preterm neonates to respiratory distress syndrome (RDS) and subsequent chronic lung disease. Supplementary oxygen and ventilatory support (either invasive or non-invasive) are often required. Premature lungs are fragile and there is a high risk of pneumothorax and pulmonary

(continued)

haemorrhage. Ex-premature infants have a higher risk of respiratory syncytial virus (RSV) bronchiolitis and may require prophylactic treatment with regular intramuscular injection of monoclonal antibodies. Premature neonates are also prone to apnoeas in response to stress (for example hypoxia, hypercapnia, or acidosis) and this is worse after sedation and anaesthesia.

Cardiovascular system

After birth and inflation of the lungs, pulmonary vascular resistance (PVR) falls, the foramen ovale closes and the ductus arteriosus starts to constrict (in response to high oxygen tension and falling levels of prostaglandins—primarily PGE_2 and PGI_2). Functional closure of the ductus is normally complete within the first 24 h of independent life, although anatomical closure by fibrosis takes 2–3 weeks. If the PVR remains high (e.g. in response to hypoxia, hypercapnia, acidosis or high airway pressures) the ductus arteriosus can remain open or subsequently re-open. PDA occurs frequently in premature and low-birth-weight infants and can lead to increased pulmonary blood flow, pulmonary oedema, and heart failure. It can be closed medically with prostaglandin inhibition by treatment with NSAIDs (e.g. indomethacin) or by surgical intervention.

Persistent pulmonary hypertension of the newborn can lead to right ventricular failure and poor cardiac output. Treatment includes high FiO_2, high-frequency oscillatory ventilation and inhaled nitric oxide therapy. Extracorporeal membrane oxygenation is considered early in treatment.

Renal system

Immature renal function leads to an impaired ability to excrete large water or sodium loads. The kidneys are also less effective at retaining electrolytes, so levels need to be closely monitored. High total body water, a large surface area, and high epithelial permeability lead to large evaporative water losses.

Preterm neonates have a lower glomerular filtration rate and creatinine clearance. They are more at risk from nephrotoxic drugs, and doses should be adjusted carefully. They are at risk of acute kidney injury from hypovolaemia and poor renal blood flow.

Gastrointestinal system

Poor glycogen stores and reduced gluconeogenesis pathways make neonates prone to hypoglycaemia. Difficulty with enteral feeding can be due to poor co-ordination of sucking, swallowing, and breathing, so nasogastric or nasojejunal feeding is often required. Gastro-oesophageal reflux requiring medical treatment often occurs and may need surgical intervention, e.g. fundoplication.

NEC is seen in 5% of infants born before 33 weeks [3]. It may require surgical treatment and can lead to bowel perforation, strictures, adhesions, short gut syndrome, sepsis, and death (in up to 30%) [4].

Central nervous system

Preterm neonates are at risk of brain injury which may be related to infection, hypoxia/ischaemia, or IVH. These infants receive routine cranial ultrasound monitoring to detect periventricular leukomalacia, haemorrhage, or ventricular dilatation. IVHs are particularly prevalent in preterm infants due to the fragility of the cerebral vessels and are seen in almost half of infants born at <1000 g [5]. Brain injury in neonates can ultimately lead to cerebral palsy, developmental delay, blindness, deafness, epilepsy, hydrocephalus, or death.

Eyes

Retinopathy of prematurity occurs in partially vascularized retinas which undergo abnormal blood vessel proliferation in response to high oxygen tensions. It is seen primarily in preterm infants (especially those born at <25 weeks) and treatment includes cryotherapy or laser retinal ablation. It can lead to blindness and approximately half of those affected have poor visual acuity in childhood [6].

⊙ Expert comment Terminology

By convention, gestational age is counted in weeks from the first day of the last menstrual period. Where the date of conception is known precisely (e.g. *in-vitro* fertilization), 2 weeks should be added to the actual age to generate a theoretical gestational age. The age of preterm neonates is often expressed as postmenstrual age—this is the gestational age at birth plus the postnatal age in weeks.

Postconceptional age is a term often used interchangeably with postmenstrual age; however, conception is typically 2 weeks after the first day of the last menstrual period. The terms are therefore not synonymous and the use of postconceptional age should be avoided [7].

> **ⓘ Expert comment** Respiratory distress syndrome and bronchopulmonary dysplasia
>
> Respiratory distress syndrome (RDS) is a life-threatening condition and is seen mainly in premature infants due to surfactant deficiency. Surfactant reduces surface tension in the alveoli and without it alveoli collapse causing atelectasis and poor lung expansion. Antenatal steroids, usually betamethasone, are given to mothers at risk of delivery before 34 weeks of gestation to reduce complications of RDS and the risk of NEC, IVH, PDA, and death [8]. Early prophylactic surfactant therapy, given via the tracheal tube, significantly reduces mortality and the respiratory complications of prematurity [9].
>
> Bronchopulmonary dysplasia (BPD) is defined as the need for supplemental oxygen for at least 28 days after birth. Severity of BPD is graded according to the oxygen requirement at 36 weeks of postmenstrual age (for infants born at less than 32 weeks), or at a postnatal age of 56 days (for those born at or after 32 weeks). If a neonate no longer needs supplemental oxygen at this time, the BPD is defined as mild; a required FiO_2 of between 0.21 and 0.29 is moderate BPD; and a required FiO_2 of >0.3 or an ongoing requirement for assisted ventilation is severe BPD [10]. Treatment includes the use of protective ventilation strategies, diuretics, bronchodilators, and optimization of nutrition. Routine use of steroids is no longer recommended due to the potential for short-term complications and the risk of neurodevelopmental impairment.

After discharge home, his mother had noticed abnormal eye movements and a poor suck during bottle feeding. He had been reviewed by a consultant neurologist who found horizontal nystagmus and ordered MRI and an EEG.

The infant and his mother came to the Day of Surgery Admission Unit. The scan had already been attempted once during the previous week using the 'feed and wrap' method, but this had been abandoned as he did not fall asleep for long enough to complete the scan. His mother had many questions about the safety of general anaesthesia in her child and the risk to his development.

> **✪ Learning point** Preoperative assessment of an infant (for MRI)
>
> For important considerations in a preoperative assessment, see Table 6.1.
>
> **Table 6.1 Important considerations in a preoperative assessment**
>
> | | |
> |---|---|
> | Birth and antenatal history | Gestation, mode of delivery, initial resuscitation or support required, complications. |
> | Respiratory system | Apnoeas, respiratory support since birth, current oxygen requirement, signs of respiratory distress, and airway anatomy. Review any recent X-rays. |
> | Cardiovascular system | Examine for heart murmurs, cyanosis, evidence of heart failure (e.g. difficulty feeding, breathlessness, sweating, delayed capillary refill, or hepatomegaly). Review echocardiograph. |
> | Previous surgery | Any implanted metallic device, e.g. clips, wires, etc. |
> | Discuss starvation period: make and document a plan | 2 h for water, 4 h for breast milk, and 6 h for formula milk. Start dextrose infusion in those at risk of hypoglycaemia. |
> | Blood results | Increased risk of apnoea in presence of anaemia. There is an increased risk of nephrogenic systemic fibrosis associated with the use of gadolinium-based contrast agents and severe renal impairment. Check renal function if use of contrast is planned; there are currently no alternatives to the gadolinium-based agents. |
> | Consent | For anaesthesia, requesting team should ideally obtain consent for the MRI scan [11]. |

Conduct of anaesthesia

After a thorough preoperative assessment and examination, the anaesthetic plan was discussed with the mother. The MRI unit is in a self-contained wing of the hospital and has an anaesthetic room opposite the MRI room, as well as a separate recovery area. The mother and her child were brought down to the unit by the ward nurse and were asked a series of safety questions by the radiographer to check that it was safe to proceed to MRI. The plan was for general anaesthesia with an inhalation induction followed by tracheal intubation to provide a safe and reliable airway (supraglottic airway devices in this age group are not as reliable as for older children) and intermittent positive pressure ventilation during the scan to avoid the risk of apnoea during maintenance and to provide positive airway pressure to minimize atelectasis given his age, size, and history of BPD.

> ### ✚ Clinical tip   Preparing for anaesthesia in a remote location
>
> Many MRI or CT scanners are located in areas of the hospital remote from the main theatre complex. Guidance from the Royal College of Anaesthetists [12] on provision of anaesthetic services in remote sites emphasizes the importance of familiarity with the environment. Appropriate facilities, staff, and equipment should be available for induction, maintenance, and recovery from general anaesthesia. The preoperative anaesthetic machine, drug, and equipment checks should be thorough and comply with AAGBI guidance [13]. It is recommended that a safety briefing is performed, often as part of the World Health Organization (WHO) surgical safety checklist. Knowledge of the location of emergency equipment is vital (e.g. defibrillator, difficult airway trolley, oxygen cylinder, cardiac arrest trolley, telephone, emergency alarm, 'Quench' button (Learning point, How MRI works), fire exit, and extinguisher), while being aware that many of these may not safely enter the MRI room itself.

> ### ✚ Clinical tip   Inhalational induction
>
> Induction of anaesthesia can be intravenous or inhalational. Many paediatric anaesthetists prefer the inhalational route in neonates and small children in order to facilitate control of the airway. In neonates, especially with either difficult airways or lung disease, 100% oxygen is generally used initially and then titrated down, once control of the airway is achieved.

> ### ✚ Clinical tip   Cannulation
>
> Intravenous access can be difficult in an ex-premature infant who has been cannulated many times before. Places to check for veins include the volar aspect of the wrist, the lateral border of the foot, and the saphenous, external jugular or scalp veins. Be sure to tape the cannula securely and a 10 cm extension line with three-way tap allows drugs to be given with minimal disturbance of the cannula. In an emergency, an intraosseous (IO) needle can be inserted into the proximal tibia until intravenous access is established.

After attempted aspiration of remaining stomach contents via the nasogastric tube, the infant was placed on a forced-air warming blanket on an MR-safe tilting trolley. Because of his age and comorbidities, his mother gave him a kiss and returned to the ward with the nurse before the start of anaesthesia. Monitoring was attached (MR-safe ECG electrodes, pulse oximetry and a blood pressure cuff) and an inhalational induction was then performed with 100% oxygen and 8% sevoflurane using a neonatal facemask and an Ayre's T-piece with Jackson–Rees modification (a Mapleson F circuit). Care was taken throughout to minimize exposure of the infant and he was covered with blankets as much as possible. After siting intravenous access (24G), atracurium 0.5 mg/kg was administered and lung ventilation was assisted, with care not to inflate the stomach.

Tracheal intubation was straightforward using a straight-bladed laryngoscope (Robertshaw size 0) with external laryngeal pressure [14] to achieve a grade I view and a 3.0 mm tracheal tube was inserted to a depth of 9 cm at the lips. Lung ventilation was demonstrated by the presence of an appropriate end-tidal carbon dioxide trace, and bilateral air entry was confirmed by auscultation. A small leak was heard but ventilation was unaffected. The tracheal tube was secured using tape (with a Guedel airway *in situ*). The NG tube was aspirated to remove any insufflated air from the stomach. Bedside blood sugar was 5.7 mmol/L.

> ### ❝ Expert comment   The neonatal airway: induction and intubation
>
> - Short time to hypoxia—due to combination of high metabolic rate, low functional residual capacity, risk of apnoea during induction, difficulty of preoxygenation in an awake neonate, and potentially difficult mask ventilation. Be careful to apply pressure only on the bony part of the jaw and do not overextend the neck, so as not to obstruct the airway.
> - Large occiput and small mouth—a roll under the shoulders and keeping the head in a neutral position may aid mask ventilation and laryngoscopy.
>
> (continued)

- Long floppy epiglottis, large tongue, and anterior larynx—the best view of the cords is often achieved by using a straight blade and lifting the epiglottis. Gentle pressure on the larynx can help.
- Choice of laryngoscope—most paediatricians use the Miller blade, whereas anaesthetists may prefer a Robertshaw, Seward, or Cardiff blade (the tracheal tube can tend to slot into the channel in a Miller blade and obstruct the view of the cords). A bougie may be needed but be aware that, if advanced too far, it may cause a pneumothorax in a neonate [15].
- Size of tracheal tube—the following is a rough guide: tracheal tube size 2.5 mm internal diameter (ID) if <1 kg, 3.0 mm ID if 1–2 kg, 3.5 mm ID if 2–3 kg, and either 3.5 or 4.0 mm ID if >3 kg [16]. The tube should pass through the cords easily and should not be forced.
- The narrowest point of the airway is at the cricoid—remember that the risk of subglottic stenosis from previous tracheal intubation may necessitate a smaller tube than otherwise predicted.
- Length of tracheal tube—use the '7–8–9 rule' [17]. Add 6 to the weight of a neonate to give the length at the lips (i.e. 7 cm for a 1 kg infant, 8 cm for a 2 kg infant, and 9 cm for a 3 kg infant). Always listen for equal air entry in both axillae.
- Aspiration of stomach—it is easy to inadvertently inflate the stomach during bag mask ventilation. If this is suspected, insert an orogastric or nasogastric tube to deflate it. The correct nasogastric tube size (in French) is twice that of the tracheal tube ID (in millimetres).
- Syndromes and difficult airways—certain syndromes are associated with difficult intubation, e.g. Pierre Robin sequence, Crouzon, Apert, Treacher–Collins, and Goldenhar syndromes, as well as children with a cleft palate.

At this point, all MR-unsafe equipment was removed (in this case the pulse oximetry probe was removed, the forced-air warmer disconnected, and the laryngoscope and stethoscope left behind). The patient was transferred into the scanning room on the MR-safe trolley and then on to the MRI table. Ventilation was resumed, initially by hand ventilation via the T-piece with sevoflurane in 100% oxygen and then when bilateral air entry had been reconfirmed, using an MR conditional anaesthetic machine and a long paediatric circle system (2.4 m length). Dedicated MR-safe monitoring was attached and vital signs displayed on a monitor in the scanning room as well as on a separate slave-monitor in the MR control room. Once satisfactory vital signs had been seen, air was added to the fresh gas flow to reduce the FiO_2 to <0.6. Care was taken to ensure that the infant was well wrapped in a warmed blanket, that he was protected from the risk of burns from monitoring cables, and that ear protectors to minimize the risk of acoustic injury were in place. The table was then advanced into the MR scanner while making sure that the breathing system and monitoring cables were well secured and not under tension. The anaesthetic team then returned to the control room for the duration of the scan.

> ⊕ **Learning point** How MRI works
>
> MRI is a non-invasive imaging technique that uses the magnetic properties of atomic nuclei to produce high-resolution cross-sectional images of the body. Atoms with an unpaired proton or neutron in their nuclei have a property known as 'spin'. When placed in a strong external magnetic field, the spin vectors on these nuclei align themselves with that magnetic field. In MRI, a super-conducting magnet supplies a constant magnetic field and bursts of radiofrequency (RF) energy are used to create temporary secondary magnetic fields which displace the alignment of these nuclei. As the RF pulse is removed, the nuclei return to their original positions and energy taken up during the RF pulse is released. This emitted energy is measured and its characteristics depend on the properties of the tissue it comes from. The timing of image capture is also important, hence fat appears white (high signal) in T1-weighted images whereas in T2-weighted images water is white (and therefore CSF appears bright). As well as the permanent electromagnet, MR scanners contain three smaller gradient coils to create three-dimensional magnetic field gradients and allow spatial information to be gathered. It is these gradient coils that make the loud banging noise during a scan, and the noise level is related to the strength of both the main magnetic field and the gradient pulse.
>
> (continued)

The walls of the scanning room contain a mesh of conducting material, forming an RF shield (sometimes called a Faraday cage), in order to stop external signals from interfering with detection of the weak electromagnetic signals produced during the scan. Infusion lines (or a breathing system if the anaesthetic machine is in the control room) can be passed into the scanner through the wall via tubes known as waveguides (usually made from copper or brass).

Quenching occurs when the coils in the electromagnet cease to be superconducting (a state in which there is no electrical resistance) and become resistive. The temperature therefore rises rapidly and the liquid helium used as a coolant then boils with explosive force (1 L of liquid helium at −269°C expands to 760 L of gaseous helium, and a magnet may contain up to 800 L of liquid helium). This gaseous helium is usually vented externally through a quench pipe, although if that fails it may then be released into the scanning room, resulting in a risk of asphyxiation through oxygen displacement. Superconducting magnets can malfunction and quench unexpectedly, or a quench can be activated by MR staff in the event of an emergency such as an immediate threat to life from the magnet. Oxygen monitoring is used in scanning rooms to detect a hypoxic environment which can result from a slow leak of helium, or an unexpected quench caused by cryogenic coolant depletion.

✪ **Learning point**   MR safety (Figures 6.1 and 6.2)

The MR environment poses multiple hazards. These include risks of injury from ferromagnetic objects (such as oxygen canisters, beds, wheelchairs, laryngoscopes, pens, or scissors) becoming projectiles pulled into the magnet core; injury from dislodged ferromagnetic implants (e.g. surgical clips) or objects (e.g. metal fragments retained in eyes); burns from the inside walls of the magnet or from wires (either internal such as pacemaker wires, or external such as monitoring leads); device malfunction due to the magnetic field (e.g. pacemakers or infusion devices); noise-related injury; reaction to contrast agents; and injury from inadvertent cryogen release [18]. Of these, device malfunction is the most likely to lead to death whereas the most common injuries are burns related to ECG leads and pulse oximeter probes.

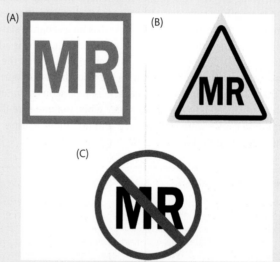

Figure 6.1 Safety signs for devices or equipment to be used in an MR environment. (A) MR safe: an item which poses no known hazard in all MR environments. (B) MR conditional: an item which poses no known hazard in a 'specified' MR environment. (C) MR unsafe: an item known to pose a hazard in the MR environment. Reprinted with permission, from *F2503-08 standard practice for marking medical devices and other items for safety in the magnetic resonance environment*, copyright © ASTM International, 100 Barr Harbor Drive, West Conshohocken, PA 19428, USA. A copy of the complete standard may be obtained from ASTM International (<http://www.astm.org>).

(continued)

Magnetic fields are measured in Tesla (T) or Gauss (G), where 1 T is equal to 10,000 G. Standard safety practice is to mark the area within which the magnetic field strength is >5 G. This 5 G line represents an exclusion zone that only staff or patients who have completed safety checks can enter; outside this zone the magnetic field is weak enough to be considered safe for everyone.

In order to minimize the risks, patients (or their parents) and new staff are questioned about metal implants, previous surgery, and implanted devices. All equipment used within the 5 G area must be either 'MR safe' or 'MR conditional'—where the specific conditions are being adhered to (e.g. used with the appropriate strength scanner, securely attached to the wall, or in a position below a certain Gauss strength). As an example, the Aestiva® 5/MRI anaesthetic machine can be used with a magnet up to 3 T and in an environment up to 300 G (Figure 6.2). A line on the floor marks the limit of proximity of the anaesthetic machine to the MRI scanner beyond which the magnetic field strength is >300 G.

MR-safe ECG electrodes and carbon ECG leads should be used (these have high resistance therefore heat less). Leads should never be looped (to avoid magnetic induction) and should not touch the patient – ideally foam or gamgee should be used as protection. MRI scans are loud and the noise can approach 130 decibels (equivalent to a military jet taking off 15 m away) therefore ear protection should be worn by the patient as well as by anyone else who stays in the room during a scan. Self-adhesive foam ear-muffs are available for neonates to wear under ear defenders.

Induction and emergence should take place in dedicated areas outside the 5 G line where the usual monitoring and equipment can be used. A high level of vigilance is required during anaesthesia for MRI as the remoteness of the patient, the reduced patient access, and interference with monitoring all increase the potential for complications. Should a critical incident occur during the scan the patient should be taken out of the scanner and definitive treatment given in a safe place beyond the 5 G line. Never attempt a resuscitation inside the scanning room as the risk of entry of unscreened staff or unsafe items is unacceptably high.

Gadolinium-based contrast agents are often used to enhance tissue differentiation. They can cause anaphylaxis although the frequency of this (~1 in 100,000) is much lower than that seen with other contrast agents. Gadolinium-based agents can also cause nephrogenic systemic fibrosis in people with severe renal impairment and are relatively contraindicated in neonates [19].

Remember that the MR radiographers are experts in MR safety; always work closely with them to ensure safe practice.

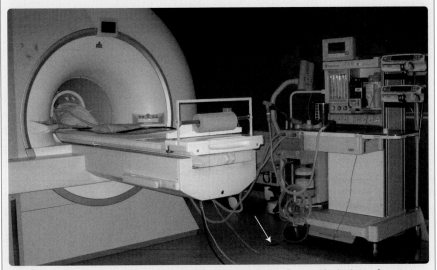

Figure 6.2 Magnetic resonance (MR) scan room—the tape on the floor marks the limit of proximity of the anaesthetic machine to the MR scanner beyond which the magnetic field strength is >300 G (arrow).

After 30 min the scan was completed, the sevoflurane turned off and ventilation reverted to hand ventilation via the T-piece with 100% oxygen. The infant was then transferred back on to the MR-safe trolley and taken back to the anaesthetic induction area. Neostigmine 50 μg/kg and glycopyrrolate 10 μg/kg were given to reverse neuromuscular blockade. His axillary temperature was measured at 36.4°C and the forced-air warmer was reattached. Hand ventilation with 100% oxygen was continued via the T-piece. A bedside blood sugar was measured again and was 5.4 mmol/L.

✪ Learning point   Temperature, glucose, and fluids

Temperature control in the neonate is extremely important (especially in ex-premature or low-birth-weight infants) and their thermoneutral zone is 32–36°C [20]. Neonates have a large surface area:weight ratio, have minimal subcutaneous fat, do not shiver, and have poorly developed vasoconstrictive mechanisms. Preterm neonates lose most heat through transepidermal evaporation and extremely premature neonates may need to be nursed in environments of up to 95% relative humidity [21]. Hypothermia-induced stress can lead to hypoglycaemia, apnoeas, and metabolic acidosis. Forced-air warmers and radiant heaters can only be used for induction and emergence outside the 5 G line. MR-safe incubators are commercially available, but most units simply cover infants with warmed blankets—the scan itself can produce a significant amount of heat and active warming is not usually required. The infant's temperature should be measured at the end of the scan and the infant warmed as appropriate.

Neonatal hypoglycaemia is defined as a glucose level <2.6 mmol/L (although there is little scientific justification for this cut-off) [22]; treatment should involve an intravenous bolus of 2 mL/kg of 10% dextrose followed by an infusion at 4 mL/kg/h. Infants at highest risk of hypoglycaemia include those who are small for gestational age, preterm, or stressed (e.g. sepsis, hypoglycaemia, seizures, etc.), as well as those who had a low birth weight (<2.5 kg), or who are on total parenteral nutrition. Infants who are on dextrose infusions already should have these continued during the scan (the easiest way is either via an MRI conditional syringe driver in the scanning room or a normal syringe driver in the control room with a long narrow-gauge giving set). All neonates should have blood sugar checked prior to the start of anaesthesia and then hourly during surgery (or for MRI simply again at the end) with treatment given as appropriate. A feed should be given as soon as possible after recovery from anaesthesia.

Intravenous fluids rarely need to be given during anaesthesia for MRI scans other than for maintenance of glucose levels as already discussed. Hartmann's, 0.9% sodium chloride or colloid (10–20 mL/kg) should be given if bolus fluid therapy is required to minimize the risk of postoperative hyponatraemia, and this fluid should be warmed.

Soon afterwards the infant started to make occasional movements (although these were not sustained) and started to make good respiratory effort. Manual ventilation was therefore stopped and he was allowed to breathe spontaneously with gentle CPAP applied via the T-piece. He did, however, have several episodes of apnoea requiring manual ventilation. As he became more awake these became less frequent although gentle pharyngeal suction still stimulated apnoea. Eventually (after ∼15 min) he was fully awake and no longer having apnoeas. His tracheal tube was removed and he confirmed that his airway was patent with a vigorous cry. He was transferred to the recovery area with facemask oxygen.

Once in recovery, however, he continued to have occasional apnoeas, although these responded to gentle stimulation and were not associated with bradycardia or desaturation. His blood sugar was measured again (5.6 mmol/L) as was his haemoglobin using HemoCue® (HemoCue Ltd, Dronfield, UK) point-of-care testing (11.8 g/dL). His axillary temperature was now 37.1°C. His respiratory rate was 54 breaths/min and oxygen saturation was 96% in air. His chest was clear on auscultation, with no added sounds. His mother was called and she breastfed him, although this did appear to result in some shortness of breath. A chest X-ray was performed and was unremarkable.

He continued to be observed in recovery, but the intermittent apnoeas did not resolve and he was referred to the neonatal intensive care unit (NICU) for further observation. Nasopharyngeal aspirates taken on admission to NICU subsequently showed RSV infection. His apnoeas resolved over the next 12 h but he went on to develop mild symptoms of bronchiolitis and required a short period of hospitalization with supplementary oxygen therapy.

✪ Expert comment   Postoperative apnoeas

Clinically significant apnoea is defined as a pause in breathing of >20 s, or a pause of >10 s if associated with bradycardia (<80 beats/min), cyanosis, or monitored desaturation (SaO₂ <80% or 85%, depending on which definition is used) [23]. Primary apnoeas are frequent in preterm neonates and are almost universal in infants weighing <1000 g. Of note, there is no clear relationship between apnoeas and sudden infant death. Apnoeas can be central, obstructive or mixed, with mixed being the most widespread—airway tone decreases rapidly after the start of a central apnoea and, when respiratory effort returns, it is often initially against a closed larynx or collapsed pharynx. Most apnoeas are self-limiting or respond to gentle stimulation, but recurrent apnoeas can be treated with methylxanthines—usually caffeine [24].

Apnoeas can also be induced by a wide variety of events including acidosis, hypoxia, hypothermia, hypoglycaemia, electrolyte disturbance, anaemia, pain, drugs (e.g. sedatives and opiates), neurological disturbance (e.g. IVH or seizures), and intercurrent illness (e.g. NEC) or infection (especially RSV). The incidence of apnoea in former preterm infants after anaesthesia is strongly related to both gestational and postmenstrual age, and the risk of apnoea after leaving recovery (in infants who do not have apnoeas in recovery) does not fall to <1% until 56 weeks of postmenstrual age [25]. Anaemia (haematocrit <30%) is a strong independent risk factor for postoperative apnoea.

When waking a neonate after general anaesthesia, it is important not to remove the tracheal tube until the infant is fully awake (eyes open and consistently moving all four limbs) and no longer responds to stimulation (such as gentle pharyngeal suction) with an apnoea.

Postoperative care for term infants up to 44 weeks of postmenstrual age should include apnoea and continuous saturation monitoring for at least 12 apnoea-free hours. As preterm infants are at greater risk of apnoeas and for a longer period, they should have this level of monitoring postoperatively up to 60 weeks of postmenstrual age (some units say 56 weeks). Anaesthesia in these infants should be on an inpatient basis only.

Discussion

Parents of infants undergoing anaesthesia are naturally anxious and frequently ask about the long-term effects of anaesthesia on their child's development – this is a normal concern but may also be related to media coverage of the effects of anaesthetics on neurodevelopment [26]. A committee of the US Food and Drug Administration met recently to discuss this issue and concluded that there was still too little information to allow any firm conclusions to be drawn regarding the safety of anaesthesia in infants, but that clinicians should summarize the current state of knowledge and uncertainty when asked by parents [27].

There is much debate regarding the effects of anaesthesia on the developing neonatal brain. Animal studies have shown that all the common anaesthetic agents and sedatives can induce neuronal apoptosis (programmed cell death) in neonatal animals, and this effect appears to be dependent on both dose and length of exposure [28]. The timing of maximum susceptibility coincides with a period of rapid synaptogenesis (thought to occur in humans between the third trimester and 3 years). There are always problems with extrapolating animal evidence to humans; however, there are significant concerns for the safety of anaesthesia in neonates.

Clinical studies have shown conflicting results [29], with some suggesting a link between anaesthetic exposure early in life and developmental/behavioural problems, but given the huge potential for confounding factors it is difficult to draw any firm conclusions. An American study found that children who had undergone hernia repair before 3 years of age had a 2.3-fold increased risk of developmental delay or behavioural problems (95% confidence interval: 1.3–4.1) [30]; however, a Dutch study looking at twins found that although those who had had surgery did indeed have lower educational achievement scores and more cognitive problems, there was no difference between twins where one twin had had surgery and the other had not, suggesting that confounding factors rather than surgery or anaesthesia may be to blame [31]. It should also be remembered that painful events in the neonatal period without anaesthesia can also lead to developmental and behavioural problems [32].

In summary, there remains insufficient evidence to know what damage occurs to the developing neonatal brain during anaesthesia, although there are large-scale studies currently being undertaken (including the PANDA and GAS studies) [33, 34]. In the meantime, it remains good practice to delay procedures that can reasonably be delayed until after the neonatal period, and ideally until after 3 years of age.

A Final Word from the Expert

It is often (somewhat unhelpfully) stated that children are not small adults; this is most true for neonates and preterm infants who can present significant challenges to the anaesthetist—in particular with respect to airway management; cannulation; temperature, glucose and fluid management; emergence; and postoperative care. Anaesthesia for neonates and preterm infants should only be undertaken by experienced, appropriately trained anaesthetists, and requires meticulous attention to detail.

All anaesthesia carries the risk of serious complications, and children aged <1 year represent a high-risk group [35]. Children in general, and neonates in particular, can deteriorate very rapidly and tolerate physiological insults poorly. In addition, the MR environment poses a unique set of challenges, and anaesthetists must be familiar with the risks associated with MRI and how to mitigate them. The unquantifiable risk of neurotoxicity to the developing neonatal brain is another ingredient to add to the balance of risk and benefit, and as anaesthetists we have a duty to make sure that people (both clinicians requesting procedures that require anaesthesia and the parents of the children involved) have an understanding of those risks. It is important that when children have comorbidities that put them at particular risk of perioperative complications, there is a mechanism whereby a discussion can take place between the referring clinician, the radiologist, the anaesthetist, and the parents to ensure that the procedure requiring anaesthesia is indeed both the most appropriate investigation and in the child's best interests.

Increasing survival rates from extreme prematurity coupled with the short- and long-term morbidity from which these children suffer mean that we will increasingly be asked to anaesthetize these patients.

References

1. Walsh M, Engle W, Laptook A, *et al.* Oxygen delivery through nasal cannulae to preterm infants: can practice be improved? *Pediatrics* 2005;116:857–61.

2. Mohangoo AD, Buitendijk SE, Szamotulska K, *et al.* Gestational age patterns of fetal and neonatal mortality in Europe: results from the Euro-Peristat Project. *PLoS One* 2011;6:e24727.

3. Yee WH, Singh Soraisham A, Shah VS, *et al.* Incidence and timing of presentation of necrotizing enterocolitis in preterm infants. *Pediatrics* 2012;128:e298–e304.

4. Fitzgibbons SC, Ching Y, Yu D, *et al.* Mortality of necrotizing enterocolitis expressed by birth weight categories. *J Pediatr Surg* 2009;44:1075–6.

5. Wilson-Costello D, Friedman H, Minich N, *et al.* Improved survival rates with increased neurodevelopmental disability for extremely low birth weight infants in the 1990s. *Pediatrics* 2005;115:997–1003.

6. Anderson C, Phelps D. Peripheral retinal ablation for threshold retinopathy of prematurity in preterm infants. *Cochrane Database Syst Rev* 1999;(3):CD001693.

7. American Academy of Pediatrics Committee on Fetus and Newborn. Age terminology during the perinatal period. *Pediatrics* 2004;114:1362–64.

8. Roberts D, Dalziel S. Antenatal steroids for accelerating fetal lung maturation for women at risk of preterm birth. *Cochrane Database Syst Rev* 2006;(3):CD004544.

9. Soll R. Early versus delayed selective surfactant treatment for neonatal respiratory distress syndrome. *Cochrane Database Syst Rev* 1999;(4):CD001456.

10. Baraldi E, Filippone M. Chronic lung disease after premature birth. *N Engl J Med* 2007;357:1946–55.

11. Wellesley H, Chong WK, Segar P. Who should obtain written consent for magnetic resonance imaging under general anaesthesia? *Pediatr Anesth* 2009;19:961–3.

12. Royal College of Anaesthetists. *Guidance for the provision of anaesthetic services.* Chapter 7. Anaesthesia services for care in the non-theatre environment. London: RCA; 2013 < http:// www.rcoa.ac.uk/system/files/GPAS-2013-07-ANTE_1.pdf >

13. Association of Anaesthetists of Great Britain and Ireland. Checking anaesthetic equipment 2012. *Anaesthesia* 2012;67:660–68.

14. Moied AS, Pal J. Cricoid pressure—a misnomer in pediatric anaesthesia. *J Emerg Trauma Shock* 2010;3:96–7.

15. Kumar S, Walker R. Bougie-related tension pneumothorax in a neonate. *Pediatr Anesth* 2009;19:800–1.

16. Wyllie J. Neonatal endotracheal intubation. *Archs Dis Childh Educn Pract* 2008;93:44–9.

17. Peterson J, Johnson N, Deakins K, *et al.* Accuracy of the 7–8–9 rule for endotracheal tube placement in the neonate. *J Perinatol* 2006;26:333–6.

18. The Joint Commission. *Sentinel event alert: preventing accidents and injuries in the MRI suite*; 14 February 2008. < http://www.jointcommission.org/assets/1/18/SEA_38.pdf >

19. Thomsen H. ESUR guideline: gadolinium-based contrast media and nephrogenic systemic fibrosis. *Eur Radiol* 2007;17:2692–6.

20. Bell E, Gray J, Weinstein M, *et al.* The effects of thermal environment on heat balance and insensible water loss in low-birth-weight infants. *J Pediatrics* 1980;96:452–9.

21. Warner L, Peacock E, O'Reagan T. *Clinical guideline: thermoregulation for neonates.* Great Ormond Street Hospital for Children; 25 March 2011. < http://www.gosh.nhs.uk/ health-professionals/clinical-guidelines/thermoregulation-for-neonates/ >

22. American Academy of Pediatrics Committee on Fetus and Newborn. Clinical report—postnatal glucose homeostasis in late-preterm and term infants. *Pediatrics* 2011;127:575–9.

23. Finer N, Higgins R, Kattwinkel J, *et al.* Summary proceedings from the apnoea of prematurity group. *Pediatrics* 2006;117:547–51.

24. Henderson-Smart D, de Paoli A. Methylxanthine treatment for apnoea in preterm infants. *Cochrane Database Syst Rev* 2010;(12):CD000140.

25. Cote C, Zaslavsky A, Downes J, *et al.* Postoperative apnea in former preterm infants after inguinal herniorrhaphy. *Anesthesiology* 1995;82:809–22.

26. Harrel E. Anesthesia: could early use affect the brain later? *Time (Health & Family)*. < http://www.time.com/time/health/article/0,8599,1934197,00.html >

27. US Food and Drug Administration. Summary minutes of the Anesthetic and Life Support Drugs Advisory Committee Meeting, 10 March 2011. Washington DC: FDA. < http://www.fda.gov/downloads/AdvisoryCommittees/CommitteesMeetingMaterials/Drugs/AnestheticAndLifeSupportDrugsAdvisoryCommittee/UCM251282.pdf >

28. Lopeke A, Soriano S. An assessment of the effects of general anesthetics on developing brain structure and neurocognitive function. *Anesth Analg* 2008;106:1681–1707.

29. Sun L. Early childhood general anaesthesia exposure and neurocognitive development. *Br J Anaesth* 2010;105(Suppl 1):i61–8.

30. DiMaggio C, Sun L, Kakvouli A, *et al.* A retrospective cohort study of the association of anesthesia and hernia repair surgery with behavioural and developmental disorders in young children. *J Neurosurg Anesthesiol* 2009;21:286–91.

31. Bartels M, Althoff R, Boomsma D. Anesthesia and cognitive performance in children: no evidence for a causal relationship. *Twin Res Hum Genet* 2009;12:246–53.

32. Anand KJ. Effects of perinatal pain and stress. *Prog Brain Res* 2000;122:117–29.

33. US Food and Drug Administration. *Pediatric anesthesia neuro-development assessment (PANDA) study.* Federal Business Opportunities. < https://www.fbo.gov/index?s = opportunity&mode = form&id = c23e20720a5aac52a3ead753ff399cfc&tab = core&_cview = 1 >

34. US National Institutes of Health. *A multi-site randomized controlled trial comparing regional and general anesthesia for effects on neurodevelopmental outcome and apnea in infants.* < http://clinicaltrials.gov/ct2/show/NCT00756600 >

35. Morray J, Geiduschek J, Ramamoorthy C, *et al.* Anesthesia-related cardiac arrest in children: initial findings of the Pediatric Perioperative Cardiac Arrest (POCA) Registry. *Anesthesiology* 2000;93:6–14.

6.2 Paediatric tonsillectomy

Rachel Homer

ⓘ **Expert Commentary** Kathy Wilkinson
CPD Matrix Code: *2D02, 3A02, 3A06, 3D00*

Case history

A 19 kg 6-year-old girl was listed for elective adenotonsillectomy. Her primary indication for tonsillectomy was recurrent tonsillitis causing her to miss several days of school over the last year. The general practitioner's referral letter also mentioned probable symptoms of obstructive sleep apnoea (OSA): 'snoring, always tired, dark circles under eyes', but she had not had a sleep study. She arrived on the children's ward of her local district hospital as a morning-of-surgery admission. She had no other past medical history, no allergies, and had not previously had a general anaesthetic. There was no family history of anaesthetic problems. It was confirmed that she had had no food since the previous evening, but a drink of water early that morning. On examination she was bright and chatty, with a normal facial appearance, although she was mouth-breathing, which, alongside the symptoms noted in the referral letter, raised further concerns of possible OSA (Figure 6.3). Although booked as an inpatient, her parents' first question upon meeting the anaesthetist was 'We will be able to take her home tonight, won't we?'

✪ Learning point Indications for (adeno)tonsillectomy

Tonsillectomy remains one of the most frequent operations in children and is most often performed in a non-specialist setting. However, there is evidence that the number of patients requiring tonsillectomy in England decreased during the period 1994–2005 [1].

In 2005 recurrent acute tonsillitis remained the most likely indication for tonsillectomy in both children and adults in the UK [2]. This is often defined as recurrent sore throat due to tonsillitis over at least one year with at least seven episodes in one year or five episodes per year for 2 years [3]. Symptoms must also be sufficiently severe to interfere with normal activities such as school attendance. OSA is a further common indication, whilst unilateral tonsillar swelling, chronic tonsillitis and past history of quinsy (tonsillar abscess) are less common indications. Both tonsillar swelling and chronic tonsillitis are most often encountered in teenagers and adults.

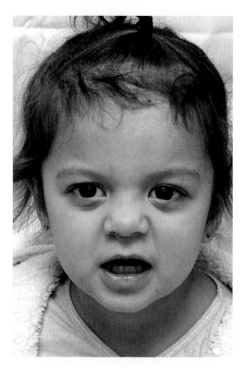

Figure 6.3 This child was mouth-breathing at preoperative assessment; OSA might reasonably be suspected, and a thorough enquiry into other signs and symptoms of OSA should therefore be made. Reproduced with permission from Medical Illustration—N&N Univ Hosp.

✪ **Learning point**   Obstructive sleep apnoea in children

Sleep-disordered breathing in children due to upper airway obstruction can be described as a spectrum of disorders of varying severity:

1. Primary snoring—not associated with daytime symptoms (occurring in 12–20% of children).
2. Obstructive hypopnoea—characterized by >50% reduction in oronasal airflow (but with some flow maintained), causing oxyhaemoglobin desaturation and/or hypercapnia. Also known as obstructive hypoventilation [4].
3. OSA (estimated to occur in 1–3% of all children [4–6])—characterized by intermittent upper airways obstruction leading to absent oronasal airflow despite continuing respiratory effort [4], with cardiovascular and/or neurobehavioural sequelae [6, 7].

Upper airway obstruction can lead to abnormal central control of breathing, and results in episodes of both hypoxaemia and hypercapnia. This may ultimately lead to pulmonary vasoconstriction and effects on the right ventricle (initially hypertrophy but later right heart failure). Clinical examination may confirm relevant comorbidity, and, in a very small number, late signs of pulmonary sequelae including pulmonary hypertension, right ventricular hypertrophy, and ultimately right ventricular failure [5, 6].

OSA may be further classified into mild, moderate, and severe, depending on frequency and duration of apnoeas and oxyhaemoglobin desaturation.

The peak prevalence of OSA is in 2–6-year-olds and there is equal gender distribution [4–6]. OSA is more common, and frequently more severe, in children who are obese, those with craniofacial or neuromuscular disorders, and in patients with Down syndrome. Many but not all children with OSA have enlarged tonsils and adenoids, and OSA is increasingly seen as a primary indication for adenotonsillectomy with resolution of symptoms in the majority of cases [4, 6]. The risks of anaesthesia are increased in younger children; respiratory complications were reported in almost 10% of children aged <3 years with documented OSA in one large series [8].

Diagnosis is suspected clinically based on a detailed history. Snoring alone is very non-specific but additional clues to the diagnosis include: increased work of breathing when asleep, restless or disturbed

(continued)

sleep, adopting unusual sleeping positions, apnoeas, enuresis, daytime sleepiness (less common than in adults with OSA), behavioural disturbance including hyperactivity or inattention, and poor school performance [5–7].

Investigations range from screening tests such as overnight oximetry to multichannnel polysomnography including carbon dioxide monitoring and video surveillance. Whereas the latter investigations can increase diagnostic sensitivity and specificity, they are often not performed due to availability, cost, invasiveness, and disagreement on diagnostic criteria [4]. If pulmonary hypertension is suspected, ECG and echocardiography are indicated. There are drivers to suggest that the diagnosis and management of sleep-disordered breathing in children should be organized on a regional network basis [9].

Sedation and analgesia

Sedative pre-medication is best avoided in children with OSA.

Children with established OSA have chronic intermittent desaturations and may also be exquisitely sensitive to the respiratory depressant effects of opioids [10, 11]. It has been shown that children with the deepest overnight saturation troughs (<70%) may also have the most pronounced increase in sensitivity, and the lowest opioid dose requirement for complete postoperative analgesia given identical pain scores [9]. In the same study, children whose saturation remained >85% overnight seemed not to be affected, e.g. those at the 'snoring-only' end of the sleep-disordered breathing spectrum. However, many patients listed for adenotonsillectomy with possible OSA will not have had overnight oximetry, thus their overnight oxyhaemoglobin saturation nadir is unknown. Therefore if OSA is suspected, despite lack of obvious risk factors, clear history or clinical signs, opioids should be administered with caution, in smaller increments than usual, and with close postoperative monitoring. Short-acting drugs such as intravenous fentanyl (1–2 µg/kg) are preferred to morphine.

As with all patients, the use of paracetamol and NSAIDs may minimize the requirement for opioids, and also reduce the occurrence of other important side-effects, e.g. nausea [2, 12, 13].

Extubation

The child with suspected OSA should be extubated awake to minimize the likelihood of airway obstruction or apnoea, the latter resulting from a disordered carbon dioxide response curve [5, 10].

Postoperative care

Regular follow-up doses of NSAIDs and paracetamol should form the mainstay of postoperative analgesia.

In 2013 the UK drug regulatory authorities recommended avoidance of codeine in all children following tonsillectomy [14]. A standard (1 mg/kg) dose of oral codeine administered regularly may well lead to severe respiratory depression in the opioid-sensitive child with severe OSA. Given the wide variation in cytochrome P450 enzyme systems, children who are rapid metabolisers can also exhibit unexpected opioid sensitivity with possible respiratory depression if given regularly administered codeine [15, 16]. If absolutely required, a carefully titrated and closely monitored small dose (25–50 µg/kg) of intravenous morphine is probably a safer alternative [6, 10, 17].

Given the increased risk of complications in a child with known or suspected OSA, consideration should be given to performing surgery in a hospital with a paediatric high dependency and/or paediatric intensive care unit (PICU) on site.

The UK multidisciplinary consensus statement [7] suggests that children with sleep-disordered breathing, but without other risk factors for respiratory complications, can safely undergo adenotonsillectomy in a district general hospital (DGH) setting. However, there are risk factors which should prompt referral to a centre with a PICU (Box 6.1).

As a minimum, overnight inpatient observation with pulse oximetry postoperatively is needed for any child with documented OSA [6, 10]. It is probably best to avoid additional use of oxygen as a minority of children with OSA rely on a hypoxic drive.

One large centre has successfully reported the use of a carefully placed nasal airway for children postoperatively, which helps relieve residual airway obstruction that has not been immediately improved

(continued)

The majority of normal children who snore do not have OSA. If there is additional information from history or clinical examination to suggest that snoring is leading to obstruction, or if the child is very young, or falls into the group with comorbidities known to be at risk, then overnight oximetry should be arranged as a primary screening investigation.

In the management of infants and children presenting for adenotonsillectomy, the recent guidance from the Working Party on Sleep Physiology and Respiratory Control Disorders in Childhood [4] has been helpful. This document also sets standards for performance and interpretation of breathing tests.

Those with positive tests (saturations <80% and/or baseline hypoxaemia and/or positive polysomnography), and children with known risk factors as listed in Box 6.1, should be cared for in a centre with ready access to a PICU.

Many centres now perform the majority of their adenotonsillectomy cases as day cases. Criteria for decision-making in advance of admission are useful, and it may be useful to screen specifically to try and avoid children with sleep-disordered breathing.

by surgery [18]. This is left in place at least for the first postoperative night, and should be kept patent by gentle regular suction.

Note also the role of steroids in OSA (see Discussion, Role of steroids in adenotonsillectomy).

Box 6.1 Factors predicting need for paediatric intensive care unit availability in children with obstructive sleep apnoea undergoing adenotonsillectomy [4, 6, 7]

Age <2 years
Weight <15 kg, or <5th centile for age and sex
Severe obesity (BMI standard deviation score >2.5, or >99th centile for age and gender)
Severe heart disease including ECG or echocardiographic abnormalities
Severe lung disease including ex-premature infants
Severe OSA on polysomnography, e.g. oxygen saturation trough <80%
Neuromuscular disease, including hypotonia and severe cerebral palsy
Craniofacial abnormalities
Mucopolysaccharidosis
Other syndromes associated with a difficult airway
Any other significant comorbidity including all patients with ASA score 3

✪ Learning point Tonsillectomy: a day-case procedure in children?

Day-case surgery is often preferred in children as much surgery is relatively minor, good home supervision is usually in place, and children prefer to be in a familiar place when they are unwell. Hospital stays should be minimized if possible to reduce psychological disruption. The main challenges of day-case tonsillectomy are managing the risks associated with bleeding, pain, and postoperative nausea and vomiting. If OSA is undiagnosed this also remains a risk factor.

Day-stay tonsillectomy is becoming more common: the National Tonsillectomy Audit [2] of cases conducted in 2003–2004 found 12% booked as day cases with another 2% discharged home on the day of tonsillectomy. More recent cohorts from individual centres in Sweden and the UK [19–22] had rates of between 69% and 100% for day-case procedures. Consistent senior input from surgical and anaesthetic consultants appears to be important in the successful programmes provided in several of these centres.

Children undergoing tonsillectomy for recurrent infections, rather than to treat sleep-disordered breathing, can be considered particularly appropriate for day-case surgery provided they have no other conditions increasing their risk of either respiratory or haemorrhagic complications [19]. Most centres have age and weight restrictions, e.g. minimum age 4 or 5 years, minimum weight 20 kg. Social criteria should also be considered, e.g. time or distance between home and hospital, availability of a private car in which the child could be returned to hospital if necessary, and confirmation of two competent carers.

Centres performing day-case tonsillectomy generally suggest that there is an appropriate observation period prior to discharge (e.g. 4–6 h), as bleeding complications are most likely to occur in the first few postoperative hours [20–22]. This can be achieved by placing the child on a morning operating list.

Prior to discharge the child should be pain free, eating and drinking confidently, and have regular analgesia prescribed and understood. Parents and carers should receive very clear instructions on what to do if bleeding is suspected; or who they should call if pain, nausea, and vomiting occur (Figure 6.4); and where in the hospital they should attend. Some centres arrange telephone follow-up at 24 h as a minimum for all cases.

In view of a potential history of OSA the decision was made to admit the child for overnight monitoring. It was explained to the parents that this was felt to be the safest option.

On the ward she received an analgesic premedication of 15 mg/kg paracetamol orally approximately an hour before surgery. In the anaesthetic room, she refused

Norfolk and Norwich University Hospitals **NHS**
NHS Foundation Trust

Day Procedure Unit

JENNY LIND
CHILDREN'S HOSPITAL

Bleeding After Tonsillectomy - Advice for Parents

Bleeding from the throat after tonsillectomy is **NOT** normal.

If you notice any bleeding from your child's throat after you have left hospital with your child, you should phone CAU (Children's Assessment Unit) on **01603 289774** and tell them your child has had atonsillectomy and is now bleeding.

If it is necessary to bring your child immediately to CAU, the map below shows the location of the Day Procedure Unit (where your child had their operation) and the location of CAU which is in the Jenny Lind Children's Department with "footsteps" indicating the closest car park for access.

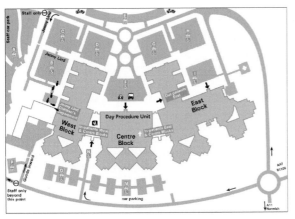

Figure 6.4 Instructions for parents of children treated as day-cases. Reproduced with kind permission from Norfolk and Norwich University Hospitals.

removal of EMLA (eutectic mixture of local anaesthetic) cream from her hands, but co-operated cheerfully with an inhalational induction of anaesthesia (50% nitrous oxide in oxygen, with sevoflurane 2% to a maximum of 8%) while seated on her mother's lap. Once lifted on to the surgical bed and routine monitoring applied (SpO_2 finger probe, ECG, blood pressure cuff), a 22G intravenous cannula was inserted and 1 microgram/kg fentanyl with 0.5 mg/kg atracurium administered to facilitate tracheal intubation. She became mildly obstructed but responded to facemask-delivered CPAP and insertion of an oropharyngeal airway. She was intubated with a 6.0 mm internal diameter preformed south-facing 'RAE' (Ring, Adair and Elwyn) tracheal tube. She was given a further 1.5 microgram/kg intravenous fentanyl, rectal diclofenac 1–2 mg/kg (25 mg), and intravenous dexamethasone and ondansetron (each 0.15 mg/kg) for control of postoperative pain (dexamethasone) and nausea (both).

> ✪ **Learning point** Routine tonsillectomy—to intubate or not to intubate?
>
> Careful placement of an operative mouth gag by the surgeon is an integral part of (adeno)tonsillectomy. This may compress or displace whatever airway device is chosen, causing partial or complete obstruction, whether spontaneous or controlled ventilation is employed [21, 23–25].
>
> Advantages of choosing a flexible laryngeal mask airway (fLMA) include:
>
> - Avoiding the choice between extubation with the child awake (which risks coughing and laryngospasm) or at a deep plane of anaesthesia (which by leaving the airway unprotected also risks laryngospasm in recovery room): the fLMA may remain in place during recovery until removed by the child, without stimulating airway reflexes as strongly as a tracheal tube. However, it is not clear that there is necessarily a lower rate of laryngospasm when using an fLMA compared with a tracheal tube [23 vs 24, 25].
> - The fLMA may be associated with less coughing than an awake extubation and earlier return of airway reflexes after device removal than extubation at a deep plane of anaesthesia.
> - Avoids the risk of endobronchial intubation occurring when the neck is extended and Boyles gag inserted, a particular problem with the RAE tube.
> - One study has reported that airway soiling may be greater with an uncuffed tracheal tube than with an fLMA [25].
>
> The disadvantages of the fLMA when compared with a preformed tracheal tube include:
>
> - A larger airway tube increasing the incidence of airway obstruction when the mouth gag is inserted to approximately 5%, most often by displacing the fLMA from its position in the airway [23, 24].
> - A larger cuff which may restrict surgical access, particularly in children with a relatively small upper airway [24, 25].
> - The possibility of dislodgement during surgical manipulation causing acute difficulty ventilating the child's lungs [25].
> - Not a technique for use in inexperienced hands (either anaesthetist or surgeon) as meticulous placement of both fLMA and gag are essential for all the reasons above.
> - Concerns regarding potential transmission of new variant Creutzfeld–Jakob disease by prions potentially present in tonsillar tissue led the Department of Health to recommend only single-use surgical and anaesthetic equipment be used for tonsillectomy, specifically mentioning LMAs [26]. This recommendation was rescinded for surgical instruments due to increased bleeding rates [27] but not for anaesthetic equipment. Single-use fLMAs may not perform so well in terms of placement or dislodgement as re-usable devices, even in experienced hands [28].

The patient was transferred into the operating room. Anaesthesia was maintained using isoflurane in 35% oxygen: 65% nitrous oxide with pressure-controlled ventilation. A 20 mL/kg bolus of Hartmann's solution was administered. Surgery proceeded uneventfully, although the surgeon did comment at one point that 'she is a little oozy'. At the end of the operation, once haemostasis was achieved, the throat was examined by direct laryngoscopy and bleeding was found to be minimal. Muscle relaxation was reversed and the patient began to breathe spontaneously. She was placed into the left lateral position, and the tracheal tube was removed as soon as airway reflexes had returned and the child was responding purposefully to minimal stimulation and breathing regularly. She had a 20 min stay in recovery, with no episodes of desaturation, apnoea or obstruction. She was transferred back to the paediatric ward with pulse oximetry to be continued overnight, and was prescribed regular ibuprofen (10 mg/kg, 8-hourly) and paracetamol (15 mg/kg 4–6-hourly) as well as ondansetron as needed.

On the ward 3 h postoperatively the child was pale, quiet, and 'not herself' but not in pain, according to her parents. Her observation chart showed tachycardia with a heart rate of 125 beats/min. She was conscious but sleepy with oxygen saturations in air of 96% and a respiratory rate of 28 breaths/min. She then vomited, covering her pillow with blood and a few clots.

The ENT registrar reviewed the child, and noted a central capillary refill time of ~3 s. An urgent anaesthetic review was requested and the ENT consultant informed, with a plan to take the child back to theatre promptly. The ENT registrar explained this to the child and parents and gained consent, having explained the risks and benefits. The anaesthetic registrar asked for oxygen to be administered and the blood pressure was checked, and was found to be a little low (85/34 mmHg). The cannula was checked for patency, and blood samples sent for urgent full blood count and blood grouping. A rapid fluid bolus of 20 mL/kg Hartmann's solution was administered by the anaesthetist, and assistance from a consultant was sought. The drugs and doses given as part of the last anaesthetic were noted along with the size of tracheal tube used, and the view at laryngoscopy (grade 1).

The planned induction sequence was discussed with theatre personnel in a preoperative discussion. The child was brought to theatre within 30 min of her first review, routine monitoring was applied, and the child preoxygenated with 100% oxygen. The mother was present and the modified induction plan briefly described including the purpose of cricoid pressure. The team performed an intravenous rapid sequence induction using propofol (2 mg/kg) and suxamethonium (2 mg/kg). Cricoid pressure was applied as soon as conciousness was lost. The child's mother stayed for the early part of induction, and helped hold and reassure her. At laryngoscopy the vocal cords were initially obscured by blood which was cleared by suction, and a 5.5 mm tracheal tube was 'snug'. A second fluid

---

✚ Clinical tip Organizing the prompt return to theatre

Assess and treat:

- Airway patent?
- Breathing adequate? (Respiratory rate, SpO_2.) Administer oxygen via facemask.
- Circulation adequate? (Heart rate, blood pressure, central capillary refill.)
- Cannula present, securely fixed and patent? If not, consider re-siting now or in anaesthetic room.
- Blood sample for urgent full blood count, group and save (may be possible to take from cannula).
- Prescribe and give a rapid 20 mL/kg isotonic fluid bolus (calculate, check, and give manually).
- Review anaesthetic chart: drugs and doses; laryngoscopy grade; tracheal tube size.

Communicate:

See Table 6.2.

Table 6.2 Post-tonsillectomy bleeding: who else needs to know?

Child and parent(s)	Parents should be informed of planned return to theatre, and intended anaesthetic management (especially nature of rapid sequence induction). Consent should be gained by the ENT team.
Child's ward nurse	Continued care, ready for transfer.
ENT surgeon	Gain consent, ensure urgent bloods sent, present in theatre.
Theatre sister/ co-ordinator	To ensure that a theatre is warm, set up, and staffed, with required instruments available, for the child's arrival. Experienced nurse to be available in anaesthetic room to receive child and parent and facilitate prompt checks with anaesthetic team.
Operating department practitioner	Ask for a second suction, extra tracheal tubes including smaller sizes than originally used, extra (checked) laryngoscopes, difficult airway trolley, and isotonic fluids (crystalloid or colloid) for ongoing resuscitation. Discuss plan for airway difficulties.
Extra, senior anaesthetist	Laryngoscopy and intubation may have become more difficult; an extra pair of hands is also important when managing hypovolaemia.
Laboratory	Prioritize blood grouping and full blood count. May also require assessment of clotting. Rapid issue cross-match as required.
Location for postoperative observation	This may be a high-dependency area on the children's ward, or a separate HDU, depending on local hospital arrangements. The child will need close monitoring for 12 h postoperatively.

bolus was commenced, and the surgeon achieved haemostasis. Near-patient testing of haemoglobin provided reassurance that transfusion was unnecessary with a haemoglobin of 10 g/dL being consistent with results from the laboratory when these became available. Fentanyl 1 µg/kg and a repeat dose of intravenous paracetamol 15 mg/kg (as it had not yet been given on the ward) was given for postoperative pain relief.

Once haemostasis had been achieved, a large-bore orogastric tube was passed under direct vision, and about 100 mL of altered blood aspirated from the stomach. As before, she was placed in the left lateral position, and extubated when breathing spontaneously with airway reflexes returned and 'awake'. Her recovery room stay was again uneventful, and after 45 min she returned to the paediatric ward for overnight pulse oximetry and hourly observations. Her regular ibuprofen prescription was cancelled.

The patient was discharged the following day and suffered no further complications.

Discussion

Role of steroids in adenotonsillectomy

Initial studies of dexamethasone administration for paediatric tonsillectomy focused on dose-finding for antiemetic and co-analgesic effects (reducing the required postoperative doses of NSAIDs and/or opiates to achieve good analgesia) thus facilitating early discharge home including potential day-case tonsillectomies [29]. There has been one published study [30] suggesting that high-dose dexamethasone may be associated with an excess bleeding rate. This study also had a somewhat high overall rate of bleeding at 10.6%; numbers in each limb of the study were small and surgical technique was not standardized. Larger and more recent studies have not found such an association [31, 32].

The recently updated (2011) Cochrane review of all studies of dexamethasone in paediatric tonsillectomy [32] concluded that it is effective in reducing nausea and vomiting post surgery, with a number needed to treat of five. Dexamethasone-treated children also returned more rapidly to normal diet, and had lower pain scores than those who had not received it. Dexamethasone doses ranging from 0.15 to 1 mg/kg have been found effective in prevention of postoperative nausea and vomiting [32]. The review did not find an increase in adverse events, especially bleeding, in children treated with dexamethasone. Both these outcomes are all-important for a successful day-case tonsillectomy service.

It has also been suggested by one centre [17] that children with severe sleep apnoea may particularly benefit from the anti-inflammatory and morphine-sparing effects of a relatively high dose of dexamethasone (0.5 mg/kg). This resulted in fewer respiratory complications in these high-risk children. The dose for co-analgesia/prevention of respiratory complications in children with OSA has not been properly defined [17]. In our practice, we use 0.15 mg/kg for routine tonsillectomy and 0.3 mg/kg to a maximum of 10 mg for OSA. As always, caution should be exercised in administering steroids to children with diabetes mellitus, or where there is any possible risk of developing tumour lysis syndrome [29].

Post-tonsillectomy bleeding

Post-tonsillectomy bleeding may be primary (within hours of surgery) or secondary (occurring generally at about 7–10 days postoperatively). Secondary bleeding is a phenomenon more of eschar detachment, possibly related to infection, than of haemostatic failure. Rates of primary haemorrhage are generally quoted as <2% [2, 19, 33] with secondary haemorrhage a little more frequent at around 3–5.5% [2, 19, 33]. Only a proportion of those who suffer primary haemorrhage will require a return to theatre for haemostasis [2, 12, 19, 33]. Very few patients with secondary haemorrhage require reoperation.

The incidence of bleeding varies most with surgical technique, particularly for primary haemorrhage [2, 12, 19, 34]. Older children and adults appear to have a higher incidence [2, 34]. In the UK National Tonsillectomy audit it was noted that children with OSA appeared to have a lower incidence [2]. It has been suggested that NSAID administration in the perioperative period could increase the rate of post-tonsillectomy bleeding due to an effect on platelet inhibition [33, 35]. However, recent studies in children including a Cochrane systematic review [12, 13] have not found a statistically significant increase either for overall bleeding rate or for likelihood of requiring return to theatre. This is in contrast to the situation in adults [36].

A large series review of anaesthetic management of post-tonsillectomy haemorrhage [33] found that almost 10% have some hypoxaemia, more frequently at emergence and extubation than at induction and intubation. Bradycardia and/or hypotension at induction occurred in 4.2% and 2.5% respectively, with a similar number (2.7%) being difficult to intubate, all of whom had previously been easy.

✪ Learning point   Post-tonsillectomy bleeding anaesthetic management

Important factors in anaesthetic management include:

1. Recognition of bleeding [21, 37].
2. Preoperative fluid resuscitation to avoid haemodynamic compromise at induction of anaesthesia [35], e.g. Hartmann's solution or 0.9% saline 20 mL/kg.
3. Prompt return to theatre, which requires clear communication with all involved (Table 6.2).
4. Intravenous rapid sequence induction of anaesthesia [33] to reduce the possibility of regurgitating swallowed blood, with consideration given to reducing the dose of induction agent, given the difficulty of estimating preoperative blood loss [33, 35].
5. Ready availability of good suction [35], and of smaller tracheal tubes than used at original operation, as there may be airway oedema as well as blood in the airway, either of which can also render laryngoscopy and intubation more difficult than previously [33, 37].
6. Gently pass a large orogastric tube once haemostasis is achieved to empty the stomach of swallowed blood.
7. Blood transfusion may be required [35], and should be guided by haemoglobin level, with near-patient testing being helpful.
8. Attention to temperature management—small child, major blood loss, rapid fluid replacement.
9. Cautious use of any further analgesia, particularly in the setting of primary haemorrhage, in particular avoiding any further NSAID in this context.
10. Extubate the child awake in the left lateral position [35], or consider sitting up if haemodynamically stable and obese; this posture improves venous drainage, facilitates airway positioning and improves respiratory function.
11. Monitor closely in a high observation facility for 12 h postoperatively.

Post-tonsillectomy bleeding: why not an inhalation induction?

This is not a situation amenable to randomized controlled trials, and opinions do vary. We suggest intravenous rapid sequence induction of anaesthesia for the following reasons:

1. A frightened child with airway bleeding will struggle to co-operate with an inhalation induction; this may encourage air-swallowing, which can make

ventilation more difficult and increase the risk of regurgitation and aspiration.

2. Better protection against regurgitation (and possible inhalation) of swallowed blood, as it is more difficult to judge timing of application of cricoid pressure in an inhalation induction. If applied too early this risks laryngospasm.

3. Fluid resuscitation should be well established prior to induction of anaesthesia, i.e. the child should have a reliable working cannula *in situ*, and small doses of induction agents should be safe.

4. Whereas a lateral position for inhalational induction with head-down tilt and without cricoid is described, in practice this is difficult to maintain and most are not skilled in induction and tracheal intubation in this position.

A Final Word from the Expert

1. Prior to induction in this situation rapid resuscitation is required and if there is doubt an additional rapid infusion of isotonic fluid is justified in the anaesthetic room using a three-way tap extension, 20 mL syringe and 'push–pull' method [38]. A pressure bag may be helpful in larger children/young people.

2. Prior to induction, 3–4 min of preoxygenation is important, with the parent on hand to keep the child calm, if necessary 'swaddling' the child to maintain position. Full monitoring is essential and skilled airway assistance mandatory.

3. Use an induction drug with which you are familiar but in a reduced dose, e.g. 1–2 mg/kg propofol or 2–3 mg/kg thiopentone. If you are familiar with ketamine for emergency anaesthesia for children this is also a good alternative in terms of cardiovascular stability, and it provides useful additional analgesia.

4. Remember that a dose of 2 mg/kg suxamethonium is required in children.

References

1. Cochrane H, Tanner S. *Trends in children's surgery 1994–2005: evidence from hospital episode statistics data*. London: Department of Health; February 2007. < http://webarchive. nationalarchives.gov.uk/20130107105354/http://www.dh.gov.uk/prod_consum_dh/groups/ dh_digitalassets/@dh/@en/documents/digitalasset/dh_066320.pdf >

2. Brown P, Ryan R, Yung M, *et al*. *National prospective tonsillectomy audit final report*. London: Royal College of Surgeons of England; 2005. < http://www.rcseng.ac.uk/surgeons/ research/surgical-research/docs/National%20Prospective%20Tonsillectomy%20Audit%20 Final%20Report%202005.pdf >

3. Scottish Intercollegiate Guidelines Network. *Management of sore throat and indications for tonsillectomy—a national clinical guideline*. Glasgow: SIGN; April 2010. < http://www.sign. ac.uk/pdf/sign117.pdf >

4. Working Party on Sleep Physiology and Respiratory Control Disorders in Childhood. *Standards for services for children with disorders of sleep physiology*. London: Royal College of Paediatrics and Child Health; September 2009. < http://www.bprs.co.uk/documents/ RCPCH_sleep_resp_cont_disorders.pdf >

5. Rudra A, Ray M, Sengupta S, Iqbal A, Maitra G, Chatterjee S. Obstructive sleep apnoea syndrome in children and anaesthesia. *Indian J Anaesth* 2010;54:18–23.

6. Lerman J. A disquisition on sleep-disordered breathing in children. *Paediatr Anaesth* 2009;19(Suppl 1):100–8.

7. Robb PJ, Bew S, Kubba H, *et al.* Tonsillectomy and adenoidectomy in children with sleep related breathing disorders: consensus statement of a UK multidisciplinary working party. *Clin Otolaryngol* 2009;34:61–3.

8. McCarty Statham M, Elluru RG, Buncher R, Kalra M. Adenotonsillectomy for obstructive sleep apnea syndrome in young children: prevalence of pulmonary complications. *Arch Otolaryngol Head Neck Surg* 2006;132:476–80.

9. Primhak R, Kingshott R. Sleep physiology and sleep-disordered breathing: the essentials. *Archs Dis Childh* 2012;97:54–8.

10. Brown KA, Laferriere A, Lakheeram I, Moss IR. Recurrent hypoxemia in children is associated with increased analgesic sensitivity to opiates. *Anesthesiology* 2006;105:665–9.

11. Lerman J. Unraveling the mysteries of sleep-disordered breathing in children. *Anesthesiology* 2006;105:645–7.

12. Jeyakumar A, Brickman TM, Williamson ME, *et al.* Nonsteroidal anti-inflammatory drugs and postoperative bleeding following adenotonsillectomy in pediatric patients. *Arch Otolaryngol Head Neck Surg* 2008;134:24–7.

13. Cardwell M, Siviter G, Smith A. Non-steroidal anti-inflammatory drugs and perioperative bleeding in paediatric tonsillectomy. *Cochrane Database Syst Rev* 2005;(2):CD003591.

14. Drug Safety Update vol 6 issue 12, July 2013: A1 http://www.mhra.gov.uk/ Safetyinformation/DrugSafetyUpdate/CON296400 accessed 21/10/13

15. William G, Hatch DJ, Howard RF. Codeine phosphate in paediatric medicine. *Br J Anaesth* 2001;86:413–21.

16. US Food and Drug Aministration. *Drug safety communication: Codeine use in certain children after tonsillectomy and/or adenoidectomy may lead to rare, but life-threatening adverse events or death.* Silver Spring, MD: US FDA; 15 August 2012. < http://www.fda. gov/Drugs/DrugSafety/ucm313631.htm >

17. Raghavendran S, Bagry H, Detheux G, Zhang X, Brouillette RT, Brown KA. An anesthetic management protocol to decrease respiratory complications after adenotonsillectomy in children with severe sleep apnea. *Anesth Analg* 2010;110:1093–1101.

18. Tweedie DJ, Skilbeck CJ, Lloyd-Thomas AR, Albert DM. The nasopharyngeal prong: an effective post operative adjunct after adenotonsillectomy for obstructive sleep apnoea. *Int J Pediatric Otorhinolaryrngol* 2007;71:563–9.

19. Attner P, Haraldsson PO, Hemlin C, HessénSoderman AC. A 4-year consecutive study of post-tonsillectomy haemorrhage. *J Otorhinolaryngol Relat Spec* 2009;71:273–8.

20. Bajaj Y, Atkinson H, Sagoo R, Bhatti I, Newbegin C. Paediatric day-case tonsillectomy: a three-year prospective audit spiral in a district hospital. *J Laryngol Otol* 2012;126:159–62.

21. Ewah BN, Robb PJ, Raw M. Postoperative pain, nausea and vomiting following paediatric day-case tonsillectomy. *Anaesthesia* 2006;61:116–22.

22. Robb PJ, Ewah BN. Post-operative nausea and vomiting following paediatric day-case tonsillectomy: audit of the Epsom protocol. *J Laryngol Otol* 2011;125:1049–52.

23. Webster AC, Morley-Forster PK, Dain S, *et al.* Anaesthesia for adenotonsillectomy: a comparison between tracheal intubation and the armoured laryngeal mask airway. *Can J Anaesth* 1993;40:1171–7.

24. Peng A, Dodson KM, Thacker LR, *et al.* Use of laryngeal mask airway in pediatric adenotonsillectomy. *Arch Otolaryngol Head Neck Surg* 2011;137:42–6.

25. Williams PJ, Bailey PM. Comparison of the reinforced laryngeal mask airway and tracheal intubation for adenotonsillectomy. *Br J Anaesth* 1993;70:30–3.

26. UK Department of Health. *Single-use instruments for tonsil and adenoid surgery.* 6 June 2001. < http://webarchive.nationalarchives.gov.uk/20130107105354/http://www.dh.gov.uk/ prod_consum_dh/groups/dh_digitalassets/@dh/@en/documents/digitalasset/dh_4014167. pdf >

27. UK Department of Health. *Re-introduction of re-usable instruments for tonsil surgery.* London: DoH; 14 December 2001. < http://webarchive.nationalarchives.gov.uk/ + /www. dh.gov.uk/en/Publicationsandstatistics/Pressreleases/DH_4011629 >

28. Clarke M, Forster P, Cook TM. Airway management for tonsillectomy: a national survey of UK practice. *Br J Anaesth* 2007;99:425–8.

29. Steward DL, Welge JA, Myer CM. Steroids for improving recovery following tonsillectomy in children. *Cochrane Database Syst Rev* 2003;(1):CD003997.

30. Czarnetzki C, Elia N, Lysakowski C, *et al.* Dexamethasone and risk of nausea and vomiting and postoperative bleeding after tonsillectomy in children: a randomized trial. *JAMA* 2008;300:2621–30.

31. Brigger MT, Cunningham MJ, Hartnick CJ. Dexamethasone administration and postoperative bleeding risk in children undergoing tonsillectomy. *Arch Otolaryngol Head Neck Surg* 2010;136:766–72.

32. Steward DL, Grisel J, Meinzen-Derr J. Steroids for improving recovery following tonsillectomy in children. *Cochrane Database Syst Rev* 2011;(8):CD003997.

33. Fields RG, Gencorelli FJ, Litman RS. Anesthetic management of the pediatric bleeding tonsil. *Paediatr Anaesth* 2010;20:982–6.

34. Gallagher TQ, Wilcox L, McGuire E, Derkay CS. Analyzing factors associated with major complications after adenotonsillectomy in 4776 patients: comparing three tonsillectomy techniques. *Arch Otolaryngol Head Neck Surg* 2010;142:886–92.

35. Allen TH, Steven IM, Sweeney DB. The bleeding tonsil—anaesthesia for control of haemorrhage after tonsillectomy. *Anaesth Intens Care* 1973;1:517–20.

36. Møiniche S, Rømsing J, Dahl JB, Tramèr MR. Nonsteroidal antiinflammatory drugs and the risk of operative site bleeding after tonsillectomy: a quantitative systematic review. *Anesth Analg* 2003;96:68–77.

37. Tokumine J, Sugahara K, Ura M, *et al.* Lingual tonsil hypertrophy with difficult airway and uncontrollable bleeding. *Anaesthesia* 2003;58:385–402.

38. Stoner MJ, Goodman DG, Cohen DM, Fernandez SA. Rapid fluid resuscitation in paediatrics; testing the American College of Critical Care Medicine guideline. *Ann Emerg Med* 2007;50:601–7.

CHAPTER 7

Acute pain management

7.1 A case for paravertebral blockade?

William Key

🕮 **Expert Commentary** Barry Nicholls

CPD Matrix Code: *1D02, 2E01, 2G01, 2G02, 3A09, 3E00*.

Case history

A 52-year-old female presented for right mastectomy and axillary node clearance for breast cancer. A breast mass had been noted on examination by her general practitioner.

Following a previous anaesthetic for a day-case laparoscopic cholecystectomy she required overnight admission with severe postoperative nausea and vomiting (PONV). She denied allergies but described sensitivity to morphine, which caused significant sedation and vomiting. Other details of note in her past medical history included type 2 diabetes mellitus, well controlled on oral hypoglycaemics, and a BMI of 35 kg/m². There was no history of cardiovascular or respiratory disease, and the patient denied symptoms of gastro-oesophageal reflux.

The patient was consented for a general anaesthetic with paravertebral blockade (PVB). Specific risks discussed included failure, pleural puncture with possible pneumothorax, and bilateral spread. The procedure was described to the patient, who expressed anxiety about being completely awake for the block, and so it was agreed that it would be performed under sedation prior to the start of surgery.

> **🗩 Expert comment**
>
> In order to gain informed consent, information (literature/discussion) concerning regional techniques should preferably be given at a preoperative assessment rather than on the day of surgery. Consent forms part of a continuum of care and is integral in the care plan of the patient. Information on techniques that carry significant, although rare, complications delivered on the day of surgery will cause unnecessary anxiety to the patient and increase the likelihood of patient refusal.

> **✪ Learning point** Alternatives to opioids
>
> In this case it is clearly desirable to avoid or minimize opioid use and a multimodal approach to analgesia should be used, including judicious use of local or regional anaesthetic techniques. These techniques could include local infiltration, intercostal blocks, intrapleural blocks, thoracic epidural and PVB. In addition to these well-established techniques Blanco described the 'Pecs block', a novel interfascial plane block placed between pectoralis major and minor muscles just inferior to the clavicle under ultrasound guidance, anaesthetizing the lateral and medial pectoral nerves [1]. This technique is particularly useful in patients receiving breast expanders and subpectoral prostheses where distension of the muscles can be very painful. More recently a modification of the Pecs block (Pecs II) has been described which aims additionally to block the intercostobrachial, intercostals nerves III–VI, and the long thoracic nerve. Local anaesthetic is injected between pectoralis minor and serratus anterior at the level of the third rib. This broadens the indications for the block to include lumpectomies, wide local excisions, and axillary clearances. Both techniques are awaiting more formal evaluation of efficacy and safety [2].
>
> PVB has a number of advantages. Several studies have compared general anaesthesia with PVB either as sole technique or in combination with general anaesthesia for breast surgery. The results have shown a reduction in acute postoperative pain scores, opiate consumption [3–10], PONV [6, 7, 9–11], recovery times, and time to discharge [9, 10].
>
> (continued)

Continuous wound infiltration after breast surgery can provide good analgesia postoperatively and does not require specialist skill, but early postoperative pain is significantly worse, when compared with PVB, and there is a higher incidence of PONV [12].

Using evidence from thoracic surgery comparing PVB with thoracic epidural, there is evidence of a reduced incidence of hypotension and urinary retention, better suppression of the stress response to surgery [13], minimal risk of neuropathy and less complicated ward management [14]. Similarly PVB can result in a more profound and longer-lasting block than an interpleural block, which also leads to more variable blood concentrations of local anaesthetic. Preservation of pulmonary function following thoracotomy is better with a PVB compared with an interpleural block; this may be due to pooling of local anaesthetic around the diaphragm when patients are upright. There is also a greater risk of pneumothorax with interpleural block [15].

Intercostal blocks require an injection for each intercostal space and there is a greater risk of pneumothorax. Injection into the paravertebral space allows caudal and cephalad spread, meaning that fewer injections of larger volumes can provide a block across a number of dermatomes.

✪ Learning point Anatomy of the paravertebral space

There are a number of approaches to PVB described. Whichever technique is used, a sound knowledge and understanding of the anatomy of the paravertebral space is paramount to ensure correct needle placement and avoidance of the potential complications (see Figure 7.1).

Borders

The thoracic paravertebral space is a wedge-shaped compartment. Its medial border is defined by the vertebral bodies, foramina, and intervertebral discs. Its posterior border is defined by the superior costotransverse ligament, the transverse processes, and the head and neck of the ribs which lie slightly

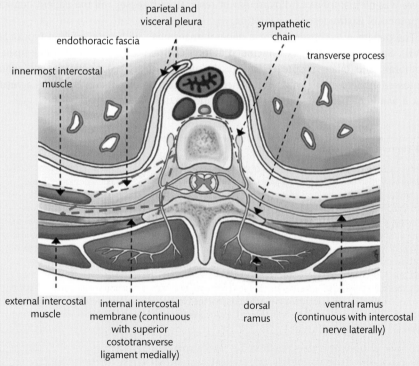

Figure 7.1 Anatomy of the paravertebral space. Reproduced with kind permission of Professor Vincent Chan. Shibata Y, Chin K. J, Thoracic Paravertebral Block. Available at: http:www.usra.ca/tpbanatomy.php (accessed: 21st Jan 2012)

(continued)

superior and deep to the transverse processes. Anterolaterally the border is defined by the parietal pleura and innermost intercostal membrane.

The endothoracic fascia splits the paravertebral space into anterior and posterior compartments, but the clinical significance of this is unclear [17].

Contents

The paravertebral space contains the spinal nerves, which are not invested in the tight fascial layer that becomes a feature more peripherally; this allows them to be blocked more readily. Other structures include the sympathetic chain, the white and grey rami communicantes, the intercostal vessels and adipose tissue.

Communications

The paravertebral space is continuous cranially and caudally, allowing multiple segments to be blocked from a single injection of adequate volume. The space also communicates laterally with the intercostal spaces, and medially with the epidural space through the intervertebral foramina. Contralateral spread may occur either via the epidural route or prevertebrally (posterior to the anterior longitudinal ligament, and the endothoracic and subserous fascia) [18].

The World Health Organization (WHO) sign in was performed on arrival in the anaesthetic room. This included confirmation with the patient of operative site and side, and consent for surgery and nerve block before positioning or administration of sedative drugs.

Following the application of routine monitoring (non-invasive blood pressure, ECG and oximetry) the patient was positioned in the left lateral position (operative side up) breathing oxygen and 2 mg midazolam was administered. Incremental doses of fentanyl were titrated to provide analgesia during the procedure.

The upper border of the spinous processes at the levels T1 and T4 were marked and a point 2.5 cm laterally on the operative side was also marked as the point of introduction of the block needle (Figure 7.2).

The block was performed under aseptic conditions with the operator wearing a hat and mask with sterile gown and gloves. The skin was prepared with 2% chlorhexidine in 70% alcohol solution and the area draped. Prior to needle insertion a further

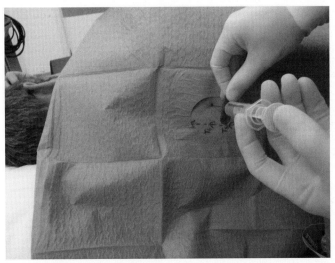

Figure 7.2 Paravertebral block: upper borders of T3, T4 and T5 spinous processes marked. Insertion point 2.5 cm lateral on operative side.

➕ Clinical tip Needle direction

In the thoracic region the neck of the rib sits superior and deep to the transverse process. If the rib is contacted initially the needle tip will be deeper and subsequently closer to the pleura than the operator envisages. By walking the needle caudally the more superficial transverse process will be encountered, alerting the operator to its actual depth and position. For this reason many practitioners advocate redirecting the needle caudally rather than cranially.

check was undertaken with the anaesthetic assistant to verify that the surgical site was marked and that it corresponded with the proposed site of the block. A 23G needle was used to infiltrate the skin and subcutaneous tissue with 1% lignocaine. A graduated 18G Tuohy needle was inserted perpendicular to all planes at the T4 level directly down to contact the transverse process, which was encountered 3.5 cm deep to the skin. The needle was then walked off the lower border of the transverse process while ensuring that the angulation of the needle was changed as little as possible. The needle was then advanced a short distance into the superior costotransverse ligament and at this point an epidural loss of resistance syringe was attached to the Tuohy needle. The paravertebral space was found by loss of resistance to saline ~1 cm deep to the transverse process.

✪ Learning point Wrong-sided block

Unintentional wrong-sided nerve block is a relatively rare event; however, the actual incidence is unknown, and with the increase in popularity of regional anaesthesia concerted efforts are being made to try to eliminate these events altogether [19].

Administering a regional anaesthetic block to the incorrect side can have serious consequences as it exposes the patient to the risks associated with a block such as nerve damage, local anaesthetic toxicity, delayed hospital discharge and even progression to incorrect site surgery, without any of the benefits.

A number of processes have been explored in an attempt to minimize the risk of wrong-sided block.

The WHO surgical safety checklist sign-in procedure includes a check by the anaesthetist and the anaesthetic assistant with the patient of the planned surgery and any nerve blocks which are then cross-referenced with the consent form, operating list, and the surgical mark. Despite this process wrong-sided blocks still occur, particularly when a delay occurs between the sign-in and a nerve block, where the patient is repositioned and when the surgical site and mark are distant to the block site. The distraction of a busy anaesthetic room has also been highlighted as a risk factor.

The 'Stop Before You Block' campaign (<http://www.rcoa.ac.uk/node/346>), endorsed by the Safer Anaesthetic Liaison Group (SALG) and Regional Anaesthesia UK (RA-UK), aimed to raise the profile of these events and involves a 'stop' moment immediately prior to needle insertion and separate from the sign-in to recheck the surgical mark and the side and site of the block [20]; even this extra check has not entirely prevented wrong-site blocks.

Other strategies include marking the block site with a different colour and symbol to the surgical mark to ensure that it remains visible during the block procedure.

All of these processes require engagement of the anaesthetist and anaesthetic assistant in embedding such processes into everyday practice to produce a change in behaviour and culture, and reduce the likelihood of these events.

✪ Learning point Depth of the paravertebral space

Since the transverse process is neither visible nor palpable when using the described technique its location is unknown until the block needle encounters the bone. Difficulty in performing the block can therefore increase when the surface landmarks themselves are difficult to locate accurately, especially in obese patients.

If bone is not encountered as the needle is advanced, the needle tip can be advanced beyond the paravertebral space causing pleural puncture and potentially a pneumothorax. Attention to landmark location and some knowledge of the expected depth to the transverse process and paravertebral space can reduce this risk.

Several studies in the literature have looked at the possible relationship between the depth of the transverse process or paravertebral space and other parameters such as weight, BMI, gender, age, and spinal level.

(continued)

Naja *et al.* used a nerve stimulator technique to identify the paravertebral space, and measured needle depth in 186 patients and 527 PVBs between the levels T1–T12 [21]. The depth of the paravertebral space varied with thoracic level, being greatest at the higher and lower levels and least at levels T7–T9. BMI significantly influenced depth for all levels other than T7–T9. The mean depth of the T4 paravertebral space increased from 46 to 60 mm as BMI rose from <25 to <30 kg/m². It should be noted these were measurements of the depth to the nerves within the paravertebral space rather than the point of first entry into the space, which may account for the greater depths compared with other studies.

In 2008, a retrospective cohort study by Chelly *et al.* examined the impact of multiple factors on the depth of the paravertebral space in 589 patients undergoing 1,318 PVBs at levels T4–T12 [22]. Whereas the associations were rather complex, in general depth increased linearly towards lower thoracic levels, and was also greater in the young and in those with higher BMI.

These studies indicate that significant variability makes prediction of depth to the paravertebral space difficult, especially in the higher thoracic region (T8 and above) where blockade for breast surgery is required. Factors influencing depth include thoracic level, BMI (weight more specifically), age, and sex. For example, in a 50 kg octogenarian the depth of the paravertebral space may be just over 2 cm at T5; whereas in a 110 kg 20-year-old the space may be encountered at 6 cm at T6 [22].

⊗ **Learning point** Use of ultrasound

Ultrasound has been used in an attempt to enhance the safety and efficacy of thoracic PVBs by determining the location and depth of the transverse process and the parietal pleura. Other identifiable structures include the rib and the superior costotranverse ligament. The paravertebral space itself cannot be seen directly with ultrasound but the anterior and posterior borders can (i.e. the superior costotransverse ligament and the pleura). Pusch *et al.* performed a pre-procedure scan noting depth to transverse process and parietal pleura, then performed thoracic PVBs in the conventional fashion using a loss-of-resistance technique: there was a good correlation between measured depth and actual depth to the transverse process [23]. Hara *et al.* imaged the transverse process in a longitudinal parasagittal plane during block performance with the needle out-of-plane and using loss-of-resistance as the endpoint for needle placement [24]. Shibata *et al.* described an intercostal in-plane approach to the paravertebral space allowing visualization of the needle as well as local anaesthetic spread [25]. Although these techniques are developing, to date no study has shown ultrasound to improve efficacy or safety.

❝ **Expert comment**

Ultrasound can offer distinct advantages both for single-shot and catheter placement. At present there are various approaches, the most popular being a lateral intercostal approach, in which the needle is positioned beneath the internal intercostal membrane into the posterior intercostal space, which communicates medially with the paravertebral space [26–28]. In more recent studies a medial approach using the bony landmarks of the junction of transverse process and lamina may offer a more consistent approach for catheter placement [29, 30].

❝ **Expert comment**

It is important to inform patients that they may experience a tight sensation in the chest during injection of local anaesthetic. Patients should be encouraged to take slow breaths. In the sitting position there is an increased incidence of vasovagal events, and pre-treatment with atropine or glycopyrronium should be considered.

Once in the space, aspiration confirmed that the needle tip had not entered a blood vessel, pleura, or the subarachnoid space, and 10 mL of 0.5% levobupivacaine was injected slowly with minimal resistance to injection. The patient was warned prior to injection that some discomfort might be experienced and should be short-lived.

The process was repeated at the T1 level although some difficulty was experienced locating the transverse process at a depth of 4 cm. After confirming that the needle was perpendicular to all planes the insertion point was moved caudally by 5 mm and bone was contacted at 4 cm.

Induction of general anaesthesia then followed with administration of fentanyl 100 µg and a propofol target-controlled infusion delivering plasma levels between 3 and 4 microgram/mL which was also used for maintenance of anaesthesia. The airway was secured with an LMA and spontaneous respiration was maintained breathing an oxygen:air mixture. Dexamethasone 8 mg was administered soon after induction and ondansetron 4 mg 15 min before the end of surgery for prophylaxis against PONV.

Surgery proceeded uneventfully with minimal heart rate or blood pressure response to surgical stimulus and no patient movement.

Expert comment

The superior analgesia obtained with PVB compared with epidural analgesia may in some way be accounted for by the more complete and profound sympathetic block achieved with a paravertebral technique. The somatosensory evoked potentials are completely abolished by a PVB by contrast with central neuraxial techniques using the same concentration of local anaesthetic [13].

Clinical tip Horner's syndrome

Horner's syndrome is a frequent side-effect of nerve and plexus blocks in the neck and upper thoracic region including cervical plexus and interscalene brachial plexus blocks, stellate ganglion blocks and PVBs. Incidence following PVB is between 5% and 20%. It is generally short-lived (8–10 h) and of no clinical consequence, but patients should be warned preoperatively. It results from the blockade of the T1 and T2 sympathetic innervation to the eye on the ipsilateral side resulting in unopposed parasympathetic activity with ipsilateral miosis, partial ptosis, anhidrosis (absence of sweating) and chemosis [31].

Expert comment

Early complications such as Horner's syndrome and bilateral spread occur early enough to be seen in the recovery unit. Clinically significant pneumothorax is uncommon, but will usually become apparent within the following 24 h.

Following surgery, in recovery the patient was comfortable and required no supplementary analgesia or additional antiemetic. It was noted by the recovery staff that the patient had unequal pupils and on examination her right eye was slightly bloodshot with a constricted pupil and a partial ptosis. A diagnosis of Horner's syndrome was made and the patient reassured.

The patient made a good recovery during her inpatient stay and was discharged on the second postoperative day. She was prescribed regular paracetamol and ibuprofen, with tramadol for breakthrough pain.

During a follow-up clinic 2 months after surgery the patient mentioned to the surgeon that she was experiencing some pain from her surgery and had noticed a numb patch over the inside of her right upper arm. Although this was not causing any functional deficit the patient was anxious about the underlying cause. She was referred on to the pain clinic with a provisional diagnosis of post-mastectomy pain syndrome.

During her pain clinic consultation it transpired that the pain and numb patch were not concerning her, but rather her fear that the cancer had recurred. On examination there was demonstrable loss of sensation in the distribution of the intercostobrachial nerve. The patient was reassured that this nerve is often impossible to spare during the axillary dissection. At a subsequent surgical follow-up appointment she was reassured as all further tests showed no sign of recurrence.

Learning point Effect of regional anaesthesia on chronic post-surgical pain

Chronic pain following breast surgery is increasingly recognized as a significant problem with a reported incidence of 25–50% [32]. This manifests as both nociceptive and neuropathic pain and can occur in the chest wall, axilla and upper arm with phantom breast symptoms also being reported.

Jung et al. classified neuropathic pain following breast cancer surgery into four subgroups [33]:

1. Phantom breast pain
2. Intercostobrachial neuralgia and post-mastectomy pain syndrome
3. Neuroma pain
4. Other nerve injury pain

Risk factors for development of chronic pain include [34]:

- younger age
- severe postoperative pain
- surgery for cancer
- extensive surgery (especially axillary clearance and reconstructive surgery)
- postoperative radiotherapy

A study by Ioholm et al. evaluated the influence of continuous PVB for 48 h and simple analgesics versus standard postoperative opioid-based analgesia on the development of chronic post-surgical pain and nitric oxide production following breast surgery in 29 patients. Postoperative pain over the first 5 days was significantly less in the PVB group. At 10 weeks, 12 of 15 patients in the standard treatment group had chronic post-surgical pain compared with none in the PVB group ($P < 0.01$) [5].

Kairaluoma et al. showed that preincisional PVB provided significant postoperative analgesia and a reduction in prevalence of pain symptoms, motion-related pain, and rest pain intensity 12 months after breast cancer surgery [35].

PVB gives high-quality dermatomal block with a high degree of afferent blockade, and is one strategy to optimize postoperative analgesia and reduce the development of chronic pain [13].

> **⊗ Learning point** Effect of regional blockade on cancer recurrence
>
> Surgical removal of primary breast cancer can give the best prospect of a good prognosis. Although complete excision of all disease is the aim of surgical treatment, some residual disease is probably unavoidable, usually in the form of micrometastases and scattered tumour cells. Metastatic recurrence is the main cause of breast cancer-related deaths. A number of factors will influence whether this residual disease ultimately results in clinically important recurrence or metastases, and it is likely that the immune competence of the patient will have a bearing on this. In the perioperative period three significant factors that influence immune response may have an impact on likelihood of recurrence [36, 37]:
>
> 1. Surgical stress response—the neuroendocrine stress response to surgery impairs numerous immune functions including the activity of natural killer cells.
> 2. Anaesthesia impairs numerous immune functions, including those of neutrophils, macrophages, dendritic cells, T-cells, and natural killer cells, but to a considerably lesser extent than the surgical stress response.
> 3. Opioid analgesics (particularly morphine) inhibit both cellular and humoral immune function in humans, increase tumour angiogenesis, and promote the release of factors that increase cancer cell survival and augment breast tumour growth in rodents.
>
> Natural killer cells (a lymphocyte subtype) are thought to play a central role in preventing tumour dissemination and establishment. Experimental studies in rats show that surgical stress is attenuated better by regional than by general anaesthesia; consequently, natural killer cell function is better preserved and metastatic load to the lungs is reduced [38]. It has been shown that regional anaesthesia and optimum postoperative analgesia independently reduce the metastatic burden in animals inoculated with breast adenocarcinoma cells following surgery [38–40].
>
> A retrospective non-randomized study reviewed recurrence and metastasis-free survival in the three years following breast cancer surgery in patients who had received general anaesthesia and morphine ($n = 79$) compared with general anaesthesia and PVB ($n = 50$). They found that more patients in the PVB group were recurrence free at 24 months (94% vs 82%, $P < 0.05$) and at 36 months (94% vs 77%, $P < 0.01$) [36]. There are inherent limitations of this observational retrospective study, including lack of randomization or standardized clinical care, which may have introduced bias. To address this issue, Sessler *et al.* are undertaking a multicentre prospective randomized trial comparing the cancer recurrence rate in 1,100 breast surgery patients treated with either sevoflurane and opioids or PVB or thoracic epidural [41].

Discussion

There is good evidence that PVBs can be opioid-sparing and reduce PONV. Some evidence also suggests a reduction in chronic pain development following major breast surgery.

Ultrasound-guided PVB can be technically difficult, especially in less experienced hands, and a good knowledge of the anatomy is required for operators to know exactly what they are looking at. Its use for identification of the transverse process and pleura can improve safety margins when using a loss-of-resistance technique.

PVB is regarded as a relatively safe and effective regional block and compares favourably to alternative regional and local techniques. It can be used in conjunction with a general anaesthetic or as a sole technique in high-risk patients.

There is some evidence from retrospective cohort studies that PVB may reduce the incidence of cancer recurrence and metastases, though this has methodological limitations. A multicentre prospective randomized study is underway to ascertain the extent, if any, of these effects.

> **❝ Expert comment**
>
> It is not possible in every case to be able to perform a regional technique either due to patient refusal, challenging anatomy or operator inexperience. Simple local anaesthetic techniques such as infiltration will always have some effect on opioid use though this may be small. In such instances, a case can be made for the use of adjuvant analgesia such as perioperative gabapentin/pregabalin, intraoperative ketamine [42] or even intravenous lidocaine [43] coupled with total intravenous anaesthesia (TIVA) to reduce opioid use and PONV.

A Final Word from the Expert

Thoracic PVB was first described by Hugo Selheim (Leipzig, 1905) and reached its zenith in the 1910-1920s when it was used for major thoracic and abdominal surgery. This was the 'golden era' of regional anaesthesia, typified by the development of all major plexus and nerve block techniques [44, 45]. With the subsequent development of safer general anaesthesia, peridural and spinal techniques, thoracic PVB fell into disuse. Its modern revival relates to the interest in its use in analgesia for thoracic surgery in the 1970-1980s [46]. More recently this interest has included breast surgery, which is the most popular indication at present for thoracic PVBs.

The resurgence in the use of PVB can be attributed to the high quality of analgesia, reduced hypotension and side-effects compared with thoracic epidurals. The specific unilateral nature of the technique enhances its use in breast surgery and single-sided thoracic and abdominal surgery. As in the case described, this technique can be used with good effect for analgesia but it is also suitable as a sole anaesthetic technique. The recent increasing trend in day-case mastectomy and onco-plastic reconstructive breast surgery lends itself ideally to thoracic PVB, both as single shot, continuous local anaesthetic infusion via a catheter, or in some indications bilateral techniques [47]. The relevance of local anaesthetic techniques in the pathophysiology and outcomes in cancer-related surgery has yet to be robustly confirmed.

The landmark technique has a low incidence of side-effects and is easy to learn, but it does have a failure rate of ≥10%, which can be improved with experience and additional technical support, e.g. peripheral nerve stimulator. Ultrasound guidance would appear to have an advantage in improving success and reducing side-effects. One must temper this with the knowledge that in certain individuals it is difficult and sometimes impossible to obtain adequate images of the relevant structures. This, coupled with poor needling technique, can change a relatively easy landmark technique into a difficult ultrasound-guided technique.

Thoracic paravertebral anaesthesia has stood the test of time from its beginning in the early 1900s to today: offering excellent analgesia, reduced opiate consumption, improved PONV and perhaps even less chronic post-surgical pain, and can be considered an essential component in the armamentarium of a 'regional anaesthetist'.

References

1. Blanco R. The 'pecs block': a novel technique for providing analgesia after breast surgery. *Anaesthesia* correspondence website: < http://www.respond2articles.com/ANA/forums/post/833.aspx >
2. Blanco R, Fajardo M, Parras Maldonado T. Ultrasound description of Pecs II (modified Pecs I): a novel approach to breast surgery. *Rev Esp Anestesiol Reanim* 2012;59:470–5.
3. Buggy DJ, Kerin MJ. Paravertebral analgesia with levobupivacaine increases postoperative flap tissue oxygen tension after immediate latissimus dorsi breast reconstruction compared with intravenous opioid analgesia. *Anesthesiology* 2004;100:375–80.
4. Burlacu CL, Frizelle HP, Moriarty DC, Buggy DJ. Fentanyl and clonidine as adjunctive analgesics with levobupivacaine in paravertebral analgesia for breast surgery. *Anaesthesia* 2006;61:932–7.
5. Iohom G, Abdalla H, O'Brien J, *et al.* The associations between severity of early postoperative pain, chronic postsurgical pain and plasma concentration of stable nitric oxide products after breast surgery. *Anesth Analg* 2006;103:995–1000.

6. Kairaluoma PM, Bachmann MS, Korpinen AK, Rosenberg PH, Pere PJ. Single-injection paravertebral block before general anesthesia enhances analgesia after breast cancer surgery with and without associated lymph node biopsy. *Anesth Analg* 2004;99:1837–43.

7. Moller JF, Nikolajsen L, Rodt SA, Ronning H, Carlsson PS. Thoracic paravertebral block for breast cancer surgery: a randomized double-blind study. *Anesth Analg* 2007;105:1848–51.

8. Klein SM, Bergh A, Steele SM, Georgiade GS, Greengrass RA. Thoracic paravertebral block for breast surgery. *Anesth Analg* 2000;90:1402–5.

9. Naja MZ, Ziade MF, Lonnqvist PA. Nerve-stimulator guided paravertebral blockade vs. general anaesthesia for breast surgery: a prospective randomized trial. *Eur J Anaesthesiol* 2003;20:897–903.

10. Pusch F, Freitag H, Weinstabl C, Obwegeser R, Huber E, Wildling E. Single-injection paravertebral block compared to general anaesthesia in breast surgery. *Acta Anaesthesiol Scand* 1999;43:770.

11. Thavaneswaran P, Rudkin GE, Cooter RD, Moyes DG, Perera CL, Maddern GJ. Paravertebral block for anesthesia: a systematic review. *Anesth Analg* 2010;110:1740–4.

12. Sidiropoulou T, Buonomo O, Fabbi E, *et al.* A prospective comparison of continuous wound infiltration with ropivacaine versus single-injection paravertebral block after modified radical mastectomy. International Anesthesia Research Society. *Anesth Analg* 2008;106:997–1001.

13. Richardson J, Jones J, Atkinson R. The effect of thoracic paravertebral blockade on intercostal somatosensory evoked potentials. *Anesth Analg* 1998;87:373–6.

14. Richardson J, Lonnqvist PA. Thoracic paravertebral block. *Br J Anaesth* 1998;83:387–92.

15. Richardson J, Sabanathan S, Mearns AJ, Shah RD, Goulden C. A prospective, randomized comparison of interpleural and paravertebral analgesia in thoracic surgery. *Br J Anaesth* 1995;75:405–8.

16. Sarhadi NS, Shaw Dunn J, Lee FD, Soutar DS. An anatomical study of the nerve supply to the breast, including nipple and areola. *Br J Plast Surg* 1996;49:156–64.

17. Karmakar MK, Kwok WH, Kew J. Thoracic paravertebral block: radiological evidence of contralateral spread anterior to the vertebral bodies. *Br J Anaesth* 2000;84:263–5.

18. Karmaker KM. Thoracic paravertebral block. *Anesthesiology* 2001;95:771–80.

19. Rupp SM. Unintentional wrong-sided peripheral nerve block. *Reg Anesth Pain Med* 2008;33:95–7.

20. Royal College of Anaesthetists. *Wrong site block.* < http://www.rcoa.ac.uk/node/346 >

21. Naja MZ, Gustafsson AC, Ziade MF, *et al.* Distance between the skin and the thoracic paravertebral space. *Anaesthesia* 2005;60:680–4.

22. Chelly JE, Uskova A, Merman R, Szczodry D. A multifactorial approach to the factors influencing determination of paravertebral depth. *Can J Anaesth* 2008;55:587–94.

23. Pusch F, Wildling E, Klimscha W, Weinstabl C. Sonographic measurement of needle insertion depth in paravertebral blocks in women. *Br J Anaesth* 2000;85:841–3.

24. Hara K, Sakura S, Nomura T, Saito Y. Ultrasound guided thoracic paravertebral block in breast surgery. *Anaesthesia* 2009;64:223–5.

25. Shibata Y, Nishiwaki K. Letter to the editor. Ultrasound-guided intercostal approach to thoracic paravertebral block. *Anesth Analg* 2009;109:996–7.

26. Cowie B, McGlade D, Ivanusic J, Barrington MJ. Ultrasound-guided thoracic paravertebral blockade: a cadaveric study. *Anesth Analg* 2010;110:1735–9.

27. Marhofer P, Kettner SC, Hajbok L, Dubsky P, Fleischmann E. Lateral ultrasound-guided paravertebral blockade: an anatomical-based description of a new technique. *Br J Anaesth* 2010;105:526–32.

28. Renes SH, Bruhn J, Gielen MJ, Scheffer GJ, van Geffen GJ. In-plane ultrasound-guided thoracic paravertebral block. A preliminary report of 36 cases with radiologic confirmation of catheter position. *Reg Anest Pain Med* 2010;35:212–16.

29. Luyet C, Herrmann G, Ross S, *et al.* Ultrasound-guided paravertebral puncture and placement of catheters in human cadavers; where do catheters go? *Br J Anaesth* 2011;106:246–54.

30. Luyet C, Meyer C, Herrmann G, Hatch GM, Ross S, Eichenberger U. Placement of coiled catheters into the paravertebral space. *Anaesthesia* 2012;67:250–5.

31. Schnable A, Reichl SU, Kranke P, Porgatzki-Zahn EM, Zahn PK. Efficacy and safety of paravertebral blocks in breast surgery: a meta-analysis of randomized controlled trials. *Br J Anaesth* 2010;105:842–52.

32. Gartner R, Jensen MB, Nielsen J, Ewertz M, Kroman N, Kehlet H. Prevalence of and factors associated with persistent pain following breast cancer surgery. *J Am Med Assoc* 2009;302:1985–92.

33. Jung B, Ahrendt G, Oaklander A, Dworkin R. Neuropathic pain following breast cancer surgery: proposed classification and research update. *Pain* 2003;104:1–13.

34. Poleshuck EL, Katz J, Andrus CH, *et al*. Risk factors for chronic pain following breast cancer surgery: a prospective study. *J Pain* 2006;7:626–34.

35. Kairaluoma PM, Bachmann MS, Rosenberg PH, Pere PJ. Preincisional paravertebral block reduces the prevalence of chronic pain after breast surgery. *Anesth Analg* 2006;103:703–8.

36. Exadaktylos AK, Buggy DJ, Moriarty DC, Mascha E, Sessler DI. Can anesthetic technique for primary breast cancer surgery affect recurrence or metastasis? *Anesthesiology* 2006;105:660–4.

37. Deegan CA, Murray D, Doran P, Ecimovic P, Moriarty DC, Buggy DJ. Effect of anaesthetic technique on oestrogen receptor-negative breast cancer cell function in vitro. *Br J Anaesth* 2009;103:685–90.

38. Bar-Yosef S, Melamed R, Page GG, Shakhar G, Shakhar K, Ben-Eliyahu S. Attenuation of the tumor-promoting effect of surgery by spinal blockade in rats. *Anesthesiology* 2001;94:1066–73.

39. Ben-Eliyahu S, Shakhar G, Rosenne E, Levinson Y, Beilin B. Hypothermia in barbiturate-anesthetized rats suppresses natural killer cell activity and compromises resistance to tumor metastasis: a role for adrenergic mechanisms. *Anesthesiology* 1999;91:732–40.

40. Page GG, Blakely WP, Ben-Eliyahu S. Evidence that postoperative pain is a mediator of the tumor-promoting effects of surgery in rats. *Pain* 2001;90:191–9.

41. Outcomes Research Consortium. *Regional anesthesia and breast cancer recurrence.* < http://www.clinicaltrial.gov/ct2/show/record/NCT00418457 >

42. Weinbroum AA. Non-opioid adjuvants in the perioperative period. Pharmacological and clinical aspects of ketamine and gabapentoids. *Pharmacol Res* 2012;65:411–29.

43. McCarthy GC, Megalla SA, Habib AS. Impact of intravenous lidocaine infusion on postoperative analgesia and recovery from surgery: a systemic review of randomized controlled trials. *Drugs* 2010;70:1149–63.

44. Pauchet V, Sourdat P. *L'anesthesie regionale.* Paris: O Doin et fils; 1914.

45. Labat G. *Regional anesthesia: its techniques and clinical application.* Philadelphia: WB Saunders; 1922.

46. Eason MJ, Wyatt R. Paravertebral thoracic block—a reappraisal. *Anaesthesia* 1979;34:638–42.

47. Richardson J, Lonnqvist PA, Naja Z. Bilateral thoracic paravertebral block: potential and practice. *Br J Anaesth* 2011;106:164–71.

7.2 Achieving postoperative pain control

Simon Law

Expert Commentary Jeremy Cashman

CPD Matrix Code: *1D02, 2E01, 2G01, 2G02, 3A09, 3E00*

Case history

A previously healthy 43-year-old man was brought into the emergency department after he had been involved in a motor vehicle collision. The patient was the driver of a motorcycle which collided with a stationary car at a junction while travelling at an estimated 30 mph. He sustained a high-velocity impact to the left side of his body, was conscious at the scene, and was transferred by air ambulance. History-taking revealed only a vague recollection of events, although witnesses described a collision between the patient's motorcycle and a car with the patient thrown 10 feet. He had no past medical history of note, he was taking no regular medications, and had no history of recent alcohol or previous opioid use.

The trauma team was assembled following a pre-alert call from the ambulance crew. On arrival, he had a patent airway with oxygen saturations of 99% breathing in 15 L of oxygen and a respiratory rate of 28 breaths/min. His blood pressure was 121/77 mmHg and his pulse was 117 beats/min.

The patient described two painful areas as a result of the trauma: his right proximal thigh and the left upper thorax with radiation posteriorly. Verbal descriptors were used to assess pain severity. Despite 10 mg of intravenous morphine given in the air ambulance the patient described severe chest pain, worse on inspiration, and a background pain that was 'moderate' and 'nagging' in the upper thigh. Movement made all pain worse.

On examination, there was decreased air entry on the left side of the chest associated with bruising; abdominal and pelvic examination were unremarkable but he had a deformity of the right upper thigh. His GCS was 15/15. Routine bloods were sent including a group and save; results were within normal limits (Table 7.1). In view of the mechanism of injury a trauma series (CT) scan was performed, covering: head, cervical and thoracolumbar spine, chest, abdomen and pelvis. Head, abdominal, pelvic and spinal images demonstrated no injuries. He had fractures of the left 4th and 5th ribs anteriorly with a left pneumothorax, for which an intercostal drain was inserted. X-rays of his right leg demonstrated a closed fracture of the right femur.

For management of his pain a further 10 mg of morphine was administered intravenously titrated carefully over 10 min in 2 mg aliquots. This reduced his global pain score from 3 to 1 as assessed by the nursing staff using a verbal numerical rating scale (VNRS) of 0–3.

Expert comment

Injury following major trauma is associated with clinical signs that can be confused with those of acute pain, e.g. tachycardia, tachypnoea, hypo- or hypertension. It can therefore be difficult to distinguish between them.

One of the difficulties in managing pain after trauma is that, as in this case, there may be multiple distinct injuries, compared with postoperative pain management when there is usually only one site of injury. This adds complexity especially when regional analgesia is planned, as regional anaesthesia techniques may need to be modified in the light of use of other analgesics required to manage pain elsewhere, and vice versa.

⊕ Clinical tip Trauma team

The benefits of a structured trauma call include time for preparation and adequate staffing for simultaneous assessment of multiple systems. In this case the anaesthetist allocated to 'A' for airway assessment (with cervical spine control) had drawn up morphine (10 mg diluted to 1 mg/mL) before the patient's arrival. Having established that the patient had a patent airway (with spine immobilized) and no neurological deficit, pain assessment was rapidly undertaken ensuring minimal delay to treatment.

❝ Expert comment

Verbal pain descriptors are simple to explain but require patient co-operation and understanding. Trauma patients with diminished levels of consciousness may not be able to give an accurate score. The pain descriptors 'none', 'mild', 'moderate' or 'severe' would equate to 0, 1, 2, 3 on a four-point numerical scale.

⊕ Clinical tip Indicators of pain

The patient's self-report is the single most reliable indicator of pain; normal vital signs should not be considered a barrier to administering further analgesia in patients describing pain [1]. For analgesia here, it is appropriate to administer additional opioids carefully titrated to effect with the severity of injuries as a guide.

⊕ Clinical tip Goals

Whatever the tool used, it should be clearly documented and appropriate for the patient and the team following the patient up. The reduction of pain intensity to 'no pain', 'mild pain', 0–1 out of 3, or ≤3 out of 10, are appropriate goals.

Table 7.1 Blood test results on admission to the emergency department

Haematology	Biochemistry
Haemoglobin 14.2 g/dL (11.5–16.0)	Na 140 mmol/L (135–145)
White cell count 8.3 × 10^9/L (4.0–11.0)	K 4.1 mmol/L (3.5–5.0)
Platelets 297 × 10^9/L (150–400)	Urea 4.8 mmol/L (<7.5)
INR 1.1 (0.9–1.2)	Creatinine 94 µmol/L (35–125)
APTT 39 s (30–45)	

INR, international normalized ratio (prothrombin time); APTT, activated partial thromboplastin time.

✪ Learning point Unidimensional self-report scales

Several pain measurement tools are in widespread use. These include:

- Verbal descriptor scales: intensity reflected by a scale of adjectives, usually 'none', 'mild', 'moderate' and 'severe'; additional words used in these scales may include 'awful' or 'excruciating'.
- Verbal numeric rating scales (VNRS): pain is rated on a scale of 0–10, or 0–3, with 0 representing 'no pain' and the highest score being the 'worst pain imaginable'.
- Visual analogue scales: similar to VNRS except that the patient marks on a line (usually 10 cm in length) the ends of which are marked 'no pain' and 'worst imaginable pain'; there are numerous variations.

Knowledge of the insult (traumatic, pathological or surgical) can also give an indication of the likely severity of pain and therefore clues as to which analgesic strategies might be needed. In this case, knowledge of a >30 mph collision leading to fracture of the femur and multiple ribs (with widespread soft-tissue injury also inevitable) predicts severe pain. However, as individual responses both to injury and analgesia vary considerably, individualized pain management is necessary.

Regular consistent assessment of pain is fundamental to its management, as measurement of pain and response to pain relief underpins effective and safe individualized pain relief.

✪ Learning point Definitions

The International Association of the Study of Pain updated pain terminology in 2011 as follows [2]:

- Pain: an unpleasant sensory and emotional experience associated with actual or potential tissue damage.
- Nociceptive pain: pain that arises from actual or threatened damage to non-neural tissue and is due to activation of nociceptors.
- Neuropathic pain: pain caused by a lesion or disease of the somatosensory nervous system.

Most acute and postoperative pain is nociceptive pain. It can be present all the time as 'background pain' or present only on activity, in which case it is known as 'incident pain'. Acute neuropathic pain is less frequent but may coexist in acute trauma or surgical injury. Its recognition and management require careful assessment.

❝ Expert comment

Verbal rating scales (VRS) use words to describe pain intensity and it is usual to assign each descriptor with a numerical value. But it should be remembered that the intervals between descriptors are non-linear. Numerical rating scales (NRS) are an alternative and show good correlation with visual analogue scales (VAS). Approximately 85% of patients report moderate pain score ≤4/10 on NRS (30 mm on VAS) with an overall mean score of 5/10, whereas for severe pain 85% of patients report ≤6/10 on NRS and a median score 7.5/10 (75 mm) [3].

Table 7.2 FLACC Behavioural Scale

Categories	Scoring		
	0	1	2
Face	No particular expression or smile	Occasional grimace or frown, withdrawn, disinterested	Frequent to constant frown, clenched jaw, quivering chin
Legs	Normal position or relaxed	Uneasy, restless, tense	Kicking, or legs drawn up
Activity	Lying quietly, normal position, moves easily	Squirming, shifting back and forth, tense	Arched, rigid, or jerking
Cry	No cry (awake or asleep)	Moans or whimpers, occasional complaint	Crying steadily, screams or sobs, frequent complaints
Consolability	Content, relaxed	Reassured by occasional touching, hugging or being talked to, distractable	Difficult to console or comfort

Whenever feasible, behavioural measurement of pain should be used in conjunction with self-report. When self-report is not possible, interpretation of pain behaviours can be used to measure pain severity. Each category is scored on the 0-2 scale which results in a total score of 0-10: 0 = relaxed and comfortable; 1-3 = mild discomfort; 4-6 = moderate pain; 7-10 = severe discomfort/pain [5].
Each of the five categories (F, Face; L, Legs; A, Activity; C, Cry; C, Consolability) is scored from 0 to 2, which results in a total score between zero and 10.
© 2002, The Regents of the University of Michigan. All Rights Reserved.

Femoral nailing was undertaken 4 h later under general anaesthesia. An epidural catheter was inserted atraumatically at the first attempt at the L3–L4 interlaminar space using a 16G Tuohy needle under full asepsis. Due to anticipated pain on positioning this was done following induction of general anaesthesia. Consent for the epidural had been obtained on the ward following a discussion of the different postoperative treatment options for pain. A review of the discussion was documented on the anaesthetic chart. The epidural was loaded before starting the operation with plain 0.5% bupivacaine. An epidural infusion of 0.1% bupivacaine with 2 μg/mL of fentanyl was started at a rate of 6 mL/h to maintain analgesia both during and after the operation. Intravenous paracetamol and fentanyl were administered during the operation for intra- and postoperative analgesic effect. Regular paracetamol was also prescribed on the drug chart. The patient remained stable throughout and was discharged to the ward from recovery with a pain score of 0.

⊕ Clinical tip Prevention of chronic pain

Knowledge about chronic pain following trauma is extrapolated from data about chronic pain following surgery. Rates of chronic pain vary depending on type of surgery: 10% after inguinal hernia repair, 40% following thoracotomy. Factors which influence the development of chronic postsurgical pain include surgical damage to nerves, postoperative moderate or severe pain, pre-existing pain, psychological vulnerability, anxiety, and depression [8].

Some consider that postoperative pain relief can usefully start before the operation. Preoperative analgesic treatment may be more effective than identical treatment during or after surgery. This attractive option is known as 'pre-emptive' analgesia. Although positive studies for pre-emptive epidural analgesia for thoracic surgery have been published, others demonstrate no effect and whether pre-emptive analgesia produces a clinically meaningful reduction in pain intensity or duration is currently unclear [9].

Acute pain leads to physical and chemical changes in the central nervous system (CNS plasticity) including in the dorsal horn of the spinal column and via the release of inflammatory mediators. In cases of trauma where severe pain has already occurred, true pre-emptive analgesia is not possible; however, early effective analgesia may minimize CNS hypersensitivity. Patients who wake from surgery/anaesthesia in pain may also require more analgesia postoperatively. Overall, the earlier that effective analgesia is established the greater the effect on postoperative pain [10].

When chronic pain does occur after acute injury it can be difficult to treat and often has a neuropathic component. Symptoms and signs that suggest neuropathic pain should be actively sought (shooting or burning pain, sensory loss, hypersensitivity, spontaneous pain) since the treatment differs from that of nociceptive pain. Suitable therapeutic agents in the acute phase include amitriptyline, gabapentin, pregabalin, clonidine and ketamine.

The patient was discharged to an orthopaedic ward where appropriately trained nurses provided the necessary monitoring of analgesia and surveillance for potential epidural and opioid-related complications. He was automatically referred to the acute pain service (APS) for daily review. When he was reviewed by a member of the APS the following morning, he was found to have pain scores of 2–3 on a 4-point VNRS. The effective analgesic level of the epidural block was assessed by noting the level at which ethyl chloride was not felt to be cold and the block was found to be T10–S5 bilaterally. He had minimal weakness of his legs (Bromage Score 1 out of 4). The epidural was providing effective lower limb analgesia with no safety concerns. Above this level, however, the patient had severe incident pain over the rib fractures.

⊕ Clinical tip Bromage Scale

The Bromage Scale was developed as a research tool to assess motor block during labour epidurals [12]. It is a graduated scale from 1 to 4 based on free lower limb movement which is used as a guide to the extent of motor block: 1 = free movement of legs and feet (no block); 2 = just able to flex knees with free movement of feet (partial block); 3 = unable to flex knees but with free movement of feet (almost complete block); 4 = unable to move legs or feet (complete block). Opioids are now routinely added to local anaesthetic to augment analgesia, thus sparing the dense motor block associated with higher concentrations of local anaesthetic. Originally developed as a method to assess efficacy of blocks, its relevance to clinical practice is now in surveillance for complications. The Bromage Scale should not be confused with the Medical Research Council grading of muscle weakness/strength, which is a 6-point scale with high numbers indicating greater muscle power.

This table was published in *Epidural Anaesthesia*, Philip Bromage, p. 144, Copyright Elsevier.

⭐ **Learning point** Multimodal analgesia

As acute traumatic pain (following surgery or injury) is the result of different mechanisms (nociception, inflammation, CNS sensitization, cytokine release), analgesia is optimal when it is multimodal.

Definition

There is no universally agreed definition, but multimodal analgesia is the use of a number of drugs in combination to achieve the best possible pain relief and avoidance of drug-induced side-effects.

Background

Early concepts of pain transmission were often oversimplified. We now know that pain transmission is complex and involves many sophisticated pathways. As this system has many physiological relays in the transmission of pain from its origin to the brain, it may allow multiple points of pharmacological access.

Concept

One systematic approach to multimodal analgesia may involve the pharmacological modification of the following pathways:

1. Decreasing overall pain perception centrally with drugs such as ketamine or opioids.
2. Increasing descending inhibitory pathways from higher centres, e.g. by the use of tramadol or clonidine.
3. Decreasing ascending pain signals by the use of local anaesthetic nerve blocks or systemic NSAIDs.

Using multiple drugs acting at multiple points in the pathway can achieve effective pain relief and decrease the dose and side-effects that would be needed if a single analgesic drug were used. Simple adjunctive measures such as cooling, elevation, and psychological assurance may also be used effectively in acute pain.

Evidence

Reduced postoperative opiate consumption has been demonstrated with combinations of analgesics and use of regional techniques [14]. Other techniques are emerging which may improve multimodal analgesia, including patient-controlled regional analgesia using local anaesthetic infiltrative wound catheters [15].

💬 **Expert comment**

Rib fractures are common in cases of multiple trauma. However, the pain associated with multiple rib fractures can be extremely difficult to control and requires a multimodal approach to pain therapy. In elderly patients with blunt chest trauma PCA and use of an NSAID both impart survival benefit [13]. Patients with multiple rib fractures whose pain is not controlled by intravenous opioids may benefit from thoracic epidural or paravertebral infusions of local anaesthetic to reduce opioid requirements and side-effects.

The patient's analgesic prescription consisted of regular paracetamol and the epidural infusion; with tramadol for breakthrough pain. Doses of parenteral opioids had been withheld due to the presence of an opioid in the epidural infusate to avoid the risk of respiratory depression. To address the inadequate pain relief, the epidural infusate was changed to bupivacaine 0.1% without any opioid. Parenteral morphine was administered in aliquots until the patient was comfortable and then a morphine PCA device with standard settings of 1 mg demand bolus with 5 min lockout time was connected. The device was explained to the patient and ward staff. There was no background infusion and the 4 h limit was set at 30 mg. The method of analgesia, pain score, vital signs, and side-effects were recorded on the patient's observation chart, and daily review was scheduled by the APS. As the risk of major bleeding was now low, a regular NSAID (ibuprofen) was also prescribed.

⭐ **Learning point** Epidural analgesia

Continuous epidural analgesia is the provision of pain relief by administration of agents into the epidural space via an indwelling catheter.

Efficacy

The efficacy of epidural analgesia is well documented for a wide range of surgical procedures. In trauma, as here, it reduces incident pain and is known to reduce hospital-acquired infections in rib fractures, although only if sited in the thoracic region [16].

(continued)

Infusate

Local anaesthetic and opioid combinations provide better analgesia compared with either agent alone [17].

Treatment failure

There are many reasons for failure of epidural analgesia (e.g. inability to site the block, epidural inserted at the wrong level, catheter sited into a neural foramen rather than the epidural space, anatomical variation, inadequate dosing, failure to reload after interruption to infusion, and inadvertent leakage from, or displacement of, the epidural catheter). In a large prospective audit 22% of patients had termination of infusion for inadequate analgesia [18]. This reinforces the need for regular pain assessment, use of co-analgesics, an escalation plan, and regular APS review to support advanced postoperative pain control. Many units would expect a failure rate closer to 5%. Although there is no standard APS design, routine APS review has consistently shown improved postoperative pain control [19].

Respiratory depression

In a review of audit data and case reports, the rate of respiratory depression with opiate-containing epidural infusions ranged from 1.1% to 15.1%. Although this was dependent on infusion type and definition of respiratory depression, it is remarkably similar to that found with an opiate PCA analgesia. This review covered several decades and it is hoped that increased awareness of the potential problem combined with better management and surveillance would reduce these numbers considerably. In order to avoid cumulative effects of analgesic modalities on respiratory depression, epidural and systemic opiates should not be given at the same time, except in highly monitored environments such as an intensive care unit [20]. Careful co-administration of systemic tramadol with appropriate monitoring is considered safe.

Awake versus asleep epidural

This is an issue of much debate. It may be best practice to perform epidurals awake when a patient can report symptoms warning of potential nerve injury; in some circumstances it may only be practicable, as here, if it is done asleep. Although strong views are expressed and awake is the norm, there is a lack of robust evidence and where circumstances dictate it is reasonable to perform an asleep epidural.

The following morning ward nursing staff requested an early review by the APS since his pain scores were unsatisfactory at 2 or 3 on a 4-point VNRS. Epidural analgesia in the lower limbs remained effective, Bromage scores were low and the epidural site was clean. Vital signs were within normal limits and no new medications had been started. Clinical examination and routine bloods were unremarkable. On questioning he did not understand the PCA device and seemed unclear about its benefits despite previous and repeated explanations. This raised concerns over the benefits of self-administered morphine. He also complained of nausea directly associated with PCA activation and he lacked appetite. Analysis of PCA usage data from the previous 24 h showed 49 demands from which he had received 39 boluses of morphine. This low level of self-administered morphine (well below 2 mg/h) in the presence of continuing severe pain was indicative of PCA failure. The APS suggested a diagnosis of postoperative confusion exacerbated or caused by opioids. To gain analgesic control, reassurance was given and an explanation of PCA goals was reinforced. Regular antiemetics were prescribed and PCA morphine was replaced by PCA oxycodone.

✪ Learning point Patient-controlled analgesia (PCA)

Broadly, the efficacy and safety of intravenous PCA opioid analgesia requires a careful balance of pain relief versus side-effects. Full explanation of how to use it and its inherent safety is needed before administration to avoid fears of overdose or addiction, leading to underdosing and inadequate pain

(continued)

relief. This requires not only education by the APS but careful monitoring and reinforcement by the ward team, who should be regularly educated themselves.

The successful use of PCA requires normal cognitive function. The incidence of confusion with morphine PCA is ~2%, which is significantly less than the 18% reported in patients using intramuscular morphine [21]. Confusion should trigger a search for an identifiable and reversible cause, and, if none is found, opioid switching may be considered. There is little evidence to suggest major differences in efficacy or side-effect profile between the different opioids used in PCA devices [22]. However, individual response may vary and if side-effects do not resolve with conventional treatment there may be benefit from switching to a different opioid. Here oxycodone was substituted: fentanyl would be another suitable alternative.

Nausea is a common side-effect with all opioids. PONV is associated with other well known risk factors (female sex, a prior history of PONV or motion sickness, non-smoker) and may be a consequence of other iatrogenic influences (e.g. volatile anaesthetics or nitrous oxide). Even opiate-sparing analgesic techniques are still associated with significant nausea [23]. Good practice requires that antiemetics are prescribed routinely to manage PONV and that where necessary they are administered promptly.

The side-effect of PCA that causes the most concern is respiratory depression. Broadly, audit figures estimate the risk of respiratory depression from PCA opioid analgesia to be 1.2 to 11.5%. This incidence increases if the patient is elderly, hypovolaemic, has a pulmonary disorder, is receiving additional opiates such as a background infusion (which more than doubles the incidence alone), or is receiving concurrent sedation [20].

The most usual PCA regime used for opioid-naïve adult patients is a 1 mg morphine bolus dose with a 5 min lockout period, without a background infusion. Generally, a shorter lockout period can result in opiate 'stacking' as additional opiate doses are delivered before maximum analgesia has been reached.

⊗ **Learning point**   Ketamine in acute pain

Ketamine, a phencyclidine derivative, is a non-competitive antagonist at the N-methyl-D-aspartate receptor. It has both anaesthetic and analgesic properties. There has long been interest in subanaesthetic doses of ketamine, particularly when combined with morphine, for postoperative pain.

When ketamine is added to a postoperative morphine PCA there is a demonstrable reduction in morphine consumption in the first 24 h. In this setting ketamine in addition to morphine PCA results in less PONV.

The demand bolus dose of ketamine in morphine-containing PCA can range from 0.4 to 1.0 mg, or ketamine can run as a separate continuous infusion for 24 h (example analgesic dose range: 0.05–0.15 mg/kg/h). There is a ceiling effect on morphine reduction beyond 30 mg in 24 h [24].

A reduction in morphine use does not always equate to improved analgesia. However, it is appropriate to consider ketamine, in addition to morphine PCA, when a patient is especially sensitive to opioids or an injury is deemed to be particularly painful, in order to limit morphine use and its side-effects. Ketamine may also be considered for the same reasons in complex non-opioid-naïve patients with severe pain. Side-effects of ketamine infusions increase as dose rises, and include sedation, nausea and vomiting, and bad dreams.

The patient was followed up later that day when he reported a reduction in his pain and was less confused. His intercostal chest drain was removed later that evening after pre-treatment of anticipated pain with a morphine bolus.

The following morning his pain scores ranged from 0 to 1 and he reported no nausea. Vital signs were within normal limits. His epidural wound site was clear and his lower limbs neurologically intact. A recent full blood count was normal. The epidural infusion had been inadvertently switched off during the night and in spite of this there was no increase in his pain score. Prophylactic low-molecular-weight heparin had not been administered for > 12 h and therefore the epidural catheter was removed. The oxycodone PCA was continued.

The patient commented to the acute pain nurse that he had an area of numbness in the left anterior thigh: on examination the affected area approximated to the L2–L3 dermatome. Neurological examination revealed normal muscle power, tone, and reflexes. Straight leg raise was maintained, but there was a residual area of decreased sensation to light touch unilaterally. Bladder and bowel functions were undisturbed and temperature was 36.5°C. There were no epidural 'red flags' to indicate high risk of vertebral canal compression.

> **✪ Learning point** Neuraxial 'red flags'
>
> The presence of 'red flags' should prompt investigation to exclude a vertebral canal compression from haematoma or abscess. The gold standard investigation should be MRI. Investigation and treatment is required as soon as possible to enable completion of treatment within 8–12 h of identifying a 'red flag' to maximize the chances of recovery for the patient [26]:
>
> - significant motor block with a thoracic epidural
> - unexpectedly dense motor block, including unilateral block
> - markedly increasing motor block during epidural infusion
> - motor block that does not regress when an epidural is stopped
> - recurrent unexpected motor block after restarting an epidural infusion that was stopped because of motor block

The deficit was explained by diffuse local paraesthesia secondary to trauma. A decision was made to observe and review with a plan for lumbar spine MRI if there was persisting doubt regarding an epidural complication.

The patient had resumed eating and drinking, and, as 24 h equivalent morphine usage was < 30 mg per day, the oxycodone PCA was disconnected. The analgesic regimen was stepped down to paracetamol, ibuprofen and tramadol regularly with 10 mg oxycodone 2-hourly as required for breakthrough pain.

> **✪ Learning point** 3rd National Audit Project (NAP3) [26]
>
> Optimal postoperative pain control leads to a better patient outcome after surgery. The most clearly defined benefit of epidural analgesia is improved analgesia, and beyond reasonable doubt, a functioning epidural provides better analgesia than all other forms of postoperative analgesia. NAP3 was the largest study performed on major adverse events of central neural blockade (CNB). It involved >700,000 episodes of CNB and demonstrated:
>
> - An overall (pessimistic) risk of permanent injury from all types of CNB for all indications of 1/24,000 (95% CI: 1 in 16,400–34,500).
> - Half of the morbidity was attributable to perioperative epidurals, which accounted for <15% of the total blockade episodes.
>
> However, the data do not allow conclusions as to whether perioperative epidurals are intrinsically risky or whether it is the high-risk nature of such patients that accounts for the higher incidence of complications. The benefits of epidural analgesia, beyond improved analgesia, may also be greater in higher-risk patients than others. The benefits of epidurals and the complications of other techniques were not measured in NAP3. Weighing up adverse events is difficult, particularly since NAP3 also showed:
>
> (continued)

- No deaths from epidural analgesia.
- The majority of reported adverse events resolved.
- Delay in diagnosis and treatment as a frequent theme underlying permanent harm: this was often due to factors such as inexpert review, failure to respond to signs indicating developing complications, poor communication, and organizational delays.

A known incidence of harm does not make perioperative epidurals inappropriate. The risk in each case must be judged individually. In this case, the insertion was atraumatic, performed under aseptic conditions, and the clotting profile was normal. Superior analgesic profile (compared with its omission or with the opioid-based alternatives) and the presence of a mechanism for prompt diagnosis of complications with appropriate follow-up made it an appropriate choice to reduce the negative consequences of surgery.

❝ Expert comment

Vivid nightmares are a rare side-effect of tramadol, occurring in only 0.37% of patients, predominantly on commencement of treatment [27].

The APS was called 2 h later to review the patient due to persisting concerns over leg numbness. MRI of his lumbar spine was arranged to rule out any potential epidural-related cause for the lower limb neurology; the result was reassuring (Figure 7.3). The patient's assessment of his background pain was now 'mild to moderate' for which he had a regular analgesic plan to match his level of pain. Ward staff were advised that he could step this down to a single agent and then no analgesia as his pain levels decreased to 0–1 on an NRS. Opioids were to be used for anticipated severe incident pain, particularly on mobilization, or if unanticipated breakthrough pain occurred.

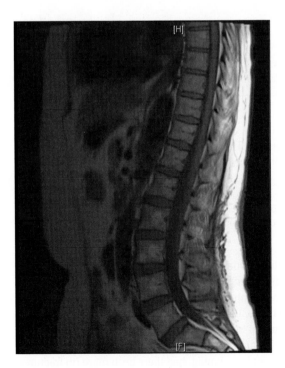

Figure 7.3 Sagittal T1-weighted MRI scan of the lumbar region, demonstrating a spacious vertebral canal with no nerve or cord compression. T1 refers to the relaxation times during MRI and allows differentiation of fat- and water-containing tissues.

> ★ **Learning point** The Pain Ladder [28]
>
> The World Health Organization's (WHO) 'Pain Ladder' was introduced in 1986 to specifically address cancer pain, although it is now widely used for most types of pain (Figure 7.4). The principle is to start at the first step on the ladder and then climb to subsequent steps if pain is not well controlled. Analgesia should be taken regularly or 'by the clock' as opposed to *pro re nata* (p.r.n.), or on a rescue basis. It is rare for more than one-quarter of the maximum dose of analgesia prescribed p.r.n. to be given, even when pain persists.
>
> One of the defining characteristics of acute pain is that it is at its worst during the first days. Therefore the analgesic ladder is more often 'stepped down' over time, as opposed to 'stepped up'. Not all pain is responsive to classical analgesic drugs, and drugs not usually considered as analgesics may be used concurrently at any stage, e.g. amitriptyline. Part of the effectiveness of the ladder is derived from the way different drugs are sequentially added. In this way pain is addressed 'multimodally' and different drugs are combined for maximal effectiveness. A single agent is not relied upon to provide analgesia, and the use of strong opioids on the higher rungs with their incumbent side-effects may be minimized.
>
>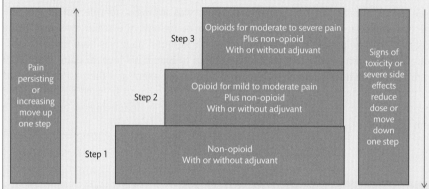
>
> **Figure 7.4** Adapted WHO Pain Ladder. At each stage the lower level is prescribed regularly and the stronger drug prescribed on a p.r.n. basis. Drugs are thus added rather than substituted. Adjuvant analgesia and other drugs such as laxatives are also part of the ladder. Reproduced with permission from the World Health Organization, http://www.who.int/cancer/palliative/painladder/en, Accessed 19th September 2013.

The APS discharged the patient from routine review—though the ward had direct access to the APS should it be required. The patient and his general practitioner were also supplied with a letter documenting the use of an epidural catheter, detailing signs and symptoms that should cause concern and contact details for the on-call anaesthetist.

Discussion

The multiple sites of injury make this a complex case. No regional block would provide analgesia for both sites. For this case a decision was made to manage the femoral fracture with an epidural and the thoracic injury with parenteral analgesia. The opposite decision might equally have been made, using a thoracic epidural for the rib fractures and parenteral analgesia for the femoral injury. In this case only two rib fractures were present, underlying lung injury was minimal and the patient was young and without respiratory disease. Had the patient not been young, had there been more rib fractures, acute lung injury, or chronic lung disease, the best option might well have switched to thoracic epidural to prevent significant respiratory complications.

There is some controversy about the use of NSAIDs for patients with bone fracture or undergoing orthopaedic surgery. NSAIDs inhibit prostaglandin formation and it is feasible that, as prostaglandins favour bone formation, NSAIDs may have an adverse effect on bone healing. There is not much in the way of good-quality evidence for this in humans, however. Small studies of bone healing in animals suggest an inhibitory effect on bone formation [29] but a meta-analysis of case–control and cohort studies in humans found no statistically significant association between NSAID exposure and non-union when lower-quality studies were excluded [30].

Confounding factors that affect bone-healing and that may have an additive effect when combined with NSAID treatment include diabetes and cigarette smoking. Further research is warranted but until then the use of NSAIDs to improve analgesia in those with fracture needs to be made on an individual basis. In this case, achieving adequate analgesia was challenging and the patient had no other factors likely to affect bone healing, so the use of a short-acting NSAID was judged to be reasonable.

The provision of good postoperative pain relief is an important component of anaesthetic practice. It is cost-effective and increases the likelihood of satisfied patients. This might be considered an easy task since most surgery leads to predictable tissue disruption and numerous drugs and clinicians are available to provide analgesia. In spite of this, postoperative pain control is often poor. In a seminal UK survey of 3000 inpatients in the mid-1990s more than half of the patients had had episodes of unrelieved moderate or severe acute pain [31]. More recent surveys in the USA [32] and Germany [33] have reported similar results. Whereas the causes are not certain, the consequences of this from an individual and financial viewpoint are profound. Improving the evidence base and application of available evidence in acute pain management remains a priority.

From the known trials of drugs in acute pain, effective postoperative analgesia is often defined as 50% relief of pain following medication. Using this measure of efficacy, a number needed to treat (NNT) can be derived, i.e. the number of patients needed to treat for one patient to gain 50% pain relief. The advantage of these numbers is that they allow comparison and benchmarking of analgesia. An analgesic with NNT < 6 is broadly said to be clinically useful [34, 35]. Unfortunately the NNT does have caveats. It is often derived from trial data from simple surgical operations which use only single doses of analgesics as the intervention (e.g. dental extractions). Although this information is useful, it fails to guide the clinician's choice in more complex cases such as when to start multiple drugs and how to switch from one drug type to another. Nonetheless, a 2011 Cochrane review on acute pain combined the results from 35 individual Cochrane reviews which included 45,000 postoperative patients [36]. This review has identified some guiding principles for postoperative analgesia:

Variability of effectiveness and available evidence

There is substantial variability of effectiveness of drugs and no one drug can produce consistently high levels of pain relief in all who receive it. The better drugs achieve pain relief in 70% of participants and the worst only 30%. Paracetamol alone produced pain relief in only 40% of participants but when combined with ibuprofen 70% of participants achieved effective pain relief. Referring this evidence to this particular case, it reinforces the drive to initiate multimodal analgesia with the prescription of regular paracetamol and NSAID.

There is also substantial variability in the available evidence for single and composite analgesic treatments. Some analgesics are well studied and proven to produce good analgesia; 1 g of paracetamol alone has an NNT value of 3.2 but when combined with 60 mg of codeine the NNT decreases to 2.2. By contrast there is inadequate data to allow a comparison with drugs such as indomethacin where the NNT value is unknown. Analgesics should be chosen in clinical practice because they are known to work. The use of antidepressants and anticonvulsants would seem an attractive option given their efficacy in chronic pain. Anticonvulsants such as gabapentin and pregabalin have been studied in acute pain, but their efficacy is unproven in standard postoperative pain models. For pregabalin, there is only one small trial from which it is impossible to derive the NNT. In the case of gabapentin, pooled result analysis of four trials in postoperative pain derive an NNT of 11 [37]. This high NNT suggests that it is inferior to other analgesics in routine use. The efficacy of gabapentin, along with other anticonvulsants and antidepressants as single agents, therefore appears limited. In acute pain the routine use of such drugs as first-line analgesics alone would be unlikely to provide good analgesia. In practice the addition of these drugs is often considered in cases where the pain has a neuropathic component or pain control is inadequate.

Analgesic failure

It should not be a surprise if an analgesic drug does not work, as no drug produces high levels of pain relief in everyone. Review of the adequacy of analgesia and the prescription of alternative agents for breakthrough pain are essential. Adverse event rates for many drugs are largely comparable between drugs and their placebo comparator in large trials. This is not the case for opioids, and, as demonstrated here, morphine was an ineffective analgesic agent because of the side-effects. The use of multimodal analgesia to minimize opioid use can reduce the side-effect burden.

Route of administration

When considering the route of administration for analgesic drugs it seems best to give drugs by mouth. Indeed, there is little evidence to suggest that other routes of administration (for example rectal rather than oral in the case of NSAIDs) work any faster or for longer, or produce fewer side-effects [35].

A Final Word from the Expert

Whereas acute pain frequently occurs in the postoperative period, surveys have revealed repeatedly that >80% of patients admitted to hospital for whatever reason complain of pain.

Pain relief in multiple trauma patients, as presented in this case report, is a particular challenge with >60% of patients complaining of moderate pain or worse one year after injury. Acute pain management should reduce pain severity while controlling side-effects with the aim of improving long-term outcomes. Postoperative pain relief is an integral part of all anaesthetic practice, and failure to deliver it should always prompt an active search for a solution.

References

1. Ferrell B, MaCaffery M. Nurses' knowledge of pain issues. *J Pain Symptom Manage* 1987;2:207–11.
2. Merskey H, Bogduk N. *Classification of chronic pain: descriptions of chronic pain syndromes and definitions of pain terms*, 2nd ed. Seattle: IASP Press; 1994. p. 212.
3. Collins SL, Moore RA, McQuay HJ. The visual analogue pain intensity scale: what is moderate pain in millimetres? *Pain* 1997;72:95–7.
4. Wong D, Baker C. Pain in children: comparison of assessment scales. *Pediatr Nurs* 1988;14:9–17.
5. Merkel SI, Voepel-Lewis T, Shayevitz JR, Malviya S. The FLACC: a behavioral scale for scoring postoperative pain in young children. *Pediatr Nurs* 1997;23:293–7.
6. Mar GJ, Barrington MJ, McGuirk BR. Acute compartment syndrome of the lower limb and the effect of postoperative analgesia on diagnosis. *Br J Anaesth* 2009;102:3–11.
7. Karagiannis G, Hardern R. No evidence found that a femoral nerve block in cases of femoral shaft fractures can delay the diagnosis of compartment syndrome of the thigh. *Emerg Med J* 2005;22:814.
8. Beard DJ, Aldington D. Chronic pain after trauma. *Trauma* 2012;14:57–66.
9. Dahl JB, Kehlet H. Preventive analgesia. *Curr Opin Anaesthesiol* 2011;24:331–8.
10. McQuay H, Moore A, Justins D. Treating acute pain in hospital. *Br Med J* 1997;314:1531–5.
11. Rivara FP, Mackenzie EJ, Jurkovich GJ, Nathens AB, Wang J, Scharfstein DO. Prevalence of pain in patients 1 year after major trauma. *Arch Surg* 2008;143:282–7.
12. Bromage PR. *Epidural analgesia*. Philadelphia: WB Saunders; 1978.
13. Harrington DT, Phillips B, Machan J, *et al.* Factors associated with survival following blunt chest trauma in older patients: results from a large regional trauma cooperative. *Arch Surg* 2010;145:432–7.
14. Bonnet F, Marret E. Postoperative pain management and outcome after surgery. *Best Pract Res Clin Anaesthesiol* 2007;21:99–107.
15. Axelsson K, Nordenson U, Johanzon E, *et al.* Patient-controlled regional analgesia (PCRA) with ropivacaine after arthroscopic subacromial decompression. *Acta Anaesthesiol Scand* 2003;47:993–1000
16. Bulger EM, Edwards T, Klotz P, Jurkovich GJ. Epidural analgesia improves outcome after multiple rib fractures. *Surgery* 2004;136:426–30.
17. Curatolo M, Petersen-Felix S, Scaramozzino P, Zbinden AM. Epidural fentanyl, adrenaline and clonidine as adjuvants to local anaesthetics for surgical analgesia: meta-analyses of analgesia and side-effects. *Acta Anaesthesiol Scand* 1998;42:910–20.
18. Ballantyne JC, McKenna JM, Ryder E. Epidural analgesia—experience of 5628 patients in a large teaching hospital derived through audit. *Acute Pain* 2003;4:89–97.
19. Sartain JB, Barry JJ. The impact of an acute pain service on postoperative pain management. *Anaesth Intensive Care* 1999;27:375–80.
20. Cashman JN, Dolin SJ. Respiratory and haemodynamic effects of acute postoperative pain management: evidence from published data. *Br J Anaesth* 2004;93:212–23.
21. Egbert AM, Parks LH, Short LM, Burnett ML. Randomized trial of postoperative patient-controlled analgesia vs intramuscular narcotics in frail elderly men. *Arch Intern Med* 1990;150:1897–1903.
22. Collins JJ, Geake J, Grier HE, *et al.* Patient-controlled analgesia for mucositis pain in children: a three-period crossover study comparing morphine and hydromorphine. *J Pediatr* 1996;19:722–8.
23. Woodhouse A, Mather LE. Nausea and vomiting in the postoperative patient-controlled analgesia environment. *Anaesthesia* 1997;52:770–5.
24. Bell RF, Dahl JB, Moore RA, Kalso EA. Perioperative ketamine for acute postoperative pain. *Cochrane Database Syst Rev* 2006(1):CD004603.

25. Joint Working Party of the Association of Anaesthetists of Great Britain & Ireland (AAGBI), Obstetric Anaesthetists' Association (OAA) and Regional Anaesthesia UK. *Regional anaesthesia in patients with abnormalities in coagulation.* < http://www.aagbi.org/sites/default/files/RAPAC%20for%20consultation.pdf >

26. Cook TM, Counsell D, Wildsmith JAW. Major complications of central neuraxial block: report on the Third National Audit Project of The Royal College of Anaesthetists. *Br J Anaesth* 2009;102:179–90.

27. eHealthMe.com. *Does tramadol cause vivid nightmare?* Mountain View, CA: eHealthMe; 2013. < http://www.ehealthme.com/ds/tramadol/vivid + nightmare >

28. World Health Organization. *Cancer pain relief.* Geneva: WHO; 1986. < http://www.who.int/cancer/palliative/painladder/en/ >

29. Vuolteenaho K, Moilanen T, Moilanen E. Non-steroidal anti-inflammatory drugs, cyclooxygenase-2 and the bone healing process. *Basic Clin Pharmacol Toxicol* 2008;102:10–14.

30. Dodwell ER, Latorre JG, Parisini E, *et al.* NSAID exposure and risk of nonunion: a meta-analysis of case–control and cohort studies. *Calcified Tiss Int* 2010;87:193–202.

31. Bruster S, Jarman B, Bosanquet N, Weston D, Erens R, Delbanco TL. National survey of hospital patients. *Br Med J* 1994;309:1542–6.

32. Apfelbaum JL, Chen C, Mehta SS, Gan TJ. Postoperative pain experience: results from a national survey suggest postoperative pain continues to be undermanaged. *Anesth Analg* 2003;97:534–40.

33. Maier C, Nestler N, Richter H, *et al.* The quality of pain management in German hospitals. *Dtsch Arztebl Int* 2010;107:607–14.

34. Moore A, Edwards J, Barden J, McQuay H, editors. *Bandolier's little book of pain.* Oxford: Oxford University Press; 2003.

35. McQuay HK, Poon H, Derry S, Moore A. Acute pain: combination treatments and how we measure their efficacy. *Br J Anaesth* 2008;101:69–76.

36. Moore RA, Derry S, McQuay HJ, Wiffen PJ. Single dose oral analgesics for acute postoperative pain in adults. *Cochrane Database Syst Rev* 2011;(9):CD008659.

37. Straube S, Derry S, Moore RA, Wiffen PJ, McQuay HJ. Single dose oral gabapentin for established acute postoperative pain in adults. *Cochrane Database Syst Rev* 2010;(5):CD008183.

CHAPTER 8

Multiple trauma

Case 8.1	Multiple trauma and the anaesthetist

8.1 Multiple trauma and the anaesthetist

Caroline Sampson

⊕ **Expert Commentary** Michael Parr
CPD Matrix Code: *2A02, 3A10, 3C00*

Case history

23.40

A previously fit and well 23-year-old female patient was involved in a high-speed road traffic collision. She was the unrestrained driver of a car that hit a bollard at an esti-mated speed of 60 mph. The car had rolled and then hit a tree, landing on its roof. The patient was ejected from the vehicle and found ~10 m from the car, which had been extensively damaged. A second unrestrained passenger (presumed to have been the front seat passenger) was pronounced dead at the scene.

Witnesses had heard the crash and called the emergency services, which arrived at the scene within 10 min. Paramedics reported that on their arrival the patient had a patent airway, was tachypnoeic and tachycardic with a pulse rate of 125 beats/min. She responded to voice but was agitated and had an obvious right open femoral fracture. They were unable to record her blood pressure or secure venous access. She was rapidly transported to hospital with an overall scene and transport time of 50 min.

00.40: arrival at emergency department

The primary survey identified the following:

A: Airway patent, moaning. Oxygen administered via a non-rebreathing mask at 15 L/min. Triple 'spinal immobilization' precautions in place with hard cervical collar, sandbags and tape, with patient on a spinal board.

B: No obvious chest wall injuries. Good bilateral breath sounds on auscultation. No crepitus felt, central trachea. Peripheral oxygen saturation trace unrecordable.

C: Very pale, clammy. Heart rate 140 beats/min. Blood pressure unrecordable. Radial pulse not palpable—able to feel faint, thready brachial pulse. Capillary refill time 5 s. Right upper quadrant pain and guarding demonstrable.

Pelvic binder applied and massive transfusion protocol activated. Following several failed attempts at venous cannulation, intraosseous access was gained in her left tibia.

> ✪ **Clinical tip** The primary survey
>
> The primary survey is the first and key part of the assessment of trauma patients as taught by the Advanced Trauma Life Support system, during which immediately life-threatening injuries are identified and treated in a systematic way.
>
> The sequence follows the ABCDE approach: Airway (with cervical spine control), Breathing and ventilation, Circulation with haemorrhage control, Disability (neurological evaluation), and Exposure/Environment [1].

> ✪ **Learning point** Intraosseus (IO) cannulation
>
> There is a direct communication from the medullary canal of bone via Volkmann canals to periosteal blood vessels and the vascular plexus of the limb. This space is non-collapsible, even in severely shocked patients [2].
>
> (continued)

IO cannulation is not a new technique—sternal IO cannulation was standard practice for wounded soldiers in World War II, but the technique all but died out with the introduction of plastic intravenous cannulae in the 1950s [3]. There was renewed interest in the 1980s for shocked paediatric patients, but it was not until 2005 that resuscitation guidelines recommended IO access if intravenous access is unavailable in cardiac arrest; 'IO cannulation provides access to a non-collapsible venous plexus, enabling drug delivery similar to that achieved by central venous access…and is attainable in all age groups' [4]. IO cannulation therefore provides alternative access to the circulation in severely shocked trauma patients in whom peripheral intravenous access is not possible, and it is now widely used in both military and civilian trauma [1].

Sites recommended for IO cannulation in adults are sternum, proximal humerus, and proximal and distal tibia. A number of commercially available insertion kits exist. Fluid flow rates of up to 150 mL/min can be attained. Primary complications include extravasation of fluid, fracture at the insertion site and osteomyelitis. IO needles should be removed as soon as possible (within 24 h) [2].

Expert comment

Fluid resuscitation in trauma is usually achieved by upper limb venous access, often at the antecubital fossa. Central venous cannulation usually has little place in the initial resuscitation as cannulation attempts are associated with more severe complications and the cannulae used are often not ideal for large-volume resuscitation: for high flow rates, short cannulae with a large internal diameter are best. Femoral access by Seldinger or cutdown techniques are options, but, where intra-abdominal injury is considered the likely cause of blood loss, the upper limb remains the preferred route.

The first unit of O-negative blood was syringed through the IO needle. Intravenous access was achieved in the patient's right antecubital fossa—blood tests were taken and sent urgently (Tables 8.1 and 8.2). The second unit of O-negative blood was pressurized through this peripheral line. Blood pressure became recordable at 72/32 mmHg, with a tachycardia of 138 beats/min.

Table 8.1 Initial venous blood gas results (patient breathing spontaneously on a non-rebreathe mask, FiO_2 ~60%)

pH	7.28[a]
PaO_2	7.87 kPa
$PaCO_2$	4.20 kPa
Lactate	5.4 mmol/L[a]
HCO_3^-	18 mmol/L[a]
Base excess	−7.2 mEq/L[a]
Haemoglobin	11.2 g/dL
Haematocrit	0.47

[a] Abnormal results.

Table 8.2 Initial blood results

Haematology	
Haemoglobin	10.5 g/dL[a]
Haematocrit	0.43
White cell count	31.4×10^9/L[a]
Platelets	190×10^9/L
Prothrombin time	15 s[a]
APTT	29 s
Thrombin time	18 s
Fibrinogen	1.6 g/L

Biochemistry	
Na	136 mmol/L
K	3.1 mmol/L
Urea	9.4 mmol/L[a]
Creatinine	110 μmol/L[a]
Alanine aminotransferase	454 IU/L[a]
Alkaline phosphatase	88 IU/L
Bilirubin	12 μmol/L
Albumin	18 g/L[a]

[a] Abnormal results.
APTT, activated partial thromboplastin time.

The primary survey continued:

D: Agitated. Glasgow Coma Score: 9/15; Eyes 2, Verbal 2, Motor 5. Pupils equal and reactive to light. Spontaneous movement of all limbs seen.

E: Right leg deformity above and below knee with puncture wounds—likely open fractures. Temperature 34.8°C.

Chest and pelvic radiographs were taken, demonstrating a fractured right iliac wing.

⭐ **Learning point** Glasgow Coma Score

This was developed by Teasdale and Jennett in 1974 as a means of standardizing assessment of conscious level in patients with traumatic brain injury [5]. It was originally intended as a research tool to define coma. It was then used as an inclusion criterion for patients with severe head injury to an international database of cases, initially developed in Glasgow in 1968, with the aim to improve early management and prognostication in traumatic brain injury. Coma was defined as 'an inability to obey commands, to utter recognizable words, or to open the eyes' and the scale consisted of 14 levels of best verbal, motor, and eye opening responses to allow easy data inputting [6]. By 1976 a sixth response level had been added to the motor component and a numerical score was ascribed to each response level with a better response giving a higher number, thus creating a simple coma scoring system that was rapidly accepted into international clinical practice and is familiar to all healthcare professionals today as the Glasgow Coma Score [7].

It is formed of three components—best Verbal (V), Motor (M) and Eye opening (E) response, giving a score ranging from a minimum of 3 to a maximum of 15 (Table 8.3). When responses are variable during testing the *best* response should be recorded. A painful stimulus needs to be applied if there is incomplete response to speech, with nailbed pressure being the standard stimulus originally described. Sternal rub or pressure on the supraorbital ridge may be more appropriate in trauma patients, especially if there are upper limb injuries: the latter is preferred as it is more discriminating. Localization of an uninjured arm requires that the contralateral hand moves to the site of nailbed pressure or that either arm raises above the clavicle in response to supraorbital or sternal stimulus. Intubated patients should have a '1T' (tube) recorded for verbal, and patients with eyes closed due to facial trauma '1C' for eyes.

Focused assessment with sonography for trauma (FAST) scanning was undertaken which revealed free fluid in Morison's pouch.

The decision was made for immediate intubation and then transfer to theatre for laparotomy. Tranexamic acid 1 g was given as a slow bolus over 10 min, followed by an infusion of a further 1 g for a period of 8 h.

⭐ **Learning point** FAST scanning

FAST scanning was first described in the 1970s but only gained widespread acceptance during the 1990s with the introduction of portable, low-cost and high-quality ultrasound scanners. Where available it has largely replaced the more invasive and time-consuming diagnostic peritoneal lavage and can be performed at the bedside. It is now commonly considered as part of the primary survey in trauma. It is not considered a substitute for CT—but is useful to confirm an intra-abdominal source for haemodynamic instability necessitating emergent laparotomy—as in this case.

The scan aims to answer one question—does the patient have free fluid in the abdomen and/or pericardial sac (which in the context of trauma is assumed to be blood). FAST is not designed to assess visceral injuries. The three abdominal views examine the most dependent zones of peritoneum in the supine patient where free fluid is most likely to collect. Studies have demonstrated FAST that is an effective screening tool when performed by experienced sonographers. Sensitivity

(continued)

and specificity for therapeutic laparotomy (solid organ injury requiring surgical repair to achieve haemostasis) increased with the presence of hypotension, volume and number of fluid collections observed. In one study therapeutic laparotomy rates ≥90% were observed in hypotensive patients with moderate-to-large estimated volumes of fluid or the presence of three or more discrete fluid pockets [8].

Four standard views are used:

- pericardial: subxiphoid/subcostal—detects haemopericardium
- perihepatic: right upper quadrant/Morison's pouch—the space between the liver and the right kidney
- perisplenic: left upper quadrant
- suprapubic: pouch of Douglas in females/rectovesicular area in males [9, 10]

00.55

Rapid sequence intubation was undertaken. The stiff neck-collar was removed and manual in-line stabilization was maintained throughout. The patient, who was estimated to be 60 kg, was induced with ketamine 100 mg, alfentanil 1 mg and suxamethonium 100 mg as her blood pressure remained low at 83/46. Direct laryngoscopy demonstrated a modified Cormack and Lehane grade 2a view, allowing easy passage of a size 7.0 cuffed oral tracheal tube [11].

> ✪ **Learning point** Airway management in trauma
>
> It is widely accepted that trauma patients can present airway management difficulties due to direct airway trauma, haemorrhage into the airway, and the need to maintain cervical spine immobilization. Compounding factors include the risk of aspiration of stomach contents and the inability to adequately preoxygenate due to lung injury or patient agitation. Finally, trauma patients arrive with little warning at all times of the day and night, when experienced personnel may not be immediately available, yet the nature of their injuries requires emergent or urgent definitive airway management.
>
> Manual in-line stabilization (MILS) or manual in-line axial immobilization aims to apply sufficient forces to the head and neck to limit cervical spine movement during airway management. An assistant cradles the patient's mastoids and grasps their occiput so that the collar can be removed allowing mouth opening [12]. Views of the larynx are reported as being impaired in 45% of patients with MILS compared with optimum intubating position, with 22% of patients receiving MILS having Cormack and Lehane grade 3 or 4 views [11, 13]. A year-long audit examining major complications of airway management during anaesthesia in National Health Service hospitals in the UK highlighted the need for senior expertise for trauma airways, the importance of using end-tidal capnography and formulating a realistic plan for airway rescue in case of difficulty; including performing an emergency surgical airway [14]. Various airway adjuncts have been shown to improve laryngeal view and intubating success in patients with MILS including the gum elastic bougie, McCoy laryngoscope and videolaryngoscopy [13, 15, 16]. With precautions to protect the cervical spine in place, direct laryngoscopy and other airway manoeuvres appear to have a low risk of exacerbating cervical spine/cord injury.

> ❝ **Expert comment**
>
> It is possible to cause haemodynamic instability and hypotension in the hypovolaemic trauma patient with any induction agent or combination of agents. Skill and experience with a variety of agents are as important as the specific agents selected. Ketamine, however, has the advantage of potentially greater cardiovascular stability and is increasingly used as an induction agent for trauma patients.

> ✪ **Learning point** Ketamine for rapid sequence induction?
>
> Rapid sequence induction (RSI) can be hazardous in critically ill, hypovolaemic patients. Agents used for RSI should reliably provide rapid onset of anaesthesia and neuromuscular blockade to facilitate rapid tracheal intubation.
>
> (continued)

The intravenous induction agents most frequently used for induction—thiopentone and propofol—cause dose-dependent negative inotropy and arteriolar vasodilatation, respectively, which is exacerbated in hypovolaemic patients. Dose reduction is needed, but difficult to calculate, and the anaesthetist is left with the challenge of balancing the risks of awareness against precipitating cardiovascular collapse at induction. Etomidate is a frequent choice in hypovolaemic patients as it improves haemodynamic stability on induction, but it has been withdrawn from use in several countries due to concerns that it causes reversible adrenal insufficiency which may increase in-hospital mortality [17].

Ketamine, a phencyclidine derivative, is the most widely used anaesthetic agent worldwide, particularly in resource-poor environments. It produces a state of dissociative anaesthesia, described as: 'a trancelike cataleptic state characterized by profound analgesia and amnesia, with retention of protective airway reflexes, spontaneous respirations, and cardiopulmonary stability' [18]. Ketamine acts as a sympathomimetic to increase heart rate, arterial pressure and cardiac output, though it can exert a mild direct depressant effect on the myocardium (therefore hypotension is not guaranteed to be avoided). Ketamine has been advocated as the best available induction agent in hypovolaemic patients [19, 20]. Unpleasant emergence reactions which limit its use in elective work are not considered a major problem in the patient who is likely to remain sedated in intensive care for some time.

Ketamine has traditionally been avoided in patients with traumatic brain injury due to concerns that it raises ICP and therefore worsens CPP. These concerns appear to have arisen mainly from two papers published in 1972 that demonstrated a marked ICP rise associated with ketamine in small numbers of neurosurgical patients with obstructed CSF pathways [21, 22]. The authors did not demonstrate such a rise in patients with normal CSF pathways. By contrast, because of its cardiovascular stability, ketamine can improve CPP by maintaining the patient's MAP at induction. In addition, in vitro and animal studies have indicated a possible neuroprotective effect of ketamine. Proposed mechanisms include a reduction in glutamate neurotoxicity resulting from the blockade of the N-methyl-D-aspartate receptor [23]. A multicentre randomized clinical trial comparing ketamine 2 mg/kg with etomidate 0.3 mg/kg for RSI in 655 acutely ill patients (of whom 104 were trauma patients) concluded that ketamine is a safe and valuable alternative to etomidate [17]. Ketamine plus midazolam sedation on intensive care was compared with sufentanil plus midazolam sedation in 25 patients with severe traumatic brain injury and did not demonstrate a significant difference in mean daily ICP or CPP values [24]. Although there have been no prospective randomized controlled trials to prove ketamine's safety in patients with traumatic brain injury, the evidence against ketamine use appears to be based on a small number of studies which do not involve emergency management of patients with traumatic brain injury. More research in this area is warranted but ketamine may be a reasonable induction agent for patients with traumatic brain injury, especially if haemodynamic instability from other injuries coexists.

❝ Expert comment

A common pitfall in the emergency department is not placing an orogastric or nasogastric tube immediately after tracheal intubation. The gastric tube has diagnostic roles (e.g. aspiration of gastric blood, displacement by a mediastinal haematoma) and therapeutic roles (e.g. decompression of stomach air/contents (particularly important in paediatric trauma), improving ventilation attempts, and reducing aspiration risk). If not inserted at the time of intubation an extra chest X-ray may be required to confirm correct positioning.

❝ Expert comment

Fracture reduction is an important part of haemorrhage control. In the initial stages of resuscitation this may simply involve manual reduction and realignment of limb fractures and the application of a pelvic binding device for a suspected open-ring pelvic fracture.

An orogastric tube was placed immediately following intubation, and a repeat chest radiograph was taken to confirm correct placement of both tracheal and orogastric tubes.

Sedation and analgesia were maintained with midazolam and morphine infusions, each at a rate of 0.1 mg/kg/h with boluses of atracurium for muscle relaxation. Multiple boluses of metaraminol (500 µg) were necessary after intubation to maintain MAP ≥70 mmHg. Reduction and realignment of the right leg was achieved by pulling out to length, then using bandages to immobilize to her left leg following insertion of a urinary catheter.

Her blood results demonstrated lactic acidaemia, mild anaemia, a raised white cell count, mild coagulopathy and abnormalities of renal and hepatic function: the latter raising concerns over possible liver injury.

Table 8.3 Glasgow Coma Scale

Component	Best response	Score
Eyes	Open spontaneously. Indicates arousal, not necessarily awareness	4
	Open to voice	3
	Open to pain applied to limbs	2
	None[a]	1
Verbal	Oriented in Person, Place and Time (year, season, month)	5
	Confused speech	4
	Inappropriate words	3
	Incomprehensible sounds	2
	None[b]	1
Motor Response to nailbed pressure	Obeys commands. Exclude grasp reflex or postural adjustments	6
	Localizes: purposeful movement towards stimulus (i.e. hand crosses mid-line to site of nailbed pressure or moves above clavicle to supraorbital pressure)	5
	Withdraws/normal flexion of elbow	4
	Abnormal flexion with pronation of wrist, adduction of shoulder (decorticate positioning)	3
	Extension of elbow with pronation and adduction (decerebrate positioning)	2
	No response	1

[a] Where the patient's eyes are closed by injury an Eye score of 1C is recorded.
[b] Where the patient is intubated a Verbal score of 1T is recorded.
Reprinted from *The Lancet*, 304, 7872, G Teasdale and B Jennett, 'Assessment of coma and impaired consciousness: a practical scale', pp. 81–84, Copyright 1972, with permission from Elsevier.

> ⭐ **Learning point** 'Acute traumatic coagulopathy'
>
> The causes of coagulopathy in severe trauma are multifactorial and haemostatic control can prove to be very challenging in these patients. Traditionally coagulopathy was thought to be secondary to loss of coagulation factors due to consumption and bleeding, dilution from fluid and blood administration and dysfunction of the clotting cascade due to hypothermia and acidosis [25]. More recently an acute coagulopathy, present at admission and prior to significant fluid resuscitation, has been described in up to one-quarter of trauma patients and is associated with a 3–4-fold increase in mortality [26]. There are five proposed mechanisms for this 'acute traumatic coagulopathy': shock, tissue trauma, haemodilution, hypothermia, and acidaemia. Endothelial injury initiates coagulation, but, combined with the systemic hypoperfusion seen in shock, appears to result in the haemostatic system becoming relatively anticoagulant and hyperfibrinolytic, which is further exacerbated by fluid administration, hypothermia and acidaemia. At present there is limited understanding of why tissue trauma in the presence of shock causes coagulopathy, but it is likely to be a complex multifactorial process involving the endothelium, platelets, coagulation proteases, the protein C pathway, and the antifibrinolytic system [27, 28]. Irrespective of the underlying mechanism, a presenting coagulopathy represents a subset of critically ill trauma patients with a higher mortality and therefore must be identified and managed rapidly.

01.10: Transfer to theatre

01.20–03.40: Emergency theatre–damage control surgery

After arriving in theatre and once the surgical team was prepared, the pelvic binder was removed. Midline laparotomy demonstrated ~ 1000 mL free blood in the abdominal cavity—profuse bleeding was seen from a liver laceration lateral to the falcifom ligament and this was packed. The mesentery and ascending colon appeared bruised and the spleen was intact. A nasojejunal tube to facilitate early enteral feeding was passed by the anaesthetist and confirmed in position by the surgeon. Temporary closure of her abdomen was carried out using a modified Bogota bag (silastic closure) approach.

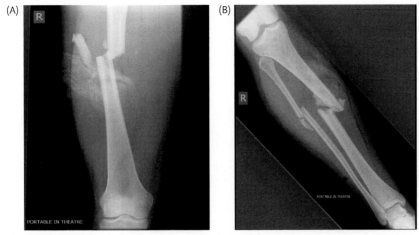

Figure 8.1 Right lower limb radiographs taken in theatre. (A) Comminuted right femoral fracture. (B) Comminuted right tibial and fibular fracture.

Damage control orthopaedic management, occurring immediately following laparotomy, involved a washout of all open fracture wounds and application of right calcaneal traction pins. Lower limb radiographs revealed open comminuted right femoral and tibial fractures with no fracture to the left lower limb (Figure 8.1).

In total the combined procedures lasted for 2 h. The patient was transfused a further six units of PRC, four units of FFP, two units of cryoprecipate, one unit of platelets and 500 mL of crystalloid solution. Standard antibiotic prophylaxis was administered prior to surgery starting. Early during the procedure a left radial arterial cannula and ultrasound-guided subclavian central line (avoiding removal of the collar) were inserted. To correct and prevent hypothermia a forced-air warming blanket and a plate fluid warmer were used, which achieved an oesophageal temperature of 35.6°C at the end of surgery. The patient was transferred for CT of her head, cervical spine, thorax, abdomen and pelvis before being transferred to the adult ICU (Figures 8.2–8.4).

Summarized CT report

- Brain: Traumatic subarachnoid haemorrhage and contusion seen in right frontal area. Signs of diffuse axonal injury with early brain swelling.
- Spine: No bony injuries detected in cervical, thoracic or lumbar spine.
- Chest: Small patchy foci of non-segmental consolidation and ground glass change in right upper and left lower lobe—likely represent contusions (Figure 8.2). No rib, sternal, or scapular fractures present or pneumothorax seen.
- Abdomen: Recent midline laparotomy with pneumoperitoneum. Haemostatic material noted beneath the midline wound and in the under-surface of the liver. Extensive liver laceration involving segments 4, 5, and 8—extending from liver surface to hilum with small subcapsular haematoma (Figure 8.3). Spleen, pancreas, adrenals and left kidney normal in appearance. Small contusion noted in the posterior cortex of the right kidney.
- Pelvis: Displaced, comminuted fracture right iliac blade (Figure 8.4).

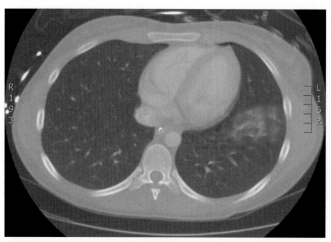

Figure 8.2 CT transverse image in thoracic region, demonstrating left lower lobe lung contusion.

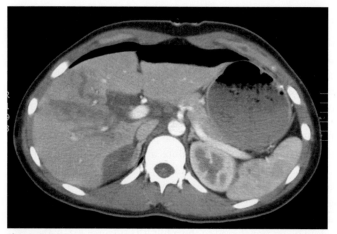

Figure 8.3 CT transverse image in upper abdominal region slice, demonstrating liver laceration and pneumoperitoneum.

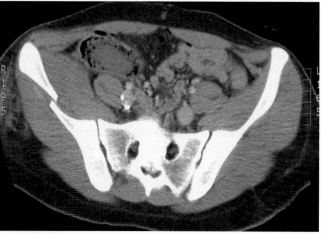

Figure 8.4 CT transverse image in pelvic region demonstrating fracture of the right iliac blade.

> **✪ Learning point**   Damage control surgery
>
> Traditional laparotomy for trauma follows the normal surgical sequence, i.e. access, exposure, haemostasis, resection, and reconstruction. Critically ill, multiply injured trauma patients are often at their physiological limit and would be unlikely to survive the combined pathophysiological insult of injury plus prolonged surgery. Therefore the concept of damage control is a planned, staged procedure—initial expeditious haemorrhage and contamination control, followed by a period of resuscitation and warming in intensive care, followed by a planned return to theatre for definitive repair [29].
>
> Indications for the damage control approach include evidence of hypovolaemic shock and:
>
> * hypothermia, acidosis, pre-existing/developing coagulopathy
> * suboptimal response to resuscitation
> * inaccessible intra-abdominal venous injury (e.g. retrohepatic) or need for radiological embolization
> * inability to perform definitive repair (physiological, manpower, equipment etc.)
> * need for time-consuming procedure
> * need to reassess intra-abdominal contents [30]

04.00: Admission to adult intensive care unit (ICU)

As the CT of the spine had cleared the cervical spine the spinal immobilization was relaxed.

> **✪ Learning point**   Clearing the cervical spine in the obtunded patient
>
> There is widespread acceptance of the EAST clinical criteria to exclude cervical spine injury in alert trauma patients without neurological deficit or distracting injury who have no neck pain or tenderness with full range cervical spine movement [31]. However, clearing the cervical spine in obtunded patients presents a significant challenge where the potential for causing considerable morbidity by missing an unstable cervical spine injury must be balanced with the complications associated with prolonged spinal immobilization. The latter includes increased ICP and risk of venous thromboembolism, difficult central venous access and airway management, increased risk of ventilator-associated pneumonia, pressure necrosis, and significantly increased staffing requirements to logroll the patient.
>
> Outdated imaging modalities include plain radiographs and dynamic fluoroscopy, and most centres either use CT or MRI. There are significant logistical and safety issues surrounding transporting unstable trauma patients for MRI in the acute setting. Advances in technology have allowed helical CT of 1 mm slices, improving detection of injuries. One retrospective review of 1,400 trauma patients demonstrated that multi-detector row CT reporting no acute bony injury and anatomic alignment had a negative predictive value of 100% for unstable cervical spine injury and 98.9% for ligament injury when compared with subsequent MRI [32]. Currently in the UK there is a lack of national guidelines and a wide variance in clinical practice [33]. All centres that receive trauma patients must therefore agree a local protocol between radiology, emergency medicine, anaesthetic, and intensive care departments. The best available evidence indicates that helical CT of the entire cervical spine with 1 mm cuts and three-dimensional reconstructions should be obtained in all obtunded trauma patients and reported by an experienced clinician (likely consultant radiologist) before spinal precautions are relaxed [34].

CT of the brain had demonstrated signs of diffuse axonal injury with early brain swelling alongside a traumatic subarachnoid haemorrhage and small frontal haematoma. An ICP monitor was inserted by the neurosurgical team and showed pressures of 14–20 mmHg. A noradrenaline infusion was commenced to maintain CPP > 60 mmHg. Her ICP was measured for a total of 4 days while she remained sedated and ventilated on ICU and remained within acceptable levels.

> **☒ Learning point** Cerebral perfusion pressure
>
> Cerebral perfusion pressure (CPP) is defined as the difference between the MAP and ICP and represents the pressure gradient driving cerebral blood flow and hence oxygen and substrate delivery to the brain.
>
> $$CPP = MAP - ICP$$
>
> In health, the brain has the capacity to autoregulate cerebral blood flow, but in certain circumstances, including following traumatic brain injury, this autoregulation may be lost and the flow varies directly with the perfusion pressure.
>
> After any primary brain injury, maintaining the CPP is the cornerstone of management—to avoid a secondary ischaemic insult to the damaged brain. Previously CPP >70 mmHg was targeted, but studies have shown an increased risk of adult respiratory distress syndrome with this goal [35], and, although optimal CPP values are still disputed, guidelines currently recommend aiming for 50–70 mmHg [36].

☒ Expert comment

Failure to correct metabolic acidosis and clear lactate are signs of ongoing blood loss or ischaemia that, if not addressed, will lead to multiple organ failure and death. Therefore the rapid improvement of acidosis and clearing of lactate are very important goals in the hours following ICU admission. Failure to improve acidosis and clear lactate must prompt repeated clinical evaluation and assessment of whether hypovolaemia has been adequately corrected and whether haemorrhage control has been achieved.

Blood tests on admission to the ICU demonstrated persistent coagulopathy and metabolic acidaemia. Continued resuscitation included transfusing a further three units of PRC, four units of FFP, and ongoing non-invasive warming. By 0900 her coagulation tests were within normal limits, her lactate had fallen to 2.6 mmol/L, base excess had improved to –4.3 mmol/L and her tympanic temperature was 36.7°C.

Progress

Later that day she returned to theatre for a planned relook laparotomy. Abdominal packs were removed and serosal tears to the ascending and transverse colon were repaired prior to primary closure of the abdominal wall. She was then transferred to the orthopaedic theatre and underwent external fixation of her left femur and tibia. She was transfused a further two units of PRC prior to being transferred back to ICU. Antibiotics were continued for 48 h in line with the hospital protocol for open fracture management.

Venous thromboembolic prophylaxis consisted of a calf compression device on her left leg, followed by low-molecular-weight heparin (enoxaparin) subcutaneously once a day at a dose of 40 mg started on day 3, as agreed by the neurosurgical team. This was withheld the evening that her ICP bolt was removed. She received an insulin sliding scale, as per the unit's protocol, to maintain blood glucose 4–10 mmol/L and was ventilated using a lung-protective strategy, with tidal volumes of 6–8 mL/kg, plateau pressures limited to < 30 cmH$_2$O and the minimal necessary inspired fractional oxygen concentration to maintain PaO$_2$ ≥10 kPa.

On day 4 the patient returned to orthopaedic theatre for distal femoral nailing of her right femur and intramedullary nailing of her right tibia. Plastic surgeons covered the defect in her right leg with a gastrocnemius muscle flap and split skin graft.

The following day her ICP monitor was removed and the noradrenaline infusion was weaned and discontinued. She initially had signs of a postoperative ileus with high nasogastric aspirates, but nasojejunal feeding was well tolerated. On day 7 she was successfully extubated and stepped down to level 2 care. By day 12 she was tolerating oral diet and fluids; the nasojejunal tube was removed and the patient was transferred to ward care.

She developed an infection in her right tibial nail which necessitated a return to theatre on day 18 to remove the nail, and place an external fixator device. Consequences of her traumatic brain injury included mild personality change and moderate memory difficulties. She was eventually discharged home on day 34 with a care package in place to await further definitive surgery on her right tibia.

Discussion

In high-income countries, trauma from road traffic collisions is the leading cause of death in all patients aged 5–29 years and is superseded only by HIV/AIDS in middle and low-income countries [37]. Anaesthetists are likely to be involved in many steps along a patient's trauma pathway—including prehospital care, initial airway and circulatory management as part of the trauma team, perioperative care for primary and any subsequent surgery and intensive care management of the polytrauma patient. This case highlights the complexity of trauma management—from initial assessment and decision for emergency laparotomy, difficulties with intravenous access in the shocked patient, ongoing resuscitation and massive transfusion in a patient with an initial coagulopathy and optimal staging of surgery.

The decision for emergency laparotomy in this patient was easy—she had obvious haemodynamic instability and signs pointing towards an intra-abdominal source. The FAST scan demonstrating free fluid supported the decision to transfer immediately to the operating theatre prior to full radiological investigation. Her initial management was made more challenging by the difficulty in securing intravenous access, a relatively frequent problem in multiply injured, shocked patients. The intraosseus route should always be considered as a viable alternative in patients of all ages and is likely to be faster than central venous cannulation.

'Damage control surgery' was a phrase coined by Rotondo *et al.* in 1993 to describe an initial trauma laparotomy for: 'control of hemorrhage and contamination followed by intraperitoneal packing and rapid closure, [which] allows for resuscitation to normal physiology in the ICU and subsequent definitive re-exploration'. They published data on 22 patients with major vascular injury and two or more visceral injuries from penetrating abdominal trauma, demonstrating a survival rate of 77% in patients undergoing damage control surgery versus 11% in those undergoing definitive laparotomy [38]. The principle is much older; as early as 1908 Pringle had advised compression and hepatic packing for portal venous haemorrhage, but this largely fell out of favour by World War II with reports of necrosis, sepsis, and haemorrhage. It was not until the number of penetrating abdominal wounds in gunshot victims in the USA escalated during the 1980s and 1990s that the technique was reconsidered. In 1983 Stone *et al.* described improvements in mortality by termination of laparotomy as rapidly as possible in patients who developed coagulopathy intraoperatively [39].

The damage control approach is now widely accepted as best practice for trauma patients close to the limits of their physiological reserve in order to combat the lethal triad of metabolic acidosis, coagulopathy, and hypothermia—the so-called 'bloody vicious cycle'. The technique of a staged approach is applicable to a variety of surgical disciplines in seriously ill patients. The first stage consists of control of haemorrhage and contamination, using the simplest and quickest means available. Temporary wound closure methods are used prior to transferring the patient to the ICU for ongoing resuscitation and warming, aiming for as near normal physiological variables as possible (specific attention to correction of lactate levels, acid–base balance, coagulation and temperature). The final stage is definitive operative management at a later date [29, 40, 41].

Damage control orthopaedics was developed in the 1990s and recognizes the fact that, as in abdominal injuries, patients undergoing prolonged operations on extremity injuries suffer an excess of complications. Long-bone fractures always have local soft tissue injury and associated haemorrhage—inflammation from the site of trauma can cause the systemic inflammatory response syndrome which may lead to multiple organ dysfunction syndrome and death. Conversely, earlier fracture management allows for better pain control and earlier mobilization. Timing of surgery is therefore crucial—the damage control approach in orthopaedics generally involves rapid external fixation of fractures early in management, followed by definitive treatment several days later, ideally after the initial pro-inflammatory response has settled [42].

Until recently, fluid resuscitation in trauma consisted of warmed crystalloid solutions, followed by PRC, with FFP and platelets started when sufficient PRC had been transfused to be considered to have caused a dilutional coagulopathy (often after 6–10 units PRC). As discussed earlier, a significant proportion of trauma patients present with a coagulopathy and these patients have a higher mortality [26]. It would therefore seem prudent to treat this coagulopathy expediently. 'Massive transfusion' does not have a standard definition, but the majority of papers refer to the transfusion of > 10 units PRC within 24 h which would therefore include the patient in this case study who received 11 units PRC in this time.

Transfusion practice has been modified in response to recent military experience of haemorrhagic shock and massive transfusion. In 2007 Borgman *et al.* published a retrospective review of 252 military combat casualties, suggesting a significant mortality benefit of using a PRC:FFP ratio of about 1:1 [43]. In the same year Holcomb *et al.* defined 'damage control resuscitation'—so-called to link resuscitation to damage control surgical techniques. Damage control resuscitation targets the 'bloody vicious cycle' of hypothermia, acidosis and coagulopathy from the moment the casualty arrives and has several components:

1. Resuscitation limited to target systolic blood pressure of 90 mmHg (permissive hypotension).
2. Early and increased use of FFP, platelets and PRC—aiming for a ratio of 1:1:1.
3. Use of fresh whole blood where available.
4. Minimizing the use of crystalloid infusions.
5. Immediate measures to combat hypothermia and acidosis.
6. Consideration of adjuncts such as tranexamic acid and recombinant activated Factor VII.
7. Early definitive haemorrhage control [44, 45].

It is debated whether data from the military can be directly applied to civilian trauma. Far fewer civilian trauma patients require massive transfusion and the pattern of injury is different, with a much greater percentage of civilian blunt trauma. Permissive hypotension is designed to allow clots to stabilize and prevent rupture of the haemostatic plug when the patient is resuscitated to normotension. However, mortality benefit has only been demonstrated in a single civilian centre prospective trial in adults with penetrating torso injuries leading to haemorrhagic shock [46]. Hypotension is associated with significant increases in morbidity and mortality in patients with severe traumatic brain injury and the role of permissive hypotension in these patients is unclear [47]. Permissive hypotension may not be appropriate in older patients, patients with ischaemic heart disease, renal insufficiency, previous cerebral vascular disease or those with established hypertension, all of which are rarely encountered among military trauma casualties—the vast majority of whom are young, fit men.

Recently several retrospective reviews undertaken in civilian trauma centres have been published; some but not all have demonstrated a reduction in mortality in severely injured patients when a higher ratio of FFP and platelets are transfused [48, 49]. However, transfusion of any blood products is not without risk: the greater the number transfused the greater the risks, which include transfusion reactions, allergic reactions, transfusion-related acute lung injury (TRALI), transmission of blood-borne viruses, and circulatory overload. At present the best ratios or combinations of blood products are unclear, although a higher ratio of clotting products to PRC appears to confer a mortality benefit in the majority of studies. This mortality benefit is only seen in the most severely injured patients. Many trauma centres, including the one in this case study, have introduced massive transfusion protocols which ensure easier access to clotting products and platelets. In total the patient described received 11 units of PRC, 8 units of FFP, one adult dose of pooled platelets, and 1 unit of cryoprecipitate.

Two adjunct medications are currently used to treat bleeding in trauma: recombinant activated Factor VII and tranexamic acid. Recombinant human coagulation Factor VIIa (rFVIIa) was introduced into clinical practice in 1988 but is only licensed for the treatment of severe bleeding episodes in patients with haemophilia A and B who develop high inhibitory antibody titres to Factors XIII and IX. Factor VIIa in combination with tissue factor, expressed on injured or ischaemic vascular subendothelium, is needed to initiate the coagulation pathway. In supranormal quantities VIIa can bind to activated platelets at the site of injury and directly activate clotting Factors IX and X, causing a thrombin burst [50, 51]. Two large multicentre clinical trials on the use of rFVIIa in traumatic haemorrhage including a total of 226 patients with penetrating trauma and 624 patients with blunt trauma demonstrated a statistically significant reduction in blood product transfusion in patients treated with rFVIIa but did not demonstrate a mortality benefit [51, 52]. Concerns have been raised that the procoagulant effect of rFVIIa could cause an increase in thromboembolic events. No differences in numbers of thromboembolic events were seen in these clinical trials, but other authors reviewing the rate of thromboembolic events in all published randomized, placebo-controlled trials of rFVIIa used on an off-label basis (4468 subjects in total) demonstrated a significantly higher rate of arterial thromboembolic events, particularly in elderly patients [53]. Lack of mortality benefit, concerns of increased thromboembolic events, high cost and lack of approved indication in trauma provide little support for rFVIIa use.

Tranexamic acid is an antifibrinolytic that prevents clot breakdown by inhibiting both plasminogen activation and plasmin activity. It was originally used to prevent bleeding in haemophilia patients undergoing dental extractions and dysfunctional uterine bleeding, but its role has been expanded to include routine use in certain elective surgical procedures including cardiac, spinal and liver transplantation surgery, where it has been shown to reduce bleeding [54]. It is inexpensive, easy to administer and appears to have a favourable side-effect profile. In 2010 the CRASH2 (Clinical Randomisation of an Antifibrinolytic in Significant Haemorrhage) trial was published—which randomized more than 20,000 trauma patients with, or at risk of, significant bleeding from 274 hospitals in 40 countries to placebo or 1 g tranexamic acid as a loading dose for a period of 10 min followed by 1 g infusion for a period of 8 h. Primary outcome was death in hospital within 4 weeks of injury and secondary outcomes were vascular occlusive events, surgical intervention and number of units of blood transfused. All-cause mortality was significantly reduced with no apparent increase in fatal or non-fatal vascular occlusive events [54]. Of interest, there was no significant difference in the amount of blood transfused, possibly implying an alternative mechanism for mortality reduction rather than reducing bleeding *per se*. A *post hoc* analysis of data demonstrated that reduction in mortality due to bleeding was highest when tranexamic acid was administered within 1 h of injury (relative risk: 0.68) and although mortality was reduced, to a lesser extent, if administered between 1 and 3 h after injury; an increase in mortality was seen with administration more than 3 h after injury [55]. The trial data have also been used to demonstrate the cost-effectiveness of early administration of tranexamic acid to bleeding trauma patients in high-, middle- and low-income countries [56]. As a result of this work, where available, tranexamic acid is routinely given early to trauma patients worldwide, and its administration by prehospital care personnel is being considered.

A more important question to be answered by future research will be how to immediately identify the severely injured civilian patient who should be treated with a damage control approach—both resuscitation and surgery. There is an urgent need to develop internationally agreed clinical guidelines for this and other aspects of trauma management. A recent study examining differences in mortality among trauma patients across 11 different countries identified that adherence to clinical guidelines for red cell transfusion, damage control surgery, and ventilatory strategies was associated with better survival following case-mix and case-management adjustment. The guideline stated that operative or radiological management for bleeding injuries should begin within 2 h of arrival to hospital and that a 'damage control' approach is initiated when the following are present:

- temperature $< 35°C$
- lactate > 4 mmol/L (or more than twice local upper limit of normal)
- corrected pH < 7.3

The guideline also emphasizes the importance of attempted temperature regulation using active warming devices to maintain core temperature $\geq 35°C$ [57]. PROMMTT (PRospective, Observational, Multi-center Massive Transfusion sTudy) of severely injured trauma patients hopes to answer this question and to determine which massive transfusion protocol is associated with better survival. Results are keenly awaited.

A Final Word from the Expert

Optimal outcomes from major trauma require a system-wide approach that begins prehospital and continues all the way through to rehabilitation. Multidisciplinary communication and teamwork are at the centre of an effective trauma system. Critical care management that is systematic and comprehensive, which aims to achieve early definitive care and minimize complications will provide the best outcomes. Whereas level 1 evidence for a lot of trauma management is lacking, current evidence supports damage control strategies (including a transfusion protocol), the use of tranexamic acid in selected patients, early feeding and glucose control, appropriate analgesia and sedation that facilitates timely weaning from ventilation, prophylaxis to reduce the risk of venous thromboembolism, meticulous infection control and antibiotic management to reduce infective complications, a restrictive approach to blood product usage after resuscitation has been achieved, and a tertiary survey to identify any missed injuries within 24 h of admission.

References

1. Commmittee on Trauma, American College of Surgeons. *Advanced trauma life support for doctors: student course manual.* 7th ed. (student edition). Chicago: ACS; 2004.
2. Day MW. Intraosseous devices for intravascular access in adult trauma patients. *Crit Care Nurse* 2011;31:76–90.
3. Goerig M, Agarwal-Koslowski K. The bone marrow as a site for the reception of infusions, transfusions and anaesthetic agents. In: Diz JC, Franco A, Bacon DR, Rupreht J, Alvarez J editors. *The history of anesthesia: proceedings of the Fifth International Symposium, Amsterdam, The Netherlands.* Amsterdam: Elsevier; 2002. p. 105–12.
4. ECC Committee, subcommittees and task forces of the American Heart Association. 2005 American Heart Association guidelines for cardiopulmonary resuscitation and emergency cardiac care, 7.2: Management of cardiac arrest. *Circulation* 2005;112:IV-58–IV-66.
5. Teasdale G, Jennett B. Assessment of coma and impaired consciousness: a practical scale. *Lancet* 1974;2:81–4.
6. Jennett B, Teasdale G, Galbraith S, *et al.* Severe head injuries in three countries. *J Neurol Neurosurg Psychiat* 1977;40:291–8.
7. Jennett B. Development of Glasgow Coma and Outcome scales. *Nepal J Neurosci* 2005;2:24–8.
8. Lee BC, Ormsby EL, McGahan JP, *et al.* The utility of sonography for the triage of blunt abdominal trauma patients to exploratory laparotomy. *Am J Roentgenol* 2007;188:415–21.
9. Rose JS. Ultrasound in abdominal trauma. *Emerg Med Clin N Am* 2004;22:581–9.
10. Gillies R. Ultrasound in perioperative and critical care clinical practice. In: Royse C, Doonan G, Royse A editors. *Pocket guide to perioperative and critical care echocardiography.* Sydney: McGraw-Hill; 2006. p. 6.
11. Yentis SM, Lee DJH. Evaluation of an improved scoring system for the grading of direct laryngoscopy. *Anaesthesia* 1998;53:1041–4.
12. Warltier DC. Airway management in adults after cervical spine trauma. *Anesthesiology* 2006;104:1293–1318.
13. Nolan JP, Wilson ME. Orotracheal intubation in patients with potential cervical spine injuries. *Anesthesia* 1993;48:630–3.
14. Cook TM, Woodall N, Harper J, Benger J. Major complications of airway management in the UK: results of the Fourth National Audit Project of the Royal College of Anaesthetists and the Difficult Airway Society. Part 2: intensive care and emergency departments. *Br J Anaesth* 2011;106:632–42.
15. Laurent SC, de Melo AE, Alexander-Williams JM. The use of the McCoy laryngoscope in patients with simulated cervical spine injuries. *Anaesthesia* 1996;51:74–5.
16. Robitaille A, Williams SR, Tremblay MH, Guilbert F, Thériault M, Drolet P. Cervical spine motion during tracheal intubation with manual in-line stabilization: direct laryngoscopy versus GlideScope® videolaryngoscopy. *Anest Analg* 2008;106:935–41.
17. Jabre P, Combres X, Lapostolie F, *et al.* Etomidate versus ketamine for rapid sequence intubation in acutely ill patients: a multicentre randomised controlled trial. *Lancet* 2009;374:293–300.
18. Green SM, Krauss B. The semantics of ketamine. *Ann Emerg Med* 2000;30:480–2.
19. Morris C, Perris A, Klein J, Mahoney P. Anaesthesia in haemodynamically compromised emergency patients: does ketamine represent the best choice of induction agent? *Anaesthesia* 2009;64:532–9.
20. Sehdev RS, Symmons DA, Kindl K. Ketamine for rapid sequence induction in patients with head injury in the emergency department. *Emerg Med Australas* 2006;18:37–44.
21. Gardner AE, Dannemiller FJ, Dean D. Intracranial cerebrospinal fluid pressure in man during ketamine anesthesia. *Anesth Analg* 1972;51:741–5.
22. Shapiro HM, Wyte SR, Harris AB. Ketamine anaesthesia in patients with intracranial pathology. *Br J Anaesth* 1972;44:1200–4.

23. Himmelseher S, Durieux ME. Revising a dogma: ketamine for patients with neurological injury? *Anesth Analg* 2005;101:524–34.
24. Bourgoin A, Albanese J, Wereszcczynski N, *et al*. Safely of sedation with ketamine in severe head injury patients: comparison with sufentanil. *Crit Care Med* 2003;31:711–17.
25. Schreiber MA. Coagulopathy in the trauma patient. *Curr Opin Crit Care* 2005;11:590–7.
26. Macleod JB, Lynn M, McKenney MG, Cohn SM, Murtha M. Early coagulopathy predicts mortality in trauma. *J Trauma* 2003;55:39–44.
27. Hess JR, Brohi K, Dutton R, *et al*. The coagulopathy of trauma. A review of mechanisms. *J Trauma* 2008;65:748–54.
28. Brohi K, Cohen MJ, Davenport RA. Acute coagulopathy of trauma: mechanism, identification and effect. *Curr Opin Crit Care* 2007;13:680–5.
29. Hoey BA, Schwab CW. Damage control surgery. *Scand J Surg* 2002;91:92–103.
30. Moore EE, Burch JM, Franciose RJ, Offner PJ, Biffl WL. Staged physiologic restoration and damage control surgery. *World J Surg* 1998;22:1184–91.
31. Como JJ, Diaz JJ, Dunham CM, *et al*. Practice management guidelines for identification of cervical spine injuries following trauma: update from the Eastern Association for the surgery of trauma practice management guidelines committee. *J Trauma* 2009;67:651–9.
32. Hogan GJ, Mirvis SE, Shanmuganathan K, Scalea TM. Exclusion of unstable cervical spine injury in obtunded patients with blunt trauma: is MR imaging needed when multi-detector row CT findings are normal? *Radiology* 2005;237:106–13.
33. Jones PS, Wadley J, Healy M. Clearing the cervical spine in unconscious adult trauma patients: a survey of practice in specialist centres in the UK. *Anaesthesia* 2004;59:1095–9.
34. Harrison P, Cairns C. Clearing the cervical spine in the unconscious patient. *Cont Edu Anaesth Crit Care Pain* 2008;8:117–20.
35. Robertson CS, Valadka AB, Hannay HJ, *et al*. Prevention of secondary ischemic insults after severe head injury. *Crit Care Med* 1999;27:2086–95.
36. Bratton SL, Chestnut RM, Ghajar J, *et al*. Brain Trauma Foundation; American Association of Neurological Surgeons; Congress of Neurological surgeons; Joint Section on Neurotrauma and Critical Care, AANS/CNS: Guidelines for the management of severe traumatic brain injury. *J Neurotrauma* 2007;24:S-59–64.
37. World Health Organization. *Injury: a leading cause of the global burden of disease*. Geneva: WHO; 2000. < http://whqlibdoc.who.int/publications/2002/9241562323.pdf >
38. Rotondo MF, Schwab CW, McGonigal MD, *et al*. 'Damage control': an approach for improved survival in exsanguinating penetrating abdominal injury. *J Trauma* 1993;35:375–82.
39. Stone HH, Strom AR, Mullins RJ. Management of the major coagulopathy with onset during laparotomy. *Ann Surg* 1983;197:532–5.
40. Sargraves SC, Toschlog EA, Rotondo MF. Damage control surgery—the intensivist's role. *J Intensive Care Med* 2006;21;5–16.
41. Schreiber MA. Damage control surgery. *Crit Care Clin* 2004;20:101–18.
42. Hilldebrand F, Giannoudis P, Krettek C, Pape HC. Damage control: extremities. *Injury* 2004;35:678–89.
43. Borgman MA, Spinella PC, Grathwohl KW, *et al*. The ratio of blood products transfused affects mortality in patients receiving massive transfusions at a combat support hospital. *J Trauma* 2007;63:805–13.
44. Holcomb JB, Jenkins D, Rhee P, *et al*. Damage control resuscitation: directly addressing the early coagulopathy of trauma. *J Trauma* 2007;62:307–10.
45. Holcomb JB. Optimal use of blood products in severely injured trauma patients. *Hematology* 2010;1:465–9.
46. Bickell WH, Wall MJ Jr, Pepe PE, *et al*. Immediate versus delayed fluid resuscitation for hypotensive patients with penetrating torso injuries. *N Engl J Med* 1994;331:1105–9.
47. Chesnut RM, Marshall LF, Klauber MR, *et al*. The role of secondary brain injury in determining outcome from severe head injury. *J Trauma* 1993;34:216–22.

48. Dente CJ, Shaz B Nicholas JM, *et al.* Improvements in early mortality and coagulopathy are sustained better in patients with blunt trauma after institution of a massive transfusion protocol in a civilian level I trauma center. *J Trauma* 2009;66:1616–24.

49. Kashuk JL, Moore EE, Johnson JL, *et al.* Post injury life-threatening coagulopathy: is 1:1 fresh frozen plasma:packed red blood cells the answer? *J Trauma* 2008;65:261–71.

50. Vincent JL, Rossaint R, Riou B, Ozier Y, Zideman D, Spahn DR. Recommendations on the use of recombinant activated factor VII as an adjunctive treatment for massive bleeding—a European perspective. *Crit Care* 2006;10:R120.

51. Hauser CJ, Boffard K, Dutton R, *et al.* Results of the CONTROL Trial: efficacy and safety of recombinant activated Factor VII in the management of refractory traumatic hemorrhage. *J Trauma* 2010;69:489–500.

52. Boffard KD, Riou B, Warren B, *et al.* Recombinant factor VIIa as adjunctive therapy for bleeding control in severely injured trauma patients; two parallel randomized, placebo-controlled, double-blind clinical trials. *J Trauma* 2005;59:8–15.

53. Levi M, Levy JH, Andersen HF, Truloff D. Safety of recombinant activated factor VII in randomized clinical trials. *N Engl J Med* 2010;363:1791–1800.

54. CRASH-2 trial collaborators. Effects of tranexamic acid on death, vascular occlusive events and blood transfusion in trauma patients with significant haemorrhage (CRASH-2): a randomised placebo-controlled trial. *Lancet* 2010;376:23–32.

55. CRASH-2 trial collaborators. The importance of early treatment with tranexamic acid in bleeding trauma patients: an exploratory analysis of the CRASH-2 randomised controlled trial. *Lancet* 2011;377(9771):1096–101, 1101.e1–2.

56. Guerriero C, Carins J, Perel P, Shakur H, Roberts I, on behalf of CRASH-2 trial collaborators. Cost-effectiveness analysis of administering tranexamic acid to bleeding trauma patients using evidence from the CRASH-2 trial. *PLoS ONE* 2011;6(5):e18987.

57. Christensen M, Parr M, Tortella B, *et al.* Global differences in causes, management and survival after severe trauma: the recombinant activated Factor VII Phase 3 Trauma Trial. *J Trauma* 2010;69:344–52.

CHAPTER 9

Cardiac disease and anaesthesia

Coronary stents and anaesthesia

Michael DeVile

Expert Commentary Pierre Foex

CPD Matrix Code: *1A02, 2A03, 2A06*

Case history

A 58-year-old woman was scheduled for elective abdominoperineal resection for a low obstructing rectal carcinoma recently diagnosed on endoscopy. Five months before this, following symptoms of crescendo angina, she had undergone percutaneous coronary intervention (PCI) comprising the insertion of two drug-eluting stents (DES) into the left anterior descending artery (LAD) and one in the left circumflex artery (LCx). Her past medical history included a 30-pack-year smoking history but good baseline pulmonary function, hypertension, type 2 diabetes and ischaemic heart disease. Medication included ramipril, amlodipine, bendroflumethiazide, gliclazide, simvastatin, aspirin, and more recently clopidogrel—commenced following PCI. Post-procedural angiography gave a thrombolysis in myocardial infarction (TIMI) flow grade of 2 (partial reperfusion) down the LAD, and because there was also a small degree of overlap with the two stents within this vessel, she had been advised to take clopidogrel for 18 months. Ventriculography during PCI revealed preserved left ventricular (LV) systolic function.

> ✪ **Learning point** Thrombolysis in myocardial infarction (TIMI) grading of coronary blood flow during PCI
>
> TIMI is the name of an Academic Research Organization based in Boston, Massachusetts. The group has conducted numerous practice-changing clinical trials in patients with, or at risk for, cardiovascular disease.
>
> They developed a grading scale for coronary blood flow during angiography, based on the visual assessment of flow of contrast through a stenosed vessel. This was originally assessed after thrombolysis following acute myocardial infarction. TIMI flow grading has since become the standard for semiquantitative evaluation of myocardial perfusion before and after coronary intervention, and gives important prognostic information in patients with acute coronary syndromes (ACS). The grades are as follows:
>
> - TIMI 0 flow (no perfusion) refers to the absence of any antegrade flow beyond a coronary occlusion.
> - TIMI 1 flow (penetration without perfusion) is faint antegrade coronary flow beyond the occlusion, with incomplete filling of the distal coronary bed.
> - TIMI 2 flow (partial reperfusion) is delayed or sluggish antegrade flow with complete filling of the distal territory.
> - TIMI 3 flow (complete perfusion) is normal flow which fills the distal coronary bed completely.
>
> Reproduced from JH Chesbro et al., 'Thrombolysis in Myocardial Infarction (TIMI) Trial, Phase I: A comparison between intravenous tissue plasminogen activator and intravenous streptokinase. Clinical findings through hospital discharge', *Circulation*, 76, 1, pp. 142–154, copyright 1987, with permission from the American Heart Association.

> ❝ **Expert comment**
>
> This patient was intolerant to beta-blockers—hence she was not treated with such an agent. Patients with coronary artery disease benefit from beta-blockade. If they are not treated and are not known to be intolerant it would be legitimate to start beta-blockers preoperatively but preferably a week before surgery and with a relatively low dose. In patients treated with beta-blockers it is important to maintain their treatment throughout the perioperative period, as withdrawal of beta-blockers is associated with a significant increase in the risk of adverse cardiac events [1].

> ❝ **Expert comment**
>
> There is growing evidence that statins offer perioperative cardiac protection [2]. This patient was already treated with statins. In this situation it is important to maintain this medication perioperatively as withdrawal increases the risk of adverse cardiac events. It is probably advisable to use a long-acting statin, such as fluvastatin, during the perioperative period. The preoperative initiation of statin therapy may be justified in patients with atheromatous disease who should be on such treatment irrespective of impending surgery. Starting treatment at least a week before surgery would be advisable.

> ✪ **Learning point**   Coronary stents
>
> There are two types of coronary stent: bare metal stents (BMS) and drug-eluting stents (DES) (Figure 9.1). DES were designed to reduce the incidence of stent re-stenosis, an inflammatory proliferation of cells migrating from the vessel media causing occlusion of the vascular lumen and recurrence of symptoms. DES minimize this by slowly releasing an antimitotic drug, such as sirolimus or paclitaxel, everolimus, or zotarolimus.

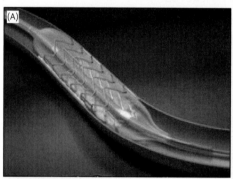 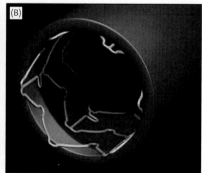

Figure 9.1 Schematic images depicting coronary stents within the arterial lumen. (A) Deployment is via a delivery catheter that has radio-opaque location markers flanking the surrounding stent to correctly traverse a target lesion. The angioplasty balloon is intermittently inflated to 8–12 atmospheres (800–1200 kPa) for 30–120 s at a time. This stretches the vessel to relieve the stenosis, and is repeated until satisfactory flow to the myocardium is restored. (B) The stent remains in the artery to maintain its patency and prevent re-stenosis, but temporarily exposes their struts to coronary blood flow until the endothelium can re-grow. The rate of re-endothelialization depends on the type of stent deployed. Reproduced with kind permission from Abbott Laboratories, Vascular Division Ltd.

⑥ Expert comment

Whereas the usual duration of DAPT after insertion of DES is 12 months, it is recognized that a longer duration may be advisable; as in this patient because of overlapping stents. Stent thrombosis has been reported beyond 1 year of insertion especially where stents have been used off-label [3, 4].

⑥ Expert comment

The introduction of stents using different antiproliferative agents, for example everolimus or zotarolimus, may shorten the need for DAPT to 6 months, as recent evidence shows that this approach does not increase the risk of stent thrombosis in daily life [5]. Lifelong aspirin would remain essential. With such stents, this patient would have been very close to the period beyond which DAPT is no longer necessary.

> ✪ **Learning point**   The need for dual antiplatelet therapy
>
> Deployment of a coronary stent using an intravascular balloon causes vessel trauma and damages the endothelium. Metal stent struts are exposed to passing coronary blood (Figure 9.1B), increasing the risk of early stent thrombosis until the endothelium can grow over the stent. Dual antiplatelet therapy (DAPT: aspirin and clopidogrel) is required for a minimum of 6 weeks after BMS insertion to allow endothelialization, followed by lifelong aspirin thereafter. However, the antiproliferative properties of DES delay growth of the endothelium, requiring patients with this type of stent to take DAPT for at least 12 months, and sometimes longer for complicated lesions, before reverting to lifelong aspirin.

Preoperative management involved discussion between the surgeon, anaesthetist, cardiologist and patient regarding her antiplatelet therapy. Given the potential for bleeding, it was decided to stop clopidogrel 5 days before surgery, admit her to hospital 2 days preoperatively, and initiate a twice daily dose of low-molecular-weight heparin (LMWH) recommended for the treatment of ACS as thrombosis prophylaxis for stent thrombosis. The morning dose of heparin was omitted on the day of surgery; aspirin was continued throughout. Given that clopidogrel would be restarted as soon as possible after the operation, an active decision was made not to perform any regional anaesthesia.

> ✪ **Learning point** Risks of undergoing non-cardiac surgery after stent insertion
>
> Non-cardiac surgery and most invasive procedures increase the risk of stent thrombosis, especially when the procedure is performed before endothelial re-growth (after 6 weeks with BMS, 12 months with DES), where the risk of thrombosis is at its highest. This may occur because the antiplatelet therapy is stopped preoperatively, and because the surgical stress response creates a prothrombotic state: as a result most cases of stent thrombosis occur in the immediate or early postoperative period.
>
> In daily life, stent thrombosis is often associated with a large myocardial infarction or death. If patients continue to take DAPT, it has an incidence of 1–2% in the first year. However, stopping both aspirin and clopidogrel during this 'high-risk' period increases the relative risk of developing thrombosis by at least 30-fold; with even greater risk if stopped during the first 3 months following insertion [6, 7].

❝ **Expert comment**

This patient was to undergo cancer surgery. This makes management decisions very difficult because the risk of stent thrombosis is increased in cancer patients [8] and in patients undergoing abdominal surgery [9], as was the case for this patient. However, as cancer surgery can be associated with significant bleeding, there is reluctance on the part of surgeons to maintain DAPT. Interruption of DAPT puts these patients at considerable risk of stent thrombosis.

The operation proceeded as planned over a period of 4 h, with stable haemodynamics throughout surgery. Invasive blood pressure monitoring and large-bore peripheral and central venous access were used. Central venous pressure and oesophageal Doppler monitoring were used to guide perioperative fluid management. Small boluses of metaraminol were required every 10–15 min to maintain a target MAP of 75 mmHg. She received 2.5 L of crystalloid and 500 mL of colloid, with an estimated blood loss of 400 mL (based on weighed swabs and measured suction volume). Her haemoglobin fell from a baseline of 13.2–10.7 g/dL. Adequate urine output was maintained throughout surgery. Perioperative three-lead ECG monitoring was employed using the CM5 (Central Manubrium 5) configuration, and showed a stable rhythm with normal ST segments and T-wave morphology. ST and T-wave analysis was used throughout surgery and did not detect any signs of ischaemia.

> ✪ **Learning point** ECG configurations during general anaesthesia
>
> Lead II is usually used during general anaesthesia, as this is the best lead for monitoring any rhythm disturbance since its axis parallels the electrical axis of the heart, giving the best visualization of the p-wave. However, it is an insensitive detector of ischaemia. About 90% of ST-segment information obtained during the exercise ECG is found in lead V_5, and this lead was therefore suggested as the most appropriate for detecting intraoperative ischaemia. Monitoring of lead V_5 requires a five-lead system, which is often used during cardiac anaesthesia.
>
> The CM5 arrangement of the three-lead ECG is a more sensitive detector of ischaemia than lead II, detecting ~90% of ST changes due to LV ischaemia. CM5 can be obtained by placing the right arm lead over the manubrium, left arm lead over V_5, and left leg lead anywhere (but traditionally clavicle) [10].

There were no immediate postoperative surgical complications. A small volume of blood was drained from a pelvic drain placed at the time of surgery. The evening dose of LMWH was withheld at the request of the operating surgeon.

Later that night the patient suffered a sudden, witnessed, cardiac arrest on the general surgical ward. She was urgently intubated, underwent one cycle of cardiopulmonary resuscitation and one direct-current (DC) shock for ventricular fibrillation (VF), which successfully converted her heart rhythm to sinus tachycardia. ECG revealed widespread anterior ST elevation (Figure 9.2) consistent with acute myocardial infarction. She was hypotensive with a blood pressure of 65/32 mmHg and needed 50 microgram boluses of adrenaline for haemodynamic support and safe transfer to the

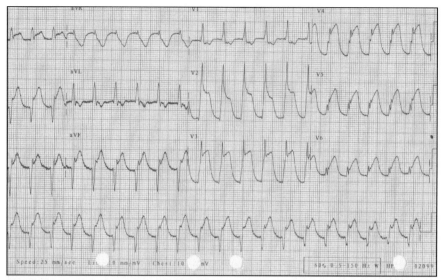

Figure 9.2 Electrocardiogram showing acute ST elevation in leads V$_2$–V$_6$, II, III and aVF due to a large anterolateral myocardial infarction following direct-current cardioversion for ventricular fibrillation. Although the changes in leads II, III, and aVF suggest additional inferior infarction (commonly due to right coronary artery occlusion), there was no evidence of this at angiography.

ICU. A propofol infusion was also started for sedation as she was opening her eyes spontaneously, coughing and localizing to the endotracheal tube prior to transfer to the ICU.

Management and progress

She required regular adrenaline boluses following her VF arrest, and was commenced on an adrenaline infusion in the ICU as this formed the logical continuation of inotropic support from the resuscitative adrenaline boluses. She was then transferred to the cardiac catheter laboratory for urgent coronary angiography. This revealed occlusion of a dominant LAD due to acute stent thrombosis (Figure 9.3A). Balloon angioplasty was performed which successfully restored flow to the anterior wall of the LV (TIMI grade 2) (Figure 9.3B). Because of continuing inotrope dependency, hypotension and likelihood of myocardial stunning, an IABP was inserted. During the procedure she was given a 5000-unit bolus of heparin, followed by an infusion targeting an activated partial thromboplastin time ratio (APTTR) of 1.5–2.0; antiplatelet therapy in the form of a tirofiban infusion was also started. Despite the fact that the procedure was less than 6 h after major surgery with a high risk of bleeding, it was judged that at that point her cardiac problems were a greater risk to her life than postoperative haemorrhage.

> ✪ **Learning point** Pharmacology of antiplatelet agents
>
> Aspirin (a salicylate) and clopidogrel (a thienopyridine) are irreversible oral antiplatelet agents. Both are prodrugs with clopidogrel requiring metabolism to its active form by the hepatic cytochrome P450 isoenzyme CYP3A4. Salicylates irreversibly inhibit the cyclo-oxygenase enzyme (COX-1); thienopyridines inhibit the P2Y$_{12}$ subtype of the ADP receptor. Since platelets do not have DNA to re-synthesize proteins, both exert their effect throughout the lifespan of the platelet, which is around 7 days. When undergoing operations in which any bleeding could cause severe morbidity (e.g. neurosurgery), patients must stop
>
> (continued)

these antiplatelet drugs at least 7 days preoperatively unless there is a particularly high risk of thrombosis and partial recovery of function is considered safer.

In cases of uncontrolled bleeding, only a platelet transfusion will reverse the effect of these agents. By contrast, tirofiban (a glycoprotein IIb/IIIa inhibitor) is a more potent but reversible intravenous antiplatelet agent. GPIIb/IIIa inhibitors have greater antiplatelet activity, as this represents the final common pathway in platelet activation. Glycoprotein IIb/IIIa, an integrin complex found on the platelet surface, binds platelets to fibrinogen, as well as each other via Von Willebrand Factor. Their expression leads to rapid platelet aggregation and thrombus formation at the site of vessel injury.

Tirofiban has a half-life of 2–5 h, with normal platelet function usually returning within 6–8 h of stopping an infusion. This allows some reversibility compared with the oral antiplatelet agents. The drug is licensed for use in unstable angina or non-ST elevation myocardial infarction (NSTEMI), and as an adjunct to PCI.

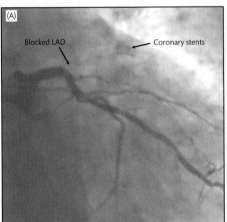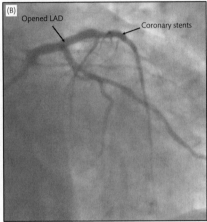

Figure 9.3 Coronary angiography following cardiac arrest on the general surgical ward. (A) AP caudal view revealing an acute stent thrombosis and blocked left anterior descending artery (LAD). (B) Following balloon angioplasty to the LAD, restoration of thrombolysis in myocardial infarction (TIMI) grade 2 flow to the anterior wall of the left ventricle. Images kindly provided by Dr Florim Cuculi and Dr Raj Kharbanda, Oxford Heart Centre, John Radcliffe Hospital, Oxford.

✪ Learning point Intra-aortic balloon counter pulsation

The intra-aortic balloon pump (IABP) is a helium-filled balloon that is typically inserted in a retrograde fashion up the femoral artery to lie in the descending aorta. Less usually, it may be inserted via the subclavian artery and advanced in an anterograde direction.

The distal end of the balloon must lie above the renal arteries to avoid compromising renal blood flow, whereas its tip lies downstream of the left subclavian artery to preserve upper limb perfusion. Anticoagulation is required, usually with heparin, targeting an APTTR of 1.5–2.5.

The balloon is typically inserted in patients with a low cardiac output, following coronary intervention or cardiac surgery, where it reduces inotrope requirements, improves coronary blood flow and reduces myocardial oxygen demand. Contraindications to insertion are severe aortic regurgitation and aortic dissection.

The balloon inflates during diastole, beginning with the closure of the aortic valve (marked by the dicrotic notch on the arterial pressure waveform). It deflates during the isovolaemic contraction phase, before ventricular ejection, to allow diastolic pressure to fall to a lower level than would occur without counter-pulsation. Systolic and diastolic pressures usually decrease slightly with IABP use, but the augmented diastolic pressure (the peak pressure produced during IABP inflation in diastole)

(continued)

> is higher—increasing coronary perfusion. Deflation of the balloon reduces afterload and reduces cardiac work and oxygen demand.
>
> Initially balloon inflation occurs with every cardiac cycle (1:1). As LV function recovers, IABP support can be weaned to every 2nd or 3rd cycle (1:2 and 1:3) before finally being removed—usually after a period of 48–72 h.

The patient remained haemodynamically stable overnight, and was successfully weaned off the adrenaline infusion. The next day intra-aortic balloon counter-pulsation was gradually reduced from 1:1 to 1:3, as there were clinical signs of improved cardiac output and organ perfusion. There were no signs of excessive surgical bleeding despite being on infusions of unfractionated heparin and tirofiban. The IABP was removed on the 2nd postoperative day, and enteral aspirin and clopidogrel were re-started. She was extubated on the 3rd postoperative day with no signs of neurological sequelae and transferred to coronary care unit on the 4th postoperative day. Her surgical progress was satisfactory, being able to tolerate free fluids with good stoma output. Serial 12-lead ECGs showed full resolution of the acute ST changes seen in Figure 9.3, which, following PCI, did not recur. However, prior to discharge from ICU, anterior Q-waves were noted. Echocardiography revealed moderate-to-severe impairment of systolic function with a hypokinetic anterior ventricular wall. She went on to make an uneventful medical and surgical recovery and was eventually discharged home.

She was subsequently reviewed in the outpatient cardiology clinic where she reported a reasonable exercise tolerance: able to walk at a moderate pace, limited largely by bilateral patellofemoral osteoarthritis rather than shortness of breath. There were no signs of cardiac failure on examination, and she remained on secondary prevention medication (aspirin, clopidogrel, statin, and angiotensin-converting enzyme (ACE) inhibitor). She remained intolerant to beta-blockers, and was advised to take both aspirin and clopidogrel for life.

Discussion

The complexity of modern medicine means that best treatment of a patient is often based on achieving a balance of risks. In this situation the patient required planned cancer surgery during a period when she was still at risk of developing early stent thrombosis 5 months after PCI. Major surgery should ideally be delayed until endothelial re-growth is established. However, this takes much longer with DES, so the probability of encountering patients needing surgery during a 'risk period' is greater with this type of stent. Furthermore the degree of re-endothelialization is variable even many months after DES insertion [11]. Therefore DAPT must be maintained for at least 12 months—longer if there are additional risk factors (Box 9.1), as in this case. The patient described here had a high thrombosis risk with overlapping stents in a major coronary vessel that supplied most of the anterior wall of the LV (Figure 9.3B), and only moderate (TIMI grade 2) post-procedural flow. Undergoing major surgery greatly increases this risk so DAPT should be maintained throughout the perioperative period whenever possible.

An important question is: 'Did the risks of important bleeding outweigh the risks of thrombosis in this case and should DAPT have been continued'? In deciding the optimal treatment for a patient it is necessary to balance the risk of re-thrombosis with the

---

Box 9.1 Risk factors for stent thrombosis

Clinical

Premature cessation of dual antiplatelet therapy (DAPT)
Prior brachytherapy[a]
Low ejection fraction
Acute coronary syndrome
Renal failure
Diabetes

Procedural

Long stents
Multiple lesions
Overlapping stents
Ostial or bifurcation lesions
Small vessels
Suboptimal angiographic results

[a] Intracoronary radiation to treat stent re-stenosis.

Source: American Heart Association, Inc.

---

risk of important bleeding. This requires an analysis of both the patient-specific risk of thrombosis and patient/operation-specific risk of bleeding. The risks of surgical bleeding associated with continuing DAPT depend on the site and extent of surgery and the patient's physiological ability to tolerate such bleeding. For example, excessive bleeding in a closed cavity such as the posterior chamber of the eye, spinal canal or cranial vault could be catastrophic. Similarly in operations where full haemostasis is difficult to achieve (e.g. transurethral prostatectomy) there is a high risk of uncontrolled haemorrhage. In these situations both aspirin and clopidogrel are generally stopped 7 days before operation, ensuring complete recovery of platelet function prior to surgery.

In other forms of non-cardiac surgery, aspirin increases neither the severity nor the mortality of bleeding complications [14]. Clopidogrel has caused greater concern among surgeons, because thienopyridines are known to have greater antiplatelet activity than salicylates, and there is firm evidence of increased bleeding following coronary artery bypass grafting (CABG) in patients who continue to take clopidogrel [15]. Epidural and spinal anaesthesia are either not recommended [9, 16] or are 'recommended against' [17] in patients who have taken clopidogrel in the previous 7 days, though this is likely based on pharmacological considerations rather than robust clinical evidence [18, 19]. Therefore interruption of DAPT solely to facilitate neuraxial

---

❝ Expert comment

Whereas untimely interruption of DAPT is known to increase markedly the risk of stent thrombosis, there is still some doubt as to whether, in the perioperative period, maintaining DAPT, as recommended whenever possible, offers complete protection against this life-threatening complication. Cases of stent thrombosis in the presence of DAPT have been reported in the literature. A study of more than 600 operations in patients with DES did not identify the withdrawal of DAPT to be a significant correlate of adverse cardiac outcome [13]. However, 260 of those 600 patients were operated on more than a year after stent insertion. At this time they were probably no longer on DAPT. This may explain why, in the whole cohort, withdrawal (or absence) of DAPT did not seem to modify outcome. These results must be interpreted cautiously and do not contradict the recommendations of all the guidelines to maintain DAPT whenever possible.

blockade is not justified unless neuraxial blockade is judged to be mandatory to optimize the chances of good outcome for the patient.

Until recently, the evidence for excessive bleeding in non-cardiac surgery due to clopidogrel was controversial: one large study reported severe bleeding in up to 20% of patients on DAPT [21], whereas another suggested only a modest increase in postoperative bleeding [22]. A recent trial involving patients undergoing (major) peripheral arterial vascular surgery showed that those taking DAPT had no increase in bleeding requiring reoperation [23]. Thus maintenance of perioperative clopidogrel, in combination with aspirin, is most likely safe in the majority of cases of non-cardiac surgery, except those involving closed cavities.

In patients with DES who are taking DAPT, an interdisciplinary discussion between surgeon, anaesthetist and cardiologist is essential and widely recommended in published guidelines [1, 24–26]. This allows the relative risks of thrombosis and bleeding to be established for each individual patient. In our case there were clearly greater risks of thrombosis compared with bleeding, and on balance DAPT should have been continued. Often if surgeons are informed that stopping DAPT may lead to a large myocardial infarction or death, they may be persuaded that the risks of thrombosis outweigh those of bleeding. If, however, this strategy is unsuccessful and clopidogrel must be stopped, bridging therapy may be used. This refers to the replacement of long-acting, irreversible antiplatelet agents with reversible and short-acting antiplatelet drugs to offer thrombosis prophylaxis during the perioperative period. In this case the patient was started on LMWH in place of clopidogrel. However, LMWH has no antiplatelet properties, with no evidence of efficacy in this context [27].

It makes more pharmacological sense to substitute clopidogrel with a reversible antiplatelet agent such as tirofiban, a glycoprotein IIb/IIIa inhibitor; something that occurred later in her clinical course. This would offer reversible antiplatelet prophylaxis that could be stopped should any bleeding occur, with normal platelet function returning within 6–8 h of stopping an infusion. One potential bridging regime that would have been better suited throughout the perioperative period would be initiation of tirofiban 4 days preoperatively (having discontinued clopidogrel at day 5), maintained until 4 h before surgery. Clopidogrel treatment, including a loading dose, could then be re-started on the first postoperative day; with aspirin continued throughout (Figure 9.4) [29]. If

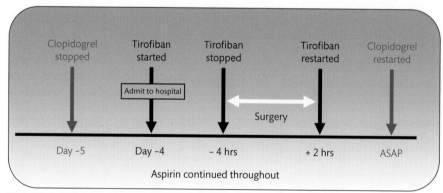

Figure 9.4 Bridging therapy as substitution of DAPT during the perioperative period. After Savonitto *et al.* [29]. ASAP, as soon as possible. Data from Savonitto S, D'Urbano M, Caracciolo M, *et al.* Urgent surgery in patients with a recently implanted coronary drug-eluting stent: a phase II study of "bridging" antiplatelet therapy with tirofiban during temporary withdrawal of clopidogrel. *British Journal of Anaesthesia.* 2010;104(3):285–291.

there are early concerns regarding postoperative bleeding, tirofiban can be resumed and clopidogrel delayed until deemed safe, or until enteral absorption returns. Although there is limited evidence and no licence for glycoprotein IIb/IIIa inhibitors in this setting, at present these are the only reversible inhibitors of platelet activity that offer a logical short-acting substitute for the prevention of stent thrombosis.

Whereas it is logistically difficult and expensive to admit patients several days before surgery, it is necessary to ensure ongoing short-term antiplatelet cover, as stopping clopidogrel leads to the emergence of functional platelets within a few days, increasing the risk of thrombosis [31, 32]. However, it should be noted that the greatest risk of thrombosis is during or soon after surgery [27]. Patients at high risk of re-thrombosis should therefore be sent to an HDU postoperatively where they can be appropriately monitored, and not the general surgical ward as happened in this case. In addition, elective or semi-elective surgery should always be performed at a centre that has the capabilities to perform emergency out-of-hours PCI should the need arise.

A summary of suggested perioperative pharmacological management [33] of antiplatelet agents during a coronary stent's high-risk period is as follows:

1. Low surgical bleeding risk: maintain DAPT. Examples: minor plastic, general, or orthopaedic surgery; tissue biopsies; tooth extraction; surgery to the anterior segment of the eye.
2. Moderate surgical bleeding risk: maintain DAPT if possible, unless surgical bleeding risk outweighs thrombosis risk. Consider bridging therapy if clopidogrel must be stopped. Examples: cardiac surgery; major orthopaedic, vascular, visceral, ENT, urological or reconstructive surgery.
3. High surgical bleeding risk: stop clopidogrel 5 days before surgery, and start bridging therapy 1–3 days preoperatively. Maintain aspirin wherever possible. Examples: intracranial and spinal surgery; surgery to the posterior segment of the eye; transurethral resection of the prostate (TURP).

New antiplatelet agents

New antiplatelet agents recently available or soon to be licensed include prasugrel, ticagrelor and cangrelor. Ticagrelor, which is taken orally, is a pentyl-triazolo-pyrimidine and is a non-competitive inhibitor of the $P2Y_{12}$ receptor; it binds to a different site to the thienopyridines [34]. The drug does not need to undergo cytochrome-dependent metabolism for activity and achieves greater inhibition of platelet activity more rapidly than clopidogrel. More importantly, its speed of offset is faster—with the majority of platelet function being restored at 3 days, compared with 5 days for clopidogrel. Furthermore, at 24–48 h, the level of inhibition for ticagrelor and clopidogrel is not significantly different [32]. Therefore patients requiring bridging therapy for surgery could be admitted 2 days preoperatively instead of 4, having stopped the drug 3 days earlier, instead of 5. This would halve the number of days patients are admitted before operation, which is considerably easier from an organizational perspective, as well as cheaper. Clinical efficacy of ticagrelor was shown in the PLATO trial (secondary prevention of cardiac events) where it resulted in significant reduction in both cardiovascular and all-cause mortality, compared with patients taking clopidogrel [35]. The number of stent re-thromboses seen in patients receiving DES was also reduced, though this finding was not statistically significant [36]. More importantly there was no significant difference in major bleeding events between the two treatment groups.

❝ Expert comment

LMWH is widely recommended for preventing deep vein thrombosis during the perioperative period. Unfortunately LMWH does not offer protection against stent thrombosis, as it does not reduce platelet adhesiveness [28]. Therefore the introduction of LMWH does not mean that DAPT can be stopped without exposing patients to an increased risk of perioperative stent thrombosis.

❝ Expert comment

Increasingly bridging therapy is mentioned in reports on the management of patients with coronary stents [25, 29, 30]. Whereas it is entirely logical there are, thus far, too few patients included in these reports to be certain that bridging therapy significantly reduces the risk of perioperative adverse cardiac events.

Prasugrel, a new thienopyridine, is also an alternative oral agent. Like clopidogrel, it is a pro-drug requiring cytochrome-dependent metabolism to an active metabolite, which irreversibly inhibits the $P2Y_{12}$ receptor. One study found that its clinical efficacy was superior to that of clopidogrel as it significantly reduced the incidence of ischaemic events, including stent thrombosis, and cardiovascular mortality [37]. However, it was also associated with increased major bleeding, including fatal haemorrhage, and would likely pose a much greater surgical bleeding risk than clopidogrel, making its perioperative continuation difficult to justify except for surgery with minor bleeding risks.

Cangrelor is an ATP analogue that is a very short-acting reversible inhibitor of the $P2Y_{12}$ receptor. Unlike the other agents, it is given by intravenous infusion and does not need conversion to an active metabolite. It has a plasma half-life of 3–5 min resulting in full recovery of platelet function within 60 min. Its clinical efficacy is not superior to clopidogrel when used instead of standard doses during PCI [38]. However, rather than replacing thienopyridines as an antiplatelet agent during coronary intervention, it would be more suited as a short-acting substitute to clopidogrel during the perioperative period. This is currently being investigated in the BRIDGE study—a phase II trial assessing the efficacy and safety of cangrelor in patients with ACS treated with DAPT, scheduled for CABG [39]. Full results are awaited.

A Final Word from the Expert

Patients with coronary stents, especially recently inserted stents, present several challenges when they need surgery. DAPT is associated with an increased risk of bleeding. However, interrupting DAPT to reduce bleeding may result in stent thrombosis. It is recommended to delay surgery until DAPT is no longer required. If surgery cannot be delayed, the management of these patients must be discussed by surgeon, cardiologist, anaesthetist and the patient to reach a consensus on the balance of risks.

References

1. Fleisher LA, Beckman JA, Brown KA, *et al.* 2009 ACCF/AHA focused update on perioperative beta blockade incorporated into the ACC/AHA 2007 guidelines on perioperative cardiovascular evaluation and care for noncardiac surgery: a report of the American College of Cardiology Foundation/American Heart Association Task Force on practice guidelines. *Circulation* 2009;120:e169–276.
2. Le Manach Y, Ibanez Esteves C, Bertrand M, *et al.* Impact of preoperative statin therapy on adverse postoperative outcomes in patients undergoing vascular surgery. *Anesthesiology* 2011;114:98–104.
3. Farb A, Boam AB. Stent thrombosis redux—the FDA perspective. *N Engl J Med* 2007;356:984–7.
4. Chieffo A, Park S-J, Meliga E, *et al.* Late and very late stent thrombosis following drug-eluting stent implantation in unprotected left main coronary artery: a multicentre registry. *Eur Heart J* 2008;29:2108–15.
5. Kandzari DE, Barker CS, Leon MB, *et al.* Dual antiplatelet therapy duration and clinical outcomes following treatment with zotarolimus-eluting stents. *J Am Coll Cardiol Cardiovasc Interv* 2011;4:1119–28.

6. Jeremias A, Sylvia B, Bridges J, *et al*. Stent thrombosis after successful sirolimus-eluting stent implantation. *Circulation* 2004;109:1930–2.

7. Iakovou I, Schmidt T, Bonizzoni E, *et al*. Incidence, predictors, and outcome of thrombosis after successful implantation of drug-eluting stents. *JAMA* 2005;293:2126–30.

8. Sherman KL, Obi SH, Aranha GV, Yao KA, Shoup MC. Heparin-coated stents do not protect cancer patients from cardiac complications after noncardiac surgery. *Am Surg* 2009;75:61–5.

9. Assali A, Vaknin-Assa H, Lev E, *et al*. The risk of cardiac complications following noncardiac surgery in patients with drug eluting stents implanted at least six months before surgery. *Catheter Cardiovasc Interv* 2009;74:837–43.

10. Edwards ND, Reilly CS. Detection of perioperative myocardial ischaemia. *Br J Anaesth*. 1994;72:104–15.

11. Joner M, Finn AV, Farb A, *et al*. Pathology of drug-eluting stents in humans: delayed healing and late thrombotic risk. *J Am Coll Cardiol* 2006;48:193–202.

12. Grines CL, Bonow RO, Casey DE, *et al*. Prevention of premature discontinuation of dual antiplatelet therapy in patients with coronary artery stents: a science advisory from the American Heart Association, American College of Cardiology, Society for Cardiovascular Angiography and Interventions, American College of Surgeons, and American Dental Association, with representation from the American College of Physicians. *Circulation* 2007;115:813–18.

13. Anwaruddin S, Askari AT, Saudye H, *et al*. Characterization of post-operative risk associated with prior drug-eluting stent use. *J Am Coll Cardiol Cardiovasc Interv* 2009;2:542–9.

14. Burger W, Chemnitius J-M, Kneissl GD, Rücker G. Low-dose aspirin for secondary cardiovascular prevention—cardiovascular risks after its perioperative withdrawal versus bleeding risks with its continuation—review and meta-analysis. *J Intern Med* 2005;257:399–414.

15. Purkayastha S. Does clopidogrel affect outcome after coronary artery bypass grafting? A meta-analysis. *Heart* 2005;92:531–2.

16. Gogarten W, Vandermeulen E, Van Aken H, *et al*. Regional anaesthesia and antithrombotic agents: recommendations of the European Society of Anaesthesiology. *Eur J Anaesthesiol* 2010;27:999–1015.

17. Horlocker TT, Wedel DJ, Rowlingson JC, *et al*. Regional anesthesia in the patient receiving antithrombotic or thrombolytic therapy. *Regional Anesth Pain Med* 2010;35:64–101.

18. Osta WA, Akbary H, Fuleihan SF. Epidural analgesia in vascular surgery patients actively taking clopidogrel. *Br J Anaesth* 2010;104:429–32.

19. Benzon HT, McCarthy RJ, Benzon HA, *et al*. Determination of residual antiplatelet activity of clopidogrel before neuraxial injections. *Br J Anaesth* 2011;107:966–71.

20. Horlocker TT, Wedel DJ, Benzon H, *et al*. Regional anesthesia in the anticoagulated patient: defining the risks (the second ASRA Consensus Conference on Neuraxial Anesthesia and Anticoagulation). *Regional Anesth Pain Med* 2003;28:172–97.

21. van Kuijk J-P, Flu W-J, Schouten O, *et al*. Timing of noncardiac surgery after coronary artery stenting with bare metal or drug-eluting stents. *Am J Cardiol* 2009;104:1229–34.

22. Rabbitts JA, Nuttall GA, Brown MJ, *et al*. Cardiac risk of noncardiac surgery after percutaneous coronary intervention with drug-eluting stents. *Anesthesiology* 2008;109:596–604.

23. Stone DH, Goodney PP, Schanzer A, *et al*. Clopidogrel is not associated with major bleeding complications during peripheral arterial surgery. *J Vasc Surg* 2011;54:779–84.

24. Savonitto S, Caracciolo M, Cattaneo M, DE Servi S. Management of patients with recently implanted coronary stents on dual antiplatelet therapy who need to undergo major surgery. *J Thromb Haemost* 2011;9:2133–42.

25. Barash P, Akhtar S. Coronary stents: factors contributing to perioperative major adverse cardiovascular events. *Br J Anaesth* 2010;105 Suppl 1:i3–15.

26. Task Force for Preoperative Cardiac Risk Assessment and Perioperative Cardiac Management in Non-cardiac Surgery, European Society of Cardiology (ESC), Poldermans D,

et al. Guidelines for pre-operative cardiac risk assessment and perioperative cardiac management in non-cardiac surgery. *Eur Heart J* 2009;30:2769–812.

27   Vicenzi MN, Meislitzer T, Heitzinger B, *et al.* Coronary artery stenting and non-cardiac surgery—a prospective outcome study. *Br J Anaesth* 2006;96:686–93.

28. Kim HJ, Levin LF. The management of patients on dual antiplatelet therapy undergoing orthopedic surgery. *Hosp Special Surg J* 2010;6:182–9.

29. Savonitto S, D'Urbano M, Caracciolo M, *et al.* Urgent surgery in patients with a recently implanted coronary drug-eluting stent: a phase II study of "bridging" antiplatelet therapy with tirofiban during temporary withdrawal of clopidogrel. *Br J Anaesth* 2010;104:285–91.

30. Broad L, Lee T, Conroy M, *et al.* Successful management of patients with a drug-eluting coronary stent presenting for elective, non-cardiac surgery. *Br J Anaesth* 2007;98:19–22.

31. Weber AA, Braun M, Hohlfeld T, *et al.* Recovery of platelet function after discontinuation of clopidogrel treatment in healthy volunteers. *Br J Clin Pharmacol* 2001;52:333–6.

32. Gurbel PA, Bliden KP, Butler K, *et al.* Randomized double-blind assessment of the ONSET and OFFSET of the antiplatelet effects of ticagrelor versus clopidogrel in patients with stable coronary artery disease: the ONSET/OFFSET study. *Circulation* 2009;120:2577–85.

33. DeVile MPJ, Foex P. Antiplatelet drugs, coronary stents, and non-cardiac surgery. *Cont Educ Anaesth Crit Care Pain* 2010;10:187–91.

34. Rosenstein R. Antiplatelet therapy in acute coronary syndromes: focus on ticagrelor. *J Blood Med* 2010:197–19.

35. Wallentin L, Becker RC, Budaj A, *et al.* Ticagrelor versus clopidogrel in patients with acute coronary syndromes. *N Engl J Med* 2009;361:1045–57.

36. Cannon CP, Harrington RA, James S, *et al.* Comparison of ticagrelor with clopidogrel in patients with a planned invasive strategy for acute coronary syndromes (PLATO): a randomised double-blind study. *Lancet* 2010;375(9711):283–93.

37. Wiviott SD, Braunwald E, McCabe CH, *et al.* Prasugrel versus clopidogrel in patients with acute coronary syndromes. *N Engl J Med* 2007;357:2001–15.

38. Harrington RA, Stone GW, McNulty S, *et al.* Platelet inhibition with cangrelor in patients undergoing PCI. *N Engl J Med* 2009;361:2318–29.

39. NCT00767507 CTGP. BRIDGE: *Maintenance of platelet inhibition with cangrelor.* < http:// www.http://clinicaltrials.gov/ct2/show/NCT00767507?term = bridge&rank = 2 >

40. Angiolillo DJ, Firstenberg MS, Price MJ, *et al.* Bridging antiplatelet therapy with cangrelor in patients undergoing cardiac surgery: a randomized controlled trial. *JAMA* 2012;307:265–74.

Post-arrest percutaneous coronary intervention: the role of the anaesthetist

Robert Jackson

⊕ **Expert Commentary** Jerry Nolan

CPD Matrix Code: *1B03, 1B04, 2A08, 2C01, 3C00*

Case history

A 55-year-old man was admitted to the emergency department having had a witnessed collapse and cardiac arrest at home. He had no previous medical history and took no medications normally, but had been experiencing episodes of chest pain over the preceding weeks which he had attributed to indigestion. He was a smoker with a 20-pack-year history, and there was a family history of hypercholesterolaemia and ischaemic heart disease.

He had been complaining of indigestion to his wife, though the pain had become more severe than usual and in fact his wife was on the telephone to the emergency services when he suddenly collapsed and became unconscious. The emergency telephone operator had advised her to perform chest compression only CPR until assisted by the emergency services, who arrived 5 min later.

The paramedics quickly confirmed cardiac arrest with VF as the initial rhythm. A 200 J biphasic shock was administered resulting in immediate return of spontaneous circulation (ROSC). An LMA was inserted for airway control, intravenous access achieved, and the patient transported to the receiving hospital. During transfer the patient was making spontaneous respiratory effort, but remained unconscious with GCS 3/15. His blood pressure was 135/65 but ECG monitoring revealed continuing ectopic activity and ST-segment elevation on lead II.

⊗ **Learning point** The burden of coronary heart disease

Despite advances in diagnosis and secondary prevention, cardiovascular disease remains the leading cause of adult death in the western world, responsible for almost half of all adult deaths. Of all deaths related to cardiovascular disease, 42% are secondary to coronary heart disease and 60% of these are in the form of sudden cardiac arrest [1]. Across Europe, 38 arrests per 100,000 population are treated annually by emergency medical services [2]. Survival to hospital discharge is ~20% for out-of-hospital VF arrests but significantly lower for all presenting rhythms (5–10%) [3].

(continued)

Expert comment

The overall survival rate from out-of-hospital cardiac arrest (OOHCA) has changed very little over the last 30 years but this statistic masks more complex changes in the epidemiology of cardiac arrest [5]. Survival rates from out-of-hospital VF cardiac arrest are improving but this success is offset by a decreasing incidence of VF as the first monitored rhythm [6]. Survival rates from non-shockable rhythms (pulseless electrical activity and asystole) are much worse than for VF but recent evidence indicates that survival is improving, even for these rhythms [7].

Major risk factors for ischaemic heart disease include:

- age (men >45 years, women >55 years)
- family history of premature coronary artery disease (in male first-degree relative aged <65 years)
- hypertension (blood pressure >140/90 mmHg or on antihypertensive medication)
- smoking
- diabetes mellitus
- hypercholesterolaemia
- low high-density lipoprotein cholesterol (<40 mg/dL)
- hypertriglyceridaemia (>200 mg/dL)
- obesity

Numerous additional risk factors and biomarkers have been identified including: presence of chronic inflammation, chronically elevated C-reactive protein, raised fibrinogen levels, renal disease, abnormal ankle/brachial blood pressure index, and many others. These factors add only moderate additional risk to the major factors listed above [4].

As the patient was brought into the resuscitation bay of the emergency department he suddenly arrested again, and was found to be in VF. The hospital resuscitation team, which included an anaesthetist, was in attendance and resuscitation commenced immediately.

Clinical tip Improving the quality of CPR

Chest compression quality should be given high priority in cardiac arrest:

- Rotate compression providers every 2 min, or more frequently.
- Continue compressions while charging the defibrillator.
- Ensure pre-shock safety checks are brief but thorough.
- Minimize all other disturbances to CPR; only perform rhythm checks at 2 min intervals.
- Use waveform capnography to confirm airway patency and effective CPR.

Learning point Management of cardiac arrest

The importance of high-quality chest compressions as a key component of successful resuscitation attempts has been demonstrated in numerous studies and is strongly emphasized in recent guidelines for the management of cardiac arrest. High-quality CPR increases the likelihood of defibrillation success; each 5 s delay between the last chest compression and defibrillation halves the chance of restoring a perfusing rhythm, and reduces survival to hospital discharge by up to 18% [8]. Furthermore, the proportion of time in arrest where no chest compressions occur (no flow) is directly linked to mortality [9].

Airway management in cardiac arrest, while important, should not be allowed to compromise the requirement for ongoing chest compressions. Tracheal intubation in arrest has not been shown to improve survival; if deemed appropriate, attempts to intubate should not be prolonged, and should not require interruption of chest compressions for more than 10 s. Supraglottic airway devices are useful for airway management in arrested patients, and may allow adequate oxygenation and ventilation.

The use of waveform capnography is now recommended during resuscitation attempts [10]. Capnography (in the presence of chest compressions) is the most reliable indicator of successful tracheal intubation in cardiac arrest, and also allows an assessment of the quality of CPR.

Expert comment

During the first 30 min of CPR adequate ventilation should generate some exhaled CO_2. If the patient has been intubated failure to detect CO_2 using waveform capnography indicates that the tube is in the oesophagus. The higher the quality of CPR, the higher the end-tidal CO_2 value recorded. After 30 min of CPR, pulmonary blood flow may reduce significantly and capnography may not be 100% reliable for detecting oesophageal intubation. During CPR, a sudden increase in the end-tidal CO_2 value suggests ROSC.

CPR was initiated and the defibrillator charged to 200 J (biphasic). A single shock was administered and CPR recommenced immediately for 2 min. During this period oxygenation was achieved using the LMA already in place and additional intravenous access was inserted. Blood samples were taken for laboratory investigations (full blood count, blood biochemistry) and arterial blood gas analysis. After 2 min a rhythm check was performed and the patient was found to be in sinus rhythm with a palpable brachial pulse. The following observations were recorded:

HR: 96
BP: 85/40
SpO_2: 99%

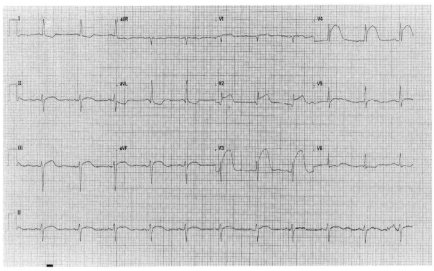

Figure 9.5 Admission electrocardiogram.

The patient was making some spontaneous respiratory effort, but was requiring assistance by manual lung ventilation, and was tolerating the LMA. Neurological assessment demonstrated no response to pain in any of the three domains (Eye opening, Motor response or Verbal), yielding GCS of 3/15.

A 12-lead ECG was recorded. This demonstrated widespread ischaemic changes consistent with an acute anterior myocardial infarction (MI), with ST-segment elevation in leads V1–V4 (Figure 9.5).

The patient was reviewed by a cardiologist who decided to take the patient to the cardiac catheterization suite for primary angioplasty. It was decided that brain CT was not required prior to this.

⊗ Learning point Indications for primary angioplasty following out-of-hospital cardiac arrest (OOHCA)

Approximately half of patients presenting with non-traumatic OOHCA will have coronary occlusion potentially amenable to revascularization. This may be attempted pharmacologically using thrombolytics or by primary PCI. Extrapolated evidence from acute MI patients who have not had a cardiac arrest suggests improved outcomes following primary PCI when compared to thrombolysis, and recent studies comparing outcomes in OOHCA patients treated with aggressive early coronary revascularization to historical controls demonstrated significantly improved hospital survival and neurological outcomes in primary PCI patients [11, 12]. Successful reperfusion is time-critical—current guidelines suggest that medical services should aim to deliver primary PCI within 90 min of presentation in appropriate patients [13]. Thrombolysis should be delivered within 30 min if primary PCI is unavailable, or unsuitable.

A normal ECG following successful resuscitation does not exclude the possibility of an occlusive coronary lesion; this may occur in more than 10% of such cases [14, 15]. Transthoracic echocardiogram may assist diagnosis in this group by demonstration of an akinetic segment of myocardium.

There should be a low threshold for performing coronary angiography in all post-arrest patients without a clear alternative diagnosis.

❝ Expert comment

As a consequence of the recognized unreliability of the 12-lead ECG after cardiac arrest, there is a trend toward taking all resuscitated OOHCA patients to the cardiac catheter laboratory unless the cause of the cardiac arrest is clearly non-cardiac. This places considerable demands on interventional cardiologists and is one of the drivers for establishing cardiac arrest centres where resources can be concentrated.

Expert comment

The proportion of OOHCAs caused by subarachnoid haemorrhage is controversial—there is marked regional variation with a study from Japan documenting an incidence of 16.2% [16], whereas a study from Vienna documented just 4% [17]. Given that most of these OOHCA patients will be cooled and in many cases anticoagulated, unless a neurological cause for cardiac arrest can be excluded confidently there is a strong argument that brain CT should be undertaken en route to the cardiac catheterization laboratory or intensive care unit.

Learning point The role of CT head scans following out-of-hospital cardiac arrest

The leading cause of non-traumatic OOHCA in the western world is ischaemic heart disease. Up to 18% of cases occur as a result of intracranial catastrophes, most frequently subarachnoid haemorrhage [16]. Distinguishing between these two groups on a clinical basis following arrival in hospital may be difficult, particularly as ECG changes consistent with MI may be present following subarachnoid haemorrhage. Clinical features such as sudden-onset headache or non-VF presenting cardiac rhythm increase the likelihood of an intracranial cause for arrest; however, these details may be unavailable during initial assessment, and lack specificity. It is common practice to perform cranial imaging (e.g. CT) to identify patients who will not benefit from attempts at coronary revascularization, and who may potentially come to harm from anticoagulant medications used during or after the procedures. Modern CT scanners are rapid, and in theory a CT head prior to coronary angiography should not delay treatment significantly; however, this is clearly determined by local facilities and staff availability. Transfers to radiology also expose a potentially unstable patient to periods of reduced monitoring and patient access in the event of an emergency. Significant haemodynamic instability post resuscitation is an indication to proceed directly to PCI rather than via CT. Local policies will currently dictate whether all, or selected at-risk groups should be scanned prior to angiography, and these policies should be assessed for their impact on door-to-balloon times.

The patient was prepared for transfer to the coronary angiography suite by the anaesthetist. A propofol infusion was commenced to maintain anaesthesia and the patient was paralysed with atracurium. The LMA was exchanged for a size 8.0 mm internal diameter cuffed oral tracheal tube, and ventilation commenced with a portable ventilator. Full standard monitoring was implemented using a portable monitor including pulse oximetry, ECG, waveform capnography, and an arterial line was inserted into the left radial artery for invasive blood pressure monitoring. Venous access was considered adequate via two functioning peripheral lines, and central

Clinical tip Preparation for transfer to the coronary angiography suite

Transferring anaesthetized patients around the hospital may be hazardous; appropriate measures should be taken to minimize the risk by ensuring that adequate monitoring, intravenous access, drugs and equipment are available. Monitoring should include pulse oximetry (SpO_2), ECG, blood pressure (non-invasive or invasive), and end-tidal capnography. Drugs must include sufficient anaesthesia for the transfer, as well as intubation drugs, and a selection of vasoactive drugs such as atropine, ephedrine and metaraminol as well as resuscitation doses of adrenaline. Keep a portable defibrillator with the patient, ideally with adhesive pads already attached. All monitors, pumps and the defibrillator should have adequate battery reserves for the journey. Additional oxygen supplies and airway equipment (facemask, self-inflating bag, rescue supraglottic airway, tracheal tube, portable suction and accessories) to enable management of a displaced airway should also accompany the transfer.

Anaesthetists should be confident that a patient is suitably prepared for transfer; however, it is important to consider the urgency of the procedure: delays in reperfusion adversely affect outcome. It may be possible to defer arterial access until arrival in the catheter laboratory, when it will be performed by the cardiologist as part of the procedure. It is also advisable to discuss the site chosen for an arterial line as the radial artery is a frequently used site for coronary angiography access. Likewise, acquiring central venous access should not be allowed to significantly delay transfer, unless it is considered vital.

In hospitals where emergency PCI is available for post-cardiac arrest patients, anaesthetists should be familiar with the equipment available in, and layout of, the coronary angiography suite. They are frequently distant from the operating department and precautions appropriate for anaesthesia in a remote location should be considered. Standards of monitoring and equipment should meet current guidelines (such as those of the Association of Anaesthetists of Great Britain and Ireland [18]), and a skilled assistant such as an ODP should be available. The angiography suite will contain motorized imaging machinery which may move in unanticipated directions; it is worth making sure that intravenous lines and monitoring cables will not become tangled and dislodged during the procedure.

venous access was not inserted. Metaraminol boluses were used to maintain a MAP of > 65 mmHg. Cooling was initiated by rapid administration of 2000 mL of cold (4°C) saline. An ODP was contacted and asked to check the anaesthetic equipment in the angiography suite.

⊗ Learning point Physiological targets during anaesthesia post-cardiac arrest

Appropriate physiological targets for the post-arrest period are not yet clearly identified. Oxygen therapy is widely used for patients suffering from acute MI, but there is limited evidence for benefit and some suggestion of harm [19]. The potential for hyperoxia to cause harm has been identified in experimental animal studies of cardiac arrest and a retrospective observational study in humans has also identified an association between high PaO_2 (>300 mmHg) after cardiac arrest and poor outcome [20]. Another observational study that included statistical adjustment for severity of illness failed to replicate this finding [21]. The latest European Resuscitation Council (ERC) guidelines recommend aiming for arterial SpO_2 of 94–96% with inspired oxygen concentrations titrated appropriately [10].

Ventilation should be titrated to achieve normocapnia. Avoidance of hypercapnia and resultant respiratory acidosis may improve cardiovascular stability. On the other hand, hypocapnia may adversely reduce cerebral perfusion and cause cerebral ischaemia.

Cardiovascular targets are also unclear. The post-arrest period is often marked by hypotension and cardiovascular instability. Identification of reversible causes is vital (such as by performing echocardiography, and correcting electrolyte abnormalities) alongside appropriate haemodynamic manipulation with fluids and vasoactive drugs. A small observational study has identified superior neurological outcome in post-arrest patients with a MAP of >100 mmHg for the 2 h post-resuscitation compared with patients with lower pressures [22]. Other studies have reported comparable mortality rates while targeting lower blood pressures [12]. The ERC guidelines suggest targeting a MAP which is associated with a urine output of 1 mL/kg/h and adequate lactate clearance, but advise adjustments for patients with chronic hypertension, and caution in interpreting urine output during therapeutic hypothermia [10].

---

❻ Expert comment

Although there is usually a brief period of hyperaemia after ROSC, cerebral oedema and intracranial hypertension is relatively rare after cardiac arrest except in those cases caused by asphyxia or where there have been very long periods of 'no flow' and 'low flow'. It is generally accepted that there is no place for ICP monitoring in post-cardiac arrest patients. Nevertheless control of ventilation is important: hypocapnia can cause significant ischaemia in the injured brain [23].

⊗ Learning point The post-cardiac arrest syndrome

The whole-body ischaemic insult which occurs during cardiac arrest acts as an initial trigger for the development of a syndrome of multi-organ dysfunction frequent in post-cardiac arrest patients. Although ischaemia initiates the process, ongoing injury occurs during reperfusion and afterwards due to activation of multiple inflammatory and apoptotic pathways. Four separate components are described:

1. Post-cardiac arrest brain injury
2. Post-cardiac arrest myocardial dysfunction
3. Systemic ischaemia/reperfusion response
4. Persisting underlying pathology

The clinical manifestations of the first three components can be variable depending on severity of insult and individual patient responses, but are generally coma, seizures, cardiovascular instability, myocardial stunning, hypotension, and multi-organ failure. Treatment should be targeted from an early stage to minimize secondary injury occurring as a result of these processes. The underlying pathology should not be overlooked, whether ischaemic heart disease or otherwise, and appropriate therapy commenced.

The patient was transferred to the coronary angiography suite without incident. He was moved across on to the imaging table, and monitoring re-instituted. The cardiologist achieved vascular access via the femoral artery and the procedure commenced. During the procedure, the patient's temperature was checked and found to be 34.8°C. Further passive cooling was achieved by removing unnecessary sheets and drapes. Blood glucose was checked and found to be 12.2 mmol/L and an insulin infusion was commenced targeting a blood glucose level < 10 mmol/L. Angiography demonstrated an acute occlusive lesion of the left anterior descending coronary artery which was successfully crossed and a BMS was deployed. Other stenoses were noted affecting other parts of the coronary circulation, and the decision was made to return at a later date if necessary to treat these lesions.

> ### ✪ Learning point Target lesion or multi-vessel PCI?
>
> Whether to perform a complete coronary revascularization in the context of an acute MI or to stent only the infarct-related artery is an unresolved controversy in interventional cardiology. The SHOCK study, which demonstrated improved survival at 6 months in acute MI patients presenting with cardiogenic shock who received aggressive revascularization compared to those who did not, can be used to justify complete revascularization for patients who remain shocked post resuscitation [24]. It is less clear how to proceed in the haemodynamically stable patient. Proponents of multi-vessel PCI point out that an acute MI involves an inflammatory process affecting the entire coronary circulation, increasing the risk of destabilizing other plaques which should therefore be dealt with when seen. The counter-opinion suggests that coronary spasm is likely post-MI, leading to inaccurate assessment of coronary lesions, and the theoretical increased risk of acute stent thrombosis in the hyperthrombotic phase which follows MI [25]. A recent study investigating this issue has suggested a reduction in major adverse cardiac events if complete revascularization is performed at the time of the MI or as a staged procedure, as opposed to target-lesion-only PCI. However, since the composite end-point included further PCI—the decision for which would have been informed by the initial procedure—the study has not fully resolved the controversy [26].
>
> Following the stenting procedure, the patient was transferred to the intensive care unit. He remained intubated and ventilated, and sedation was continued. Active cooling was commenced using external cooling pads aiming for a core temperature of 33°C (Figure 9.6). Glycaemic control was continued and enteral nutrition commenced according to the local policy. An infusion of noradrenaline was commenced in order to maintain MAP >65 mmHg. Ventilation was adjusted to maintain normocapnia, with arterial SpO$_2$ of 94–96%.
>
> The patient was kept cooled and sedated for 24 h. After this period re-warming commenced at a rate of 0.5°C per hour until normothermia was achieved. Hyperthermia was actively avoided by the use of paracetamol and further cooling measures as required. Once re-warmed, sedation was discontinued to enable assessment of neurological status.

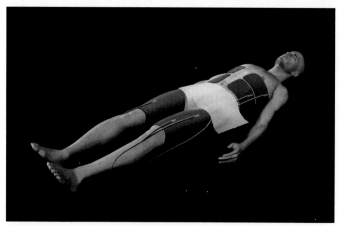

Figure 9.6 Example of a temperature management system. ArcticGel™ Pads, Medivance Inc., Louisville, CO, USA. © 2012 C. R. Bard, Inc. Used with permission. Bard is a registered trademark of C. R. Bard, Inc.

⊗ **Learning point** Post-resuscitation care

Post-resuscitation care forms the fourth link of the 'chain of survival' described in resuscitation guidelines [27]. Variation in the quality of care delivered after resuscitation between different healthcare regions, even within the same country, has a demonstrable impact upon survival and morbidity rates [3]. In patients who do not immediately regain consciousness following ROSC, admission to an intensive care unit should be strongly considered, since prognostication based on history and clinical examination at this stage is very unreliable. Up to 50% of patients admitted in this context may survive to leave hospital and achieve good neurological recovery.

Principle components of post-resuscitation care in comatose patients are:

1. Early coronary reperfusion (see 'Indications for primary angioplasty following out-of-hospital cardiac arrest')
2. Haemodynamic optimization and stabilization
3. Ventilatory optimization
4. Therapeutic hypothermia
5. Shivering prevention
6. Seizure prevention
7. Glucose control
8. Optimal cardiological management (pharmacological and interventional)
9. Prognostication

Haemodynamic and ventilatory optimization follow similar principles to those discussed in Learning point, Physiological targets during anaesthesia post-cardiac arrest.

Therapeutic hypothermia is one of very few evidence-based treatments available following cardiac arrest (see Landmark papers, Therapeutic hypothermia). Current guidelines recommend targeting a temperature of 32–34°C for a period of 12–24 h after cardiac arrest, followed by controlled re-warming at a rate of 0.25–0.5°C per hour. Avoidance of hyperthermia during and after re-warming is critically important. Cooling may cause a variety of physiological effects including: cardiovascular instability, electrolyte disturbances, hyperglycaemia, shivering, impaired immunity and reduced metabolism of drugs.

Shivering is a frequent consequence of therapeutic hypothermia, and may undermine the clinical benefits by increasing metabolic rate and decreasing cerebral oxygenation [25, 26]. Widely used approaches to reduce shivering include increasing sedative medications and use of neuromuscular blockade, but this strategy makes neurological assessment more difficult, and may prolong intensive care unit stay. An alternative stepwise approach includes skin counterwarming, regular paracetamol, normalization of serum magnesium, use of dexmedetomidine and opiates before using sedation and paralysis [30].

Seizures often occur following cardiac arrest, though they may be difficult to identify clinically, particularly in sedated patients or in those receiving neuromuscular blocking drugs. Status epilepticus is associated with a poor outcome; it is unclear whether this is a reflection of severity of generalized brain injury, or responsible for further secondary brain injury (though a retrospective study suggests the former [31]). Treatment options include phenytoin, levetiracetam, and thiopentone, though evidence for benefit is lacking. Myoclonic status is a particularly poor prognostic sign, though it may be difficult to differentiate clinically from other forms of seizure and myoclonus [32].

Glucose control is now accepted to be an important therapy on intensive care units [33]. The precise blood glucose target remains controversial; it is appropriate to apply a locally agreed protocol to patients following cardiac arrest [34]. Efforts to tightly control glucose levels to avoid hyperglycaemia must not be allowed to result in hypoglycaemia which will be rapidly harmful to the injured brain. Hyperglycaemia often occurs following arrest, and may also be influenced by cooling; regular measurement of blood glucose should be undertaken in these patients.

Optimal cardiological management is important since it may relate both to the precipitating cause of arrest (preventing further episodes in the short term) and improvement of long-term prognosis through modification of myocardial remodelling and manipulation of cardiovascular risk factors.

Prognostication following cardiac arrest is difficult. Patient factors such as age and comorbid disease, and intracardiac arrest factors such as length of arrest and initial rhythm are surprisingly poor predictors of outcome [35]. The American Academy of Neurology published practice guidance, but the evidence on

(continued)

which it is based predates the widespread use of cooling, and it is unclear what the impact of this may be [36]. Hypothermia delays clearance of sedative medication and modifies recovery of neurological function, impacting on the optimum time for neurological testing. Clinical findings which may indicate a poor prognosis include: absence of pupillary and corneal reflexes, lack of motor response to pain, or confirmed myoclonic status; additional tests including recording of somatosensory-evoked potentials and brain imaging may be helpful.

The use of standardized protocols incorporating the above components for post-resuscitation care is supported by trials demonstrating improved outcome following their implementation compared with historic controls. Survival to hospital discharge with favourable neurological outcome was 56% in one study, compared with 26% in the pre-implementation group [12].

ⓕ Expert comment

Although therapeutic hypothermia (more recently termed targeted temperature management) has now been implemented widely for the treatment of comatose patients following cardiac arrest, many knowledge gaps remain. Although animal studies indicate a much better outcome if target temperature is achieved rapidly after ROSC, we still await robust clinical data confirming this. The situation is compounded by evidence that those patients who cool spontaneously more rapidly tend to have worse outcomes than those who are more resistant to cooling (perhaps indicating less severe brain injury). Ultimately, cooling before ROSC may optimize neurological outcome, and studies involving pre-ROSC intranasal cooling are ongoing.

Intravascular cooling enables tighter temperature control compared with external techniques but there is no evidence that this results in better outcome. The optimal duration of treatment remains unknown but some 'experts' are using longer periods of cooling (up to 72 h) particularly if the time to ROSC has been long. Again these longer times are supported by some animal data but no human data so far. Slow re-warming is important—most 'experts' re-warm at 0.25°C. There is an increase in some inflammatory mediators during the re-warming phase.

It may be necessary to use the occasional bolus dose of a neuromuscular blocker during cooling and sometimes during re-warming. It is rarely necessary to use an infusion of a neuromuscular blocking drug and there is a risk that this will mask seizure activity. Consider continuous EEG monitoring if an infusion of neuromuscular blocker is used.

Seizures, myoclonus, or both occur in 30% of patients who remain comatose after cardiac arrest. Although seizures are associated with a four-fold increase in mortality, good neurological recovery has been documented in 17% of patients with seizures. Clonazepam is the most effective antimyoclonic drug.

Reliable prediction of the eventual outcome of the comatose post-cardiac arrest patient is difficult. The current consensus is that a multimodal approach should be used [37]; reliance on only clinical examination, for example, is unreliable and probably unacceptable. Use of EEG and CT is often helpful in addition to clinical examination. Somatosensory-evoked potentials provide the most reliable prediction of a poor outcome but this test is often unavailable in the UK. The use of therapeutic hypothermia delays clearance of many sedative drugs by about 30% and recovery from neurological injury is modified. Many experts recommend waiting 3 days after return to normothermia before considering withdrawal of treatment on the basis of prognostic tests [38].

ⓕ Expert comment

A recent trial of prehospital cooling with up to 2 L of 4°C normal saline versus no prehospital cooling following ROSC after all-rhythm OOHCA [39] showed no difference in hospital mortality or neurological recovery. Within the treatment arm, there were significantly more re-arrests during transport and a higher incidence of pulmonary oedema on chest X-ray. Therefore, cold intravenous fluid should not be used prehospital, but use in a closely monitored environment, such as the emergency department, may still be reasonable.

⊕ Clinical tip   Methods of delivering therapeutic hypothermia

Therapeutic hypothermia is a current cornerstone of post-resuscitation care. There is currently no clear evidence to demonstrate the optimum time to commence cooling following cardiac arrest, but it appears reasonable to do so as soon as is feasible once the patient has met appropriate criteria for cooling. Induction of cooling in a non-intensive treatment unit setting, such as the emergency department may be achieved by rapid instilling of 30 mL/kg (~2000 mL) of crystalloid cooled to 4°C. All emergency departments should provide refrigerated storage for this purpose, and have appropriate guidelines in place. This will reduce the core temperature by ~1.5°C, but additional methods will be required for further cooling and maintenance. Simple methods of cooling, including ice packs and tepid sponging, are effective, but achieve target temperatures more slowly than advanced methods [40]. Advanced methods of cooling include endovascular devices which circulate cool fluid through a

(continued)

specially adapted venous catheter, and surface devices which circulate cool fluid through heat exchanger pads applied to the torso and limbs. Both systems incorporate automated controls to achieve target core temperatures measured with oesophageal, bladder, or rectal probes. A comparison of the two methods has been performed, which demonstrated comparable performance of both systems in terms of time to achieving target temperature, and clinical outcomes [41].

⊘ Landmark papers Therapeutic hypothermia

That a period of hypothermia post-anoxic event may reduce secondary brain injury is not a new theory. As far back as the 1950s therapeutic hypothermia had been applied in post-cardiac arrest patients in an attempt to attenuate brain injury [42]. Evidence had already been accumulated from animal studies and from the operating theatre where it had been used in the context of traumatic brain injury. Usage was hampered by lack of intensive care facilities, and, although the potential was recognized, so too were the potential complications and its use declined. Animal studies conducted in the 1980s explored the physiological mechanisms which contribute to the beneficial effect of hypothermia, although these remain poorly understood. Potential mechanisms include [43]:

- prevention of apoptosis
- reduced free radical production
- reduced mitochondrial dysfunction
- reduced capillary leakage (especially the blood–brain barrier)
- reduced cell membrane leakage
- reduction of the excitotoxic cascade (induced neuronal hyperexcitability)
- reduced metabolism (makes a smaller contribution than originally thought)
- reduction in pro-inflammatory state
- reduction in cerebral 'thermopooling' (localized brain hyperthermia)
- anticoagulation (prevention of microthrombus mediated damage)
- suppression of seizure activity

Small non-randomized trials between 1997 and 2001 suggested improved neurological outcomes with hypothermia post-cardiac arrest compared with historical controls.

Two multicentre trials published in the same issue of the *New England Journal of Medicine* in 2002 refocused attention on the potential of therapeutic hypothermia to improve outcomes following cardiac arrest [44, 45].

Bernard *et al.* enrolled 43 patients to moderate hypothermia (33°C) for 12 h and 34 patients to usual care. Neurological outcomes were improved (no or moderate neurological disability in 49% vs 26%; *P* = 0.046) in the cooling group. A survival benefit was not demonstrated. Cooling was initiated rapidly during transport to hospital in this study.

The European Hypothermia after Cardiac Arrest Study Group performed a larger study, enrolling 273 patients, and demonstrated both improved neurological outcomes (55% vs 39%) and reduced mortality (41% vs 55%, relative risk: 0.74; 95% confidence interval: 0.58–0.95) in the hypothermia group. Cooling was only achieved after a mean of 8 h in this study and was continued for 24 h.

Both these studies included only patients with ventricular fibrillation/ventricular tachycardia (VF/VT) as their initial rhythm and excluded patients with persistent hypotension, hypoxia, or prolonged CPR (>1 h). Initial resuscitation guidelines recommended cooling for patients with out-of-hospital VF/VT cardiac arrest, though these recommendations are now being broadened to other initial arrest rhythms [10]. This is supported by a number of non-randomized trials and registry studies suggesting benefit in patients with any primary arrest rhythm.

A very recently published trial has questioned whether such a degree of hypothermia is beneficial [46]. 950 adults who remained unconscious following OOHCA of presumed cardiac cause (presenting rhythm was not a screening criteria) were randomized to be cooled to either 33°C or 36°C. There was no difference in mortality nor neurological outcomes between the groups at 180 days. Cooling to 33°C has been widely adopted following OOHCA, it is yet to be seen whether this significant trial is enough to change practice again.

ⓘ Expert comment

That the outcomes in the TTM trial [46] were the same in the two groups is not a reason to abandon active temperature control; hyperthermia is associated with worse neurological outcome, but means making a firm recommendation about a specific target temperature is difficult. There will be fewer physiological changes (e.g. bradycardia, electrolyte shifts, and shivering) at 36°C compared with 33°C but some post cardiac arrest patients (e.g. those with more severe neurological injury) might get better neuroprotection from the lower temperature.

The patient regained consciousness after several hours off sedation, though remained confused and combative requiring further use of sedative medications for a further 48 h. Fortunately his confusion slowly improved and he was able to follow commands allowing weaning of ventilation and extubation. He was discharged from the intensive care unit to a medical ward for medical optimization and rehabilitation, and left hospital 7 days later having made a good recovery, with no lasting neurological consequences. He continued to attend the hospital for cardiac rehabilitation as an outpatient.

A Final Word from the Expert

That the outcomes in the TTM trial [46] were the same in the two groups is not a reason to abandon active temperature control; hyperthermia is associated with worse neurological outcome, but it is difficult to make a firm recommendation about a specific target temperature. There will be fewer physiological changes (e.g. bradycardia, electrolyte shifts, and shivering) at 36°C compared with 33°C but some post cardiac arrest patients (e.g. those with more severe neurological injury) might get better neuroprotection from the lower temperature.

References

1. Myerburg RJ, Junttila MJ. Sudden cardiac death caused by coronary heart disease. *Circulation* 2012;125:1043–52.
2. Atwood C, Eisenberg MS, Herlitz J, Rea TD. Incidence of EMS-treated out-of-hospital cardiac arrest in Europe. *Resuscitation* 2005;67:75–80.
3. Nichol G, Thomas E, Callaway CW, *et al*. Regional variation in out-of-hospital cardiac arrest incidence and outcome. *JAMA* 2008;300:1423–31.
4. Wang TJ, Gona P, Larson MG, *et al*. Multiple biomarkers for the prediction of first major cardiovascular events and death. *N Engl J Med* 2006;355:2631–9.
5. Sasson C, Rogers MAM, Dahl J, Kellermann AL. Predictors of survival from out-of-hospital cardiac arrest: a systematic review and meta-analysis. *Circuln Cardiovasc Qual Outcomes* 2010;3:63–81.
6. Hollenberg J, Herlitz J, Lindqvist J, *et al*. Improved survival after out-of-hospital cardiac arrest is associated with an increase in proportion of emergency crew—witnessed cases and bystander cardiopulmonary resuscitation. *Circulation* 2008;118:389–96.
7. Kudenchuk PJ, Redshaw JD, Stubbs BA, *et al*. Impact of changes in resuscitation practice on survival and neurological outcome after out-of-hospital cardiac arrest resulting from nonshockable arrhythmias. *Circulation* 2012;125:1787–94.
8. Cheskes S, Schmicker RH, Christenson J, *et al*. Perishock pause—an independent predictor of survival from out-of-hospital shockable cardiac arrest. *Circulation* 2011;124:58–66.
9. Christenson J, Andrusiek D, Everson-Stewart S, *et al*. Chest compression fraction determines survival in patients with out-of-hospital ventricular fibrillation. *Circulation* 2009;120:1241–7.
10. Deakin CD, Nolan JP, Soar J, *et al*. European Resuscitation Council Guidelines for Resuscitation 2010: Section 4. Adult advanced life support. *Resuscitation* 2010;81:1305–52.
11. Dumas F, Cariou A, Manzo-Silberman S, *et al*. Immediate percutaneous coronary intervention is associated with better survival after out-of-hospital cardiac arrest: insights from the PROCAT (Parisian Region Out of hospital Cardiac ArresT) registry. *Circuln Cardiovasc Intervent* 2010;3:200–7.

12. Sunde K, Pytte M, Jacobsen D, *et al.* Implementation of a standardised treatment protocol for post resuscitation care after out-of-hospital cardiac arrest. *Resuscitation* 2007;73:29–39.

13. Antman EM, Anbe DT, Armstrong PW, *et al.* ACC/AHA guidelines for the management of patients with ST-elevation myocardial infarction—executive summary. A report of the American College of Cardiology/American Heart Association Task Force on Practice Guidelines (Writing Committee to revise the 1999. *J Am Coll Cardiol* 2004;44:671–719.

14. Müller D, Schnitzer L, Brandt J, Arntz H-R. The accuracy of an out-of-hospital 12-lead ECG for the detection of ST-elevation myocardial infarction immediately after resuscitation. *Ann Emerg Med* 2008;52:658–64.

15. Sideris G, Voicu S, Dillinger JG, *et al.* Value of post-resuscitation electrocardiogram in the diagnosis of acute myocardial infarction in out-of-hospital cardiac arrest patients. *Resuscitation* 2011;82:1148–53.

16. Inamasu J, Miyatake S, Tomioka H, *et al.* Subarachnoid haemorrhage as a cause of out-of-hospital cardiac arrest: a prospective computed tomography study. *Resuscitation* 2009;80:977–80.

17. Kürkciyan I, Meron G, Sterz F, *et al.* Spontaneous subarachnoid haemorrhage as a cause of out-of-hospital cardiac arrest. *Resuscitation* 2001;51:27–32.

18. Association of Anaesthetists of Great Britain and Ireland. *Recommendations for standards of monitoring during anaesthesia and recovery*; 2007 < http://www.aagbi.org/sites/default/files/standardsofmonitoring07.pdf >

19. Burls A, Cabello JB, Emparanza JI, Bayliss S, Quinn T. Oxygen therapy for acute myocardial infarction: a systematic review and meta-analysis. *Emerg Med J* 2011;28:917–23.

20. Kilgannon JH, Jones AE, Shapiro NI, *et al.* Association between arterial hyperoxia following resuscitation from cardiac arrest and in-hospital mortality. *JAMA* 2010;303:2165–71.

21. Bellomo R, Bailey M, Eastwood GM, *et al.* Arterial hyperoxia and in-hospital mortality after resuscitation from cardiac arrest. *Crit Care* 2011;15:R90.

22. Müllner M, Sterz F, Binder M, *et al.* Arterial blood pressure after human cardiac arrest and neurological recovery. *Stroke* 1996;27:59–62.

23. Curley G, Kavanagh BP, Laffey JG. Hypocapnia and the injured brain: more harm than benefit. *Crit Care Med* 2010;38:1348–59.

24. Hochman J, Sleeper L, Webb J. Early revascularization in acute myocardial infarction complicated by cardiogenic shock. *N Engl J Med* 1999;341:625–34.

25. Malik IS, Gerber RT. Justification for complete revascularisation at the time of primary angioplasty. *Heart* 2010;96:652–3.

26. Politi L, Sgura F, Rossi R, *et al.* A randomised trial of target-vessel versus multi-vessel revascularisation in ST-elevation myocardial infarction: major adverse cardiac events during long-term follow-up. *Heart* 2010;96:662–7.

27. Nolan JP, Soar J, Zideman DA, *et al.* European Resuscitation Council Guidelines for Resuscitation 2010 Section 1. Executive summary. *Resuscitation* 2010;81:1219–76.

28. Badjatia N, Strongilis E, Prescutti M, *et al.* Metabolic benefits of surface counter warming during therapeutic temperature modulation. *Crit Care Med* 2009;37:1893–7.

29. Oddo M, Frangos S, Maloney-Wilensky E, Andrew Kofke W, Le Roux P, Levine J. Effect of shivering on brain tissue oxygenation during induced normothermia in patients with severe brain injury. *Neurocrit Care* 2010;12:10–16.

30. Choi H, Ko S-B, Presciutti M, *et al.* Prevention of shivering during therapeutic temperature modulation: the Columbia anti-shivering protocol. *Neurocrit Care* 2011;14:389–94.

31. Rossetti AO, Logroscino G, Liaudet L, *et al.* Status epilepticus—an independent outcome predictor after cerebral anoxia. *Neurology* 2007;69:255–60.

32. English WA, Giffin NJ, Nolan JP. Myoclonus after cardiac arrest: pitfalls in diagnosis and prognosis. *Anaesthesia* 2009;64:908–11.

33. Van den Berghe G, Wouters P, Weekers F, *et al.* Intensive insulin therapy in critically ill patients. *N Engl J Med* 2001;345:1359–67.

34. Oksanen T, Skrifvars M, Varpula T, *et al.* Strict versus moderate glucose control after resuscitation from ventricular fibrillation. *Intens Care Med* 2007;33:2093–2100.

35. Nolan JP, Neumar RW, Adrie C, *et al.* Post-cardiac arrest syndrome: epidemiology, pathophysiology, treatment, and prognostication. A scientific statement from the International Liaison Committee on Resuscitation; the American Heart Association Emergency Cardiovascular Care Committee; the Council on Cardiovascular Surgery and Anesthesia; the Council on Cardiopulmonary, Perioperative, and Critical Care; the Council on Clinical Cardiology; the Council on Stroke. *Resuscitation* 2008;79:350–79.

36. Wijdicks EFM, Hijdra A, Young GB, Bassetti CL, Wiebe S. Practice parameter: prediction of outcome in comatose survivors after cardiopulmonary resuscitation (an evidence-based review): report of the Quality Standards Subcommittee of the American Academy of Neurology. *Neurology* 2006;67:203–10.

37. Oddo M, Rossetti AO. Predicting neurological outcome after cardiac arrest. *Curr Opin Crit Care* 2011;17:254–9.

38. Samaniego E, Persoon S, Wijman C. Prognosis after cardiac arrest and hypothermia: a new paradigm. *Curr Neurol Neurosci Rep* 2011;11:111–19.

39. Kim F, Nichol G, Maynard C, *et al.* Effect of Prehospital Induction of Mild Hypothermia on Survival and Neurological Status Among Adults With Cardiac Arrest A Randomized Clinical Trial. *JAMA* 2014; 311:45–52.

40. Hoedemaekers CW, Ezzahti M, Gerritsen A, Van der Hoeven JG. Comparison of cooling methods to induce and maintain normo- and hypothermia in intensive care unit patients: a prospective intervention study. *Crit Care* 2007;11:R91.

41. Tømte O, Drægni T, Mangschau A, Jacobsen D, Auestad B, Sunde K. A comparison of intravascular and surface cooling techniques in comatose cardiac arrest survivors. *Crit Care Med* 2010;39:443–9.

42. Williams GR, Spencer FC. The clinical use of hypothermia following cardiac arrest. *Ann Surg* 1958;148:462–8.

43. Polderman KH. Induced hypothermia and fever control for prevention and treatment of neurological injuries. *Lancet* 2008;371:1955–69.

44. Bernard SA, Gray TW, Buist MD, *et al.* Treatment of comatose survivors of out-of-hospital cardiac arrest with induced hypothermia. *N Engl J Med* 2002;346:557–63.

45. Hypothermia after Cardiac Arrest Study Group. Mild therapeutic hypothermia to improve the neurologic outcome after cardiac arrest. *N Engl J Med* 2002;346:549–56.

46. Nielsen N, Wettersley J, Cronberg T, *et al.* Targeted temperature management at 33°C versus 36°C after cardiac arrest. *N Engl J Med* 2013;369:2197–206.

INDEX